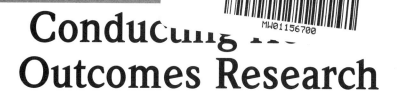

Conducting Health
Outcomes Research

Robert L. Kane, MD

Professor, School of Public Health
Minnesota Chair in Long-Term Care and Aging
Director, Minnesota Evidence-Based Practice Center
Director, University of Minnesota Clinical Outcomes Research Center
University of Minnesota
Minneapolis, Minnesota

David M. Radosevich, PhD, RN

Adjunct Assistant Professor, School of Public Health
Assistant Professor, Department of Surgery
University of Minnesota
Minneapolis, Minnesota

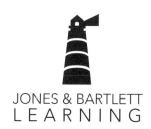

JONES & BARTLETT
L E A R N I N G

World Headquarters

Jones & Bartlett Learning	Jones & Bartlett Learning	Jones & Bartlett Learning
40 Tall Pine Drive	Canada	International
Sudbury, MA 01776	6339 Ormindale Way	Barb House, Barb Mews
978-443-5000	Mississauga, Ontario L5V 1J2	London W6 7PA
info@jblearning.com	Canada	United Kingdom
www.jblearning.com		

Jones & Bartlett Learning books and products are available through most bookstores and online booksellers. To contact Jones & Bartlett Learning directly, call 800-832-0034, fax 978-443-8000, or visit our website, www.jblearning.com.

Substantial discounts on bulk quantities of Jones & Bartlett Learning publications are available to corporations, professional associations, and other qualified organizations. For details and specific discount information, contact the special sales department at Jones & Bartlett Learning via the above contact information or send an email to specialsales@jblearning.com.

Production Credits

Publisher: Michael Brown
Associate Editor: Catie Heverling
Editorial Assistant: Teresa Reilly
Associate Production Editor: Lisa Lamenzo
Senior Marketing Manager: Sophie Fleck
Manufacturing and Inventory Control
    Supervisor: Amy Bacus

Composition: Datastream Content
    Solutions, LLC
Cover Design: Scott Moden
Cover Image: © Anette Linnea Rasmussen/
    ShutterStock, Inc.
Printing and Binding: Malloy, Inc.
Cover Printing: Malloy, Inc.

Library of Congress Cataloging-in-Publication Data

Kane, Robert L., 1940-
    Conducting health outcomes research / Robert L. Kane, David M. Radosevich.
        p. ; cm.
    Includes bibliographical references.
    ISBN 13: 978-0-7637-8677-9
    ISBN-10: 0-7637-8677-2
    1. Outcome assessment (Medical care)—Methodology. I. Radosevich, David M. II. Title.
    [DNLM: 1. Outcome Assessment (Health Care)—methods. 2. Health Services Research—methods. 3. Research Design. W 84.41 K16c 2011]
    R853.O87K35 2011
    362.1—dc22
                                    2010012082

6048
Printed in the United States of America
14 13 12   10 9 8 7 6 5 4 3

Table of Contents

Preface xi
Acknowledgments. xii
About the Authors xiii

Chapter 1   **Introduction to Outcomes Research** 1
      An Outcomes Approach 8
        Risk Adjustment. 9
        Treatment. 10
        Types of Study Designs 11
      Measuring Outcomes 15
      Conceptual Modeling. 16
      Organization of the Book. 21
      References 21

Chapter 2   **Models and Causal Thinking** 25
      Causation 25
      Conceptual Models 29
      Explanatory Models 33
      Summary 35
      References 36

Chapter 3   **Outcomes Research Study Designs** 39
      Isolating the Effect of the Intervention 39
      Threats to Validity 41
        Threats to Internal Validity 41
      Basic Research Designs. 43
      Potential Biases in Implementing a Study 46
      References 47

Chapter 4   **Measurement** **49**
The Nature of Measurement 50
Scaling 52
   Nominal Measurement.......................52
   Ordinal Measurement 54
   Interval Measurement......................55
   Ratio Measurement 56
Scaling Methods...............................56
   Rating Scales 57
   Comparative Methods 58
   Econometric Methods 60
   Item Response Theory 61
Strategic Questions in the Selection of
   Health Outcomes Measures 61
   Sensibility................................62
   Reliability................................63
   Validity 70
      The Three C's of Validity 71
   Responsiveness............................74
   Burden...................................77
   Design 78
Final Thoughts About Outcomes Measures 78
   Advantages of Multiple-Item Versus
      Single-Item Measures 78
   Other Useful Terms to Describe Measures 79
Summary 80
References 80

Chapter 5   **Generic Health Outcomes Measures**.............**85**
Why Use Generic Measures?....................86
Advantages and Disadvantages of Using
   Generic Health Outcomes Measures..............88
Health Outcome Domains......................89
   Physical Functioning 91
   Psychologic Well-Being 93
   Social Functioning.........................93

Pain 94
Cognitive Functioning. 94
Vitality. 95
Overall Well-Being. 95
Practical Considerations. 96
Choosing a Measure. 98
Conclusion. 99
References 100

Chapter 6   Health-Related Quality of Life 105
Applications for Health-Related Quality of
    Life Measures 108
Condition-Specific HRQL. 108
Examples of HRQL Measures 109
    Karnofsky Scale 109
    COOP Charts for Primary Care Practices 112
    Medical Outcomes Studies Short-
        Form Measures. 114
    Sickness Impact Profile. .115
    Quality of Well-Being Index. 118
    EuroQol 120
    World Health Organization Quality of
        Life-BREF 121
    Health Utilities Index 121
    QOL Coverage 123
    Utility Assessment 123
References 129

Chapter 7   Condition-Specific Measures 133
Condition-Specific Measures Versus Generic
    Health Status Measures. .133
Why Not Generic Health Status Measures? 134
Condition-Specific Health Status Measures 136
Physiologic Measures 137
Case Definition Disease Does Not Equal Disease. 140
Other Alternatives 140

The Choice of a Condition-Specific Measure 143
   The Conceptual Model 143
   Hierarchy of Measurement 146
The Role of Condition-Specific Versus
   Generic Measures 148
Choosing a Measure 151
Conclusion 153
References 154

Chapter 8   Satisfaction With Care **159**
The Importance of Patient Satisfaction 159
Theoretic Models of Satisfaction 160
   Interpreting Satisfaction Ratings 161
      Expectations and Psychosocial Determinants 161
      Dimensions of Satisfaction 163
      Process of Care and Satisfaction 166
      Outcomes and Satisfaction 166
   Methodology of Measuring Satisfaction 167
      Measurement Methods 167
      Methodological Issues 169
      Psychometric Testing 170
      Utilization Patterns, Survey Timing and
         Reference Group 172
      Reporting Versus Rating 173
   Importance of Satisfaction Elements 173
   Existing Satisfaction Measures 175
      Health Plan 174
      Hospital 178
      Ambulatory Care 180
      Long-Term Care 183
Literature Reviews 188
Summary 188
References 189

Chapter 9   Demographic, Psychologic, and Social Factors **199**
Demographic Factors 201
   Age 202
   Residence 202

Race 203
Marital Status 204
Social Economic Status 205
Psychologic Factors 206
Mind–Body Connection 206
Well-Being 210
Locus of Control 210
Pain 211
Stress 212
Other 212
Affect 213
Depression 216
Anxiety 216
Cognitive Function 218
Social Function 218
Social Support 219
Social Function/Adjustment 219
Summary 223
References 223

Chapter 10 Treatment and Interventions 235
Importance of Understanding Treatment 235
What is a Treatment? 235
Components of Treatment 237
Diagnosis Versus Treatment 241
Treatment Components 241
Medications 242
Procedures 242
Counseling/Education 243
Understanding the Components of Treatment 244
Does the Type of Physician Matter? 245
Isolating the Treatment of Interest 246
Statistically Isolating the Effect of Treatment 247
Variation in Treatment 248
Quality Improvement 254
Summary 254
References 255

Chapter 11 Risk Adjustment...................................**261**

Severity and Comorbidity........................262

Diagnosis-Specific Severity......................263

Generic Comorbidity Measures 264

Why Should We Measure Comorbidity

(or the Severity of Illness)? 270

Control for Selection Bias 270

Improve Prediction of Outcomes.............271

Form a Basis for Subgroup Analysis 271

Data Sources 272

Considerations in Selecting a Risk-Adjustment

Strategy 273

Statistical Performance: How Do You Evaluate the

Performance of a Risk Model? 275

Summary 277

References 277

Chapter 12 Methods for Collecting Health Outcomes and

Related Data............................**281**

Self-Report.................................282

Tailored Design 287

Designing a Survey Implementation System........288

Pretesting..................................288

Clinical Data 289

Administrative Data.........................291

Summary 294

References 294

Chapter 13 Analysis and Visual Display of Health Outcomes

Research Data...........................**297**

Considerations for Analyzing Health

Outcomes Data 297

Select the Analytic Method....................298

Threats to Validity 302

Low Statistical Power 302

Fishing and Error Rate Problems 306

Employ Acceptable Methods for Handling

Missing Data 308

Create a Database and a Data Dictionary 311
Operationalize Study Variables and
    Structure Data for Analysis. 313
Visual Display of Health Outcomes Information 315
Regulatory Demands Accompanying Health
    Outcomes Research 316
Summary 318
References 319

Chapter 14 Making Sense of It All: Interpreting the Results 323
Organizing One's Thinking 323
The Search for Simple Measures. 325
Adjusting for Case Mix. 326
Data Quality 327
Getting Follow-up Data 329
Using Extant Data Sources. 331
Basic Analysis Issues 332
Ethics. 335
Disease Management 336
Quality Improvement. 337
Operational Steps. 337
Summary 340
References 341

Index **343**

Preface

This book is, in one way, a continuation of an earlier set of efforts about outcomes research and, in another way, a totally new work. We have previously published two editions of a multi-authored text, *Understanding Health Outcomes Research*. When I was asked to consider a third edition, I opted to dramatically change the format and the content. I teamed up with my colleague, David Radosevich, who has been teaching the course on outcomes research with me at the University of Minnesota School of Public Health, to write a jointly authored text that would approach this topic afresh.

The current text, *Conducting Health Outcomes Research*, is based on our collective experience teaching this material to a diverse group of students with varying degrees of clinical and epidemiologic backgrounds. At the same time, a lot has changed. Evidence-based medicine has become the holy grail of medical care. Comparative effectiveness research has begun to blossom. There is a greater than ever need for such a text.

We have tried to make this book more practical but readily acknowledge that in many instances we draw heavily on the work of earlier chapter authors. We have acknowledged that work whenever appropriate.

Robert L. Kane, MD

Acknowledgments

Although this book is newly authored, it draws upon a number of chapters in the previous iterations of the earlier version of the book. We would like to thank Maureen Smith for her writing on satisfaction and condition-specific measures; Adam Atherly for his writing on condition-specific measures; Jeremy Holtzman for his writing on assessing treatment; Todd Rockwood for his writing on satisfaction and demographics; Melissa Constantine for her writing on demographics; and Chris Schüssler-Fiorenza for her writing on satisfaction.

About the Authors

Robert L. Kane, MD
Minnesota Chair in Long-Term Care and Aging
Division of Health Policy and Management
University of Minnesota, School of Public Health
Minneapolis, MN

Robert Kane, MD, holds an endowed chair in Long-Term Care and Aging at the University of Minnesota School of Public Health, where he was formerly the dean. He directs the University of Minnesota's Center on Aging, the Minnesota Area Geriatric Education Center, the Clinical Outcomes Research Center, and an AHRQ-funded Evidence-based Practice Center. He has conducted numerous research studies on both the clinical care and the organization of care for older persons, especially those needing long-term care. He is the author or editor of 31 books and more than 470 journal articles and book chapters on geriatrics and health services research. He has analyzed long-term systems both in this country and abroad. Recent books include *The Heart of Long-term Care, Assessing Older Persons*, the sixth edition of *Essentials of Clinical Geriatrics*, and *Meeting the Challenge of Chronic Illness*. He and his sister, Joan West, have written an account of the struggles to get adequate long-term care for their mother, titled, *It Shouldn't Be This Way*. That experience led to his founding a national organization dedicated to improving long-term care, Professionals with Personal Experience with Chronic Care (PPECC), which has over 800 members. He is a graduate of Harvard Medical School.

His current research addresses both acute and long-term care for older persons, with special attention to the role of managed care, chronic disease, and disability, as well as systematic reviews of the literature on various topics. Dr. Kane has consulted to a number of national and international agencies, including the World Health Organization's

Expert Committee on Aging. He has received the President's Award from the American Society on Aging and the Polisher Award from the Gerontological Society of America, the Enrico Greppi Prize from the Italian Society of Gerontology and Geriatrics, and the British Geriatrics Society Medal for the Relief of Suffering amongst the Aged. He was elected to the University of Minnesota's Academic Health Center's Academy for Excellence in Health Research.

David M. Radosevich, PhD, RN
Assistant Professor
Department of Surgery
University of Minnesota, School of Medicine
Minneapolis, MN

David M. Radosevich, PhD, RN is an epidemiologist and biostatistician at the University of Minnesota conducting health outcomes research in the Academic Health Center. He is a cofounder of the Health Outcomes Institute, a nonprofit organization dedicated to promoting and supporting outcomes research. He cofounded and served as the Director of Transplant Information Services and served as the deputy director of the Clinical Outcomes Research Center in the University of Minnesota, School of Public Health. He has participated in numerous projects measuring health outcomes and quality of care at the level of community, health plan, and medical group practice. In addition to collaborating in observational studies in the Division of Transplantation at the University of Minnesota and the Schultze Diabetes Institute, Dr. Radosevich works closely with studies on donor management and the donor family experience. Dr. Radosevich teaches health outcomes research in the School of Public Health.

Introduction to Outcomes Research

Several factors are responsible for the growing attention to quality of care. There is a growing sense that Americans spend too much on health care for too little value. People are beginning to demand better quality. Much has been made of the dangers of medical errors (Kohn, Corrigan, & Donaldson, 2000). Under Section 5001(c) of the Deficit Reduction Act of 2005, Medicare will no longer pay for a defined set of hospital associated complications.

Two basic strategies exist. One relies on more informed consumers who will make wiser choices if given information about quality, despite evidence that this rarely happens (Hibbard & Jewett, 1997; Hibbard, Peters, Dixon, & Tusler, 2007). The second, usually called pay for performance, is more direct; it offers incentives to clinicians and organizations for providing better care or for achieving better results (Glickman *et al.*, 2007; Lindenauer *et al.*, 2007; Rosenthal, Landon, Normand, Frank, & Epstein, 2006), but it can have perverse effects, such as encouraging providers to exclude difficult cases (Werner & Asch, 2005).

There is a new call for evidence-based practice and comparative effectiveness reviews, which compare the effectiveness of alternative treatments. All of this requires information about the outcomes of care. Much attention has been devoted to methods for assessing the quality of the medical literature and summarizing the findings from it (Juni, Altman, & Egger, 2001; Sackett, Richardson, Rosenberg, & Haynes, 1997). The Cochrane Collaborating Centers have developed a library of reports that assess the literature on various topics and make recommendations for practice.[1] The

---

[1] See http://www.cochrane.org

Agency for Healthcare Research and Quality (AHRQ) has chartered a set of Evidence-based Practice Centers to conduct systematic literature reviews and report on the findings with a direct goal of providing the bases for practice recommendations (Agency for Healthcare Research and Quality, 2002).

As a result, assessing outcomes of care has taken on new importance. Although many studies still examine outcomes like mortality and clinical parameters, the focus of much clinical research has broadened to address larger questions about the ultimate impact of care. The outcomes examined in outcomes research are more likely to approximate what one ultimately wants health care to achieve (e.g., improvements in functional status and quality of life). It is hard to get a clinical trial funded now without at least some effort to assess quality of life, and typically, health-related quality of life.

Outcomes research differs from other medical research in another important way. It is more inclusive of what can be considered an intervention. Whereas most medical research may examine the effects of a particular drug or surgical intervention, outcomes research may examine the effects of such elements as counseling or even reorganizing the way care is delivered. For example, outcomes research may not only ask "are individuals with CHD better off with angioplasty or medical therapy?" (a valid outcomes research question) but "are individuals with CHD who get their health care in HMOs better off than others?"

Like Moliere's *bourgeois gentilhomme* who suddenly discovered he had been speaking prose all his life, healthcare providers seem to have awakened to the need to examine the results of their labors. The observations about the large variation in the rates of various medical activities and utilization of care stirred interest in whether these differences had any effect on outcomes (Fisher *et al.*, 2003). The rise of managed care, with its industrial accountability and productivity models stimulated a revised way of thinking about care. As the variation data generated a press for greater consistency, which was translated into a demand for clinical guidelines, it became quickly evident that medicine does not have a vast store of empirically verified information about the relationship between what is done and the results.

Coincident with all this attention to outcomes has been a growth in outcomes research programs. Most academic medical centers now have some entity charged with leading research on the outcomes of care. Many managed care programs have such a unit, either directed at research per se or linked more closely to clinical activity under the general heading of quality improvement.

Outcomes analysis can be undertaken for several reasons:

1. *To make market decisions.* Under a scheme of what has been termed value-based purchasing, consumers looking for help in an ideal world might want to know how a given clinician has performed in treating their specific problem. Likewise, those acting on behalf of consumers (e.g., benefits managers) might want such information to help in their contracting decisions.

2. *For accountability.* Several agencies have a stake in the quality of medical care. Formal regulatory activity is vested in the government and in professional societies. Payers may also be concerned that the care they are buying is of adequate quality. In effect, the same information on the outcomes achieved can be analyzed at the level of a clinician or a clinic or a hospital (if the sample size is large enough). In conducting such analyses, however, appropriate adjustments for case mix and other relevant risk factors are needed in both cases.

3. *To improve the knowledge base of medicine.* The substrate for evidence-based medicine (EBM) is good evidence on which to base it. Solid outcomes information is the crucial building block for the EBM edifice. The enthusiasm for establishing guidelines for care has been somewhat dampened by the growing realization that the empirical database for most of these recommendations is quite weak, and they are forced to rely on clinical consensus judgments. While some would hold that the only real science comes from randomized controlled trials (RCT), much can be learned by carefully applying epidemiological analyses to large databases of well collected experiential information. Indeed, outcomes research attempts to address a particular type of medical knowledge, in other words, the knowledge of certain types of those outcomes closest to health and broader sorts of questions.

4. *For quality improvement (QI).* Medical care organizations seeking to improve their care need to know how well they are doing as a basis for choosing to intervene. Likewise they need to track outcomes to assess whether their QI is working.

5. *For marketing.* Some organizations have used quality information as a basis for distinguishing themselves from the competition. Given what appeals to most consumers, this set of outcomes data usually emphasizes satisfaction with care.

Outcomes can be expressed in different ways. Perhaps the simplest and most direct measure is survival, although some ethicists and economists might seek to complicate even this determination, arguing that all life is not equal. Economists would add a dimension of quality of life as a basis for weighting each year survived, what they call Quality Adjusted Life Years (QALYs). Clinicians are most familiar with clinical measures ranging from death to values of specific parameters like blood pressure. Outcomes can also be derived from symptoms or even the results of physical examinations. They can be the results of simple tests, like blood levels, or more complex physiological measures. Another set of outcomes relies on information collected from patients. This data usually reflects how they have experienced the illness and the effects it has had on their lives. These outcomes include measures of functioning as well as measures of affect. Satisfaction with care and with life in general can be considered part of this set of outcomes. In general, clinicians place greater faith in the data they get from laboratory tests and their own observations than what patients report, but this prejudice may not be appropriate. One cannot actually measure health in a laboratory. For example, knowing the oxygen saturation in the great toe of a person with impaired circulation may be important, but it is more salient to know that the patient still cannot walk. Patient derived information can be as valid as, or even more valid, than that obtained from a machine. For example, the results of a scale based on patient perceptions of events may be as valid as the inference placed on the results of a colorimetric reaction that is interpreted as reflecting the level of enzymatic activity.

Looking directly at the outcomes of care (as opposed to concentrating on the process of care) makes a lot of sense. In the best traditions of Willie Sutton, that is where the treasure can be found. However, using outcomes may be less satisfying than one may wish. Clinicians have difficulties with outcomes on several grounds:

1. *Joint accountability.* The outcomes of care may be due to many things, only some of which are under the clinician's control. Outcomes are rarely the product of a single individual's efforts.

Outcomes result from the collaboration and coordination of many people, working within a system. System failure is at least as deadly as individual error (Berwick, 1989). It is much more satisfying to be able to say you did all the right things, even if something bad happened. Some estimates suggest that medical care only has a limited effect on overall health of a population. Numbers in the range of 10 to 25% are bandied about. It seems reasonable to assume that the size of the effect of treatment on specific sick people is larger, but other factors will still influence the results. It is not necessary that treatment explain all (or even most) of the variance on outcomes to make it worthwhile to examine its effectiveness. One can change the risk of a successful outcome by several orders of magnitude by interventions that fail to explain even a modest amount of the variance in outcomes.

2. *No clear remedial action.* Although theory suggests that outcomes and process measures are closely linked, the relationship between process and outcomes is often weak. Hence, a poor outcome does not necessarily indicate what needs to be done differently. At best, outcomes can only suggest to an investigator where to look for more information about the process of care. In clinical practice, outcomes are often best thought of as screeners. Rather than examining the processes of care for all the care provided, a pattern of poor outcomes can suggest which types of care (or which providers) need closer scrutiny.

3. *Effort for data collection.* Outcomes information usually requires extra effort (and expense) to collect. Medical record keeping is notoriously inconsistent (Weed, 1968a, 1968b). Much information is recorded as judgments and definitions vary widely. For example, what does "within normal limits" mean? Omissions are also frequent. Medical practice does not routinely gather systematic information about the outcomes of care. At best, clinicians are generally aware of only those patients who return for further care. Rarely do they systematically follow the course of those who do not return, although these may be the outcomes of greatest interest. Even less often do clinicians systematically collect data on other variables that might influence the outcomes.

4. *Probability, not certainty.* Outcomes are essentially probability state-ments. Because outcomes can be influenced by many different factors, one should not try to judge the success of any single case. Rather, outcomes are addressed in the aggregate. The rate of success is compared. Thus, outcomes reflect the experience of a clinician, not the results of any single effort.

5. *Need for group data.* Because outcomes rely on group data, there must be enough cases to analyze. For many clinicians, the volume of cases around a specific condition is too small to permit rapid aggregation for analysis. One must either collect cases over several years or use a group of physicians as the unit of analysis. Both strategies have disadvantages.

6. *Out of date data.* Outcome results take a long time to assemble. First, you have to accumulate cases. For each case, you have to wait for the outcomes to become evident. As a result, by the time an outcomes report is available, the care reported on may have occurred some time ago. The results may no longer be up-to-date.

Given all these problems, it is little wonder that people would rather talk about outcomes than deal with them. It is much easier to test the extent to which care complies with extant orthodoxy. But we quickly run into a paradox. Despite all the attention to EBM, our beliefs about what constitutes appropriate care are still more often based on beliefs than on hard evidence. Before we endorse an orthodoxy, we would like to have bet-ter proof that a given approach really leads to better outcomes. Consensus should not be confused with wisdom. Imagine what would have happened if there had been a consensus conference in the mid-1800s on cupping and leaching. Developing such linkages means having a data system that can provide the needed grist for the analytic mill.

Three strategies are available to collect outcomes information. They are: (1) Every clinical action could be subjected to a randomized con-trolled trial. Given all the possible interventions and all the variations in practice and patients, this does not seem like a realistic strategy. (2) Routine medical practice can incorporate systematic data collection and feedback to track outcomes of care. The rise of managed care, with its improved information systems and its concerns about efficiency, may prove a catalyst for this effort. (3) Special practices can be designated to operate data collection activities under some scientific aegis that would systematically collect data on outcomes and relate them to the process of care (much the way academic centers conduct clinical trials to test new therapies). Practitioners would then rely on the validated processes for assessing their quality of care.

The first strategy relies on randomized trials, whereas the latter two use data derived from routine care. In essence, the trade-off is between fear of selection bias and of weak generalizability.

Having recognized the discrepancy between what we know and what we believe, medicine was at an impasse. One camp, anxious for fast results, pushed for creating practice guidelines based on the best available information and filling in the rest with expert opinion. They argued that, at worst, such a strategy would produce the equivalent of a higher quality textbook. The other camp maintained that enforcing arbitrary rules that were not based on empirical evidence was equivalent to codifying beliefs. They urged greater restraint until a better science base was developed.

The early experience with guideline writing confirmed the weak science base that underlies much of clinical practice (Field & Lohr, 1992). Systematic outcomes research provides an obvious remedy for the situation. However, the choice of the best research strategy remained in question.

The classical view of quality of medical care uses a framework that divides such work into structure, process, and outcome (Donabedian, 1966). Structure refers to such aspects as the training of the care providers or the equipment of the facility in which the care is provided. Process addresses what was done: Was the correct (appropriate) action taken? Was it done skillfully? Outcomes refer to the results of these actions. There is an assumption that these three aspects are directly related, but that belief has often proven hard to demonstrate empirically. One explanation is that the "lore" or medicine is just that, a set of beliefs and traditions that are poorly grounded in empirical evidence. Other interpretations include thinking the process is too complex, subject to too many factors, or that the effects of care are simply too subtle to be easily revealed by most studies, especially nonexperimental ones.

The weak relationships, often found between process and structure on the one hand and outcomes on the other, cut both ways. Investigators seeking to demonstrate the validity of their outcomes findings may turn to structural and process relationships. Turning the system on its head, one might test the validity of guidelines by assessing whether those adhering to the guidelines achieve better results than those who do not. If outcomes measures work, one would expect to find better outcomes among those providers judged by some external standard to give better care. What does it mean when care provided in teaching hospitals is no better than care offered in community hospitals? On the one hand, the measures may be insensitive; alternatively, there may be less difference than one suspects. If the results are the inverse of what is expected, there will obviously be greater cause for concern, but failure to find a difference where orthodox teaching says one should be found may raise at least as many questions about the orthodoxy as there are challenges to the validity of the observation. Ironically, one approach to addressing this dilemma would be to validate the guidelines by comparing the results of care delivered according to guidelines to care given without guidelines.

AN OUTCOMES APPROACH

An outcomes approach requires more than simply collecting data on the outcomes of care. It should be thought of in terms of an outcomes information system. Careful and complete data collection for purposes of both outcomes ascertainment and risk adjustment has to be combined with proper analyses.

The basic model for analyzing the outcomes of care is the same whether one uses an RCT or an epidemiological approach. The model can be summarized as follows:

$$Outcomes = f(baseline, patient\ clinical\ characteristics,$$
$$patient\ demographic/psychosocial\ characteristics,$$
$$treatment,\ setting)$$

This pseudo-equation indicates that clinical outcomes are the result of several factors, which can be classified as risk factors (baseline status, clinical status, and demographic/psychosocial characteristics) and treatment characteristics (treatment and setting).[2] The goal of the analysis is to isolate the relationship between the outcomes of interest and the treatment provided, by controlling for the effects of other relevant material. The latter is often referred to as risk-adjustment.

---

[2]Terminology varies a great deal with respect to the use of the term risk factors. Some people use it interchangeably with disease severity. Others use it more generically to refer to the whole set of factors that can influence the outcomes of care (even including treatment). In this book we have tried to use it consistently to refer to those factors besides treatment that can affect outcomes.

Risk Adjustment

The patient's baseline status is very important. With a few exceptions (such as plastic surgery and elective orthopedics), most medical treatment does not get a patient better than he or she was before the episode that started the need for treatment. Thus, there are really two types of baseline status information that need to be collected: (1) status at the outset of treatment, which can be used to show how much change has occurred since treatment began, and (2) usual status before the onset of the problem that requires treatment, which defines the upper bound of just how much improvement is possible, or likely. Information on baseline status basically corresponds to what will be later collected to assess outcomes.

Patient clinical characteristics cover a lot of territory. One of the reasons we make diagnoses is to group patients into classes that share a need for a given type of therapy and/or suggest an expected course. Knowing a patient's diagnosis would thus play a central role in building an outcomes data system. Many patients have more than one diagnosis, often referred to as comorbidities. It is necessary for purposes of analysis to identify one diagnosis as the primary diagnosis and to treat the others as modifiers.[3]

Diagnoses can be further refined in terms of their implications for outcomes by addressing characteristics that suggest varying prognoses. These are termed severity measures. In addition to severity, one may be concerned about other modifiers of diagnoses, such as duration of the problem and history of previous episodes. In general, it is usually safer to be as inclusive as possible. Because clinicians are especially distrustful of non-RCTs, they need a great deal of reassurance that all possible differences between groups have been considered. By including elements that seem unnecessary, the investigator may eventually gain greater acceptance for the results. Nothing is more frustrating than presenting an analysis, especially one that challenges conventional wisdom, only to have the clinical audience say: "Yes, but did you consider...?" A policy of inclusion is not an automatic talisman against rejection, but it can help avoid it. At some point, of course, the cost of collecting seemingly irrelevant data can be overwhelming. A reasonable compromise must

---

[3]It would be possible to deal with clusters of diagnoses, but the numbers of combinations could quickly become unmanageable.

be struck. If the clinician audience is involved in planning the study, at least those elements that seem most important should be covered. Other clinical information may address different risk factors (e.g., exposure to toxins, diet, habits).

The other set of patient information concerns demographic and psychosocial factors. Some obvious items, like age and gender, seem to need no justification, but even they should be thoughtfully addressed. A specific conceptual model that indicates the expected influence of each variable is a critical first step in planning an outcomes study. Others, like education and social support, may exert their effects more subtly. The relevance of specific elements may vary with the condition being examined. Other psychosocial variables, like the patient's cognitive or emotional state, may have an influence on the effects of treatment on other outcomes.

Treatment

Setting refers to both the physical location where the care is provided as well as the organization of that site. It can also address other attributes, such as the philosophy of care provided. For example, one may want to compare the same basic care provided in an inpatient and outpatient context. Alternatively, one may want to address the level of risk aversion or the extent of staffing for apparently similar models of care. One site may have a philosophy of encouraging patients to do as much as possible for themselves, whereas another may be inclined to provide a lot of services to assist patients in performing basic activities, either because the organization is concerned about safety or because they feel that doing things for patients may be faster in the long run.

At its most basic level, treatment can refer simply to gross types (e.g., does medical management work better than surgical?). It can even be simply a proxy for care given in one hospital versus another, or by one physician versus others. Measuring the effects of treatment first requires a clear, useful taxonomy for treatments. Surprisingly, little work has gone into creating such schema. One needs to think not only about formal treatments like prescribed drugs, but also about over-the-counter medications. The definition of a therapy may not be limited to what is done in a clinical setting. Informal care may play a substantial role. In some cases, the treatment may extend over several sites. For example, much of the care formerly rendered in hospitals is now provided in nursing homes and even at home.

A simple model to classify treatment can be derived from drug therapy, where one talks about such constructs as type, dosage, duration, and timing. A similar approach can be applied to other treatments like surgery. The next level of analysis might ask whether the same treatment in different hands produces different results. At this point, the issue becomes individual skill.

Treatment relates directly to Donabedian's process of care, which can be said to be composed of two basic aspects: (1) doing the right and appropriate thing and (2) doing it well (1966; 1988). The goal of outcomes research is to establish what treatment is appropriate for a given situation by isolating the effects of treatment from the effects of other factors that influence outcomes. It is harder to use outcomes to address skill compared to appropriateness, but in the end, that is the only real way. Although some may try to tease out the skill component by using some sort of direct analysis, such a strategy will not readily distinguish between skill and appropriateness. A more precise approach is first to ascertain what type of care produces the best (or at least acceptable levels of) results for a given problem (or group of patients). Then, one can apply the same deductive analytic approach to examining those cases where the appropriate care was given to look for differences across providers. Where such differences are found, they can be said to reflect differences in skill.

Types of Study Designs

There is substantial confusion about the relationship of study design to outcomes research. (This topic is discussed at length in Chapter 2.) Clinical research worships at the shrine of the RCT. The basic difference between an RCT and well conducted prospective observational study is the allocation of patients. In an RCT, the allocation is not under the control of either the medical practitioner or the patient. Although RCTs are at the top of the usual clinical science hierarchy, they have their own limitations. As their name implies, they are randomized and controlled. They utilize random assignment to treatment and control conditions (uninfluenced by either the treating clinician or the patient) and standardized treatment. But the enrollment into such trials is rarely based on a representative sample of the patient population. Indeed, most RCTs have strict inclusion and exclusion criteria. RCTs are typically conducted in specialized institutions under tightly controlled conditions. As their name further implies, great pains are taken to standardize the treatment. As a result of these conditions, questions are often raised about whether the results of an RCT are generalizable to actual practice. By contrast, so-called quasi-experimental (or observational or epidemiological) designs rely on regular practice (or perhaps care in the upper end of the quality distribution) with potential variation in who gets what kinds of treatment that reflects what happens in actual practice. As a result, the assignment of patients to treatment is not a random event but one in which clinicians (and patients) play an active role. In essence, one trades off potential selection bias against the ability to generalize the findings (Heckman, 2008). Often complex statistical techniques are used to try to counter the selection bias (Stukel *et al.*, 2007).

The science of medicine depends on matching treatment to need. The real question from the perspective of scientific study is whether some unmeasured factor might be responsible for the choice of treatment. Random assignment obviates that risk. It does not necessarily mean that the experimental and control groups are equivalent. (It is still possible to get differences by chance.) But it does mean that any differences are not systematic (i.e., they do not reflect bias). Those using observational methods are under great pressure to prove the comparability of the treated and untreated groups. Even when all measured variables are examined, there always remains the possibility of some systematic difference of an unmeasured variable.

The ability to assign subjects randomly to either experimental or control status confers an aura of science that is unsurpassed.[4] Indeed, serious questions of bias can arise whenever the decision to treat or not to treat (or how to treat) is determined by some external force. Those reviewing the results of nonrandomized studies need to be reassured that potential risk factors have been identified and addressed. Nonetheless, there remains a concern that experimental and control groups are not completely comparable, and hence unknown factors may account for differences found. A number of statistical procedures have been developed to address this issue, but the level of comfort with the results of

---

[4]Random assignment does not confer an absolute protection against bias. It simply reduces the likelihood that such bias has occurred. It is still important to examine the characteristics of the experimental and control groups to look for such bias and to consider the value of subgroup analysis where the effects of treatment may be greater with one portion of the sample than another.

these efforts varies with the discipline. Clinicians, who are usually not statistically sophisticated, need a lot of reassurance that experimental and control groups are comparable.

In recent years, biostatisticians have promoted propensity scores as a way of providing clinicians with more confidence about well conducted observational studies (D'Agostino, 1998). In essence, propensity scores identify the variables that might be associated with using or not using a given service. Clinically homogeneous risk subgroups are created on the basis of these measured variables and the results compared across each of these subgroups. Some researchers, especially economists, still worry about unmeasured variables and have developed procedures that attempt to adjust for these. One of the most common is the use of instrumental variables (IVs; Angrist, Imbens, & Rubin, 1996; Heckman, 1979; Lee, 1994). These are variables that are statistically associated with the likelihood of treatment but not with the outcomes. By using these IVs, the researchers can presumably adjust for unmeasured effects. The problem lies in finding IVs that fit the bill. In most cases, it is hard to identify a variable that is associated with getting care but not with its outcomes. The most common IVs are measures of access to care. These two approaches to addressing selection bias may yield different results (Stukel *et al.*, 2007).

RCTs may encourage false confidence. They are not a guarantee of good science. Problems with attrition, for example, may create new sources of bias. Standards for the conduct and reporting of RCTs, like CONSORT (Consolidated Standards of Reporting Trials), promote better research quality (Begg *et al.*, 1996).

RCTs have real limitations. In general, randomized trials use great care in design to specify inclusion criteria. Because RCTs are complicated and difficult to mount, they are usually restricted to very tightly targeted groups of patients. Often the investigators are not actively concerned about how the subjects are obtained and rely on random allocation to distribute any differences equally across the two groups. As a result, randomized trials often trade internal validity (tightness of comparisons) for external validity (generalizability). Thus, randomization does not provide the protective shield that some think. Even if the groups are more comparable (and such a distribution is not assured by random assignment), the pertinent analyses may still require looking at the data within subclasses. It does not seem feasible to rely exclusively on RCTs for all, or even most, of the needed empirical data linking outcomes to the process of care.

There are those who maintain that nothing but randomized controlled trials can provide real evidence of efficacy. Epidemiological models applied to observational data can never be absolutely sure that differences found were not due to unobserved variations in the two groups. Random allocation is a powerful tool, but both because of other limitations, especially with regard to examining the effectiveness of a treatment (i.e., how it actually works in practice), and simply for reasons of logistics, epidemiological (observational) studies will inevitably play a major role. It is crucial that these latter studies be carefully designed to minimize their limitations (Shadish, Cook, & Campbell, 2002). (Chapter 2 provides a more detailed discussion about the alternative approaches.)

In effect, both approaches require some level of extrapolation and inference. The RCT requires a heavy set of inferences to extrapolate the results based on extensive participant selection and fixed interventions to clinical practice. The epidemiological approach requires a substantial amount of inference in the analysis itself, but the translation to practice is thus much easier because many of the relevant variables have already been addressed.

Because the epidemiological approach is essentially a naturalistic technique that relies on data collected as part of extant practice, questions will arise about the comparability of those who receive different forms of care. The assignment to treatment groups is not based on chance. Factors, both overt and more subtle, determine who gets what care. The burden of proof lies with the investigator. In truth, no amount of evidence can absolutely guarantee comparability, but a lot of informational benefit can accrue from using carefully analyzed information derived from real practice.

A much more important problem in using clinical information is its quality. Clinical investigators quickly appreciate that clinical data is not recorded systematically or thoroughly. Patient information is entered when patients visit the system. No systematic follow-up is obtained. Much of the information recorded summarizes clinicians' summary impressions rather than capturing the presence of specific signs and symptoms. Two clinicians may opt to record quite disparate information, even when they use the same headings. Investigators seeking to mount outcomes studies will need to plan these studies to include prospective data collection and incorporate deliberate steps that attend to the quality of information at each stage. Most good observational studies require a prospective design with standardized, systematic data collection on all aspects (i.e., case mix, treatment, and outcomes).

MEASURING OUTCOMES

Outcomes come in a variety of sizes and shapes. The selection of an outcomes measure should be based on a clear sense of what one wants to measure and why. Outcomes measures can be both generic and specific to a given problem. The generic measures are useful for looking at policy issues or reflecting the bottom line effects of care on health status or even aspects of quality of life. They provide a sort of lingua franca that can be used to compare the treatments for various conditions in analyses such as cost-effectiveness.

Because much medical care can affect specific signs and symptoms but may not have a profound impact on the greater spheres of life, most clinicians are accustomed to looking at the more limited effects of care. These are more closely linked to specific interventions and hence are usually more satisfying to see. Condition-specific outcomes, as the name implies, will vary with the condition being treated, although some measures may prove useful for more than one condition.

Generic measures address larger constructs; hence, their causal links to specific treatment events may be more difficult to trace. The generic measures can include both measures of function in various sectors (e.g., self-care, social activity, emotional state) as well as satisfaction with the care provided, the way it is provided, and perhaps even the setting in which it is provided. It is not always easy to separate opinions about the quality of care from feelings about the results of treatment. While someone may feel satisfied that a clinician did his best even if the results are disappointing, it is likely that patients will be more satisfied when the results are favorable.

Both generic and condition-specific outcomes measures (as well as the other components of the outcomes equation) often need to be aggregated to create some sort of summary measure. The aggregation process is complex. There is a strong temptation to simply add raw scores to generate a total score, but such a step is foolhardy. In the simplest case, it implies an equal weighting among the components, an assumption that is not automatically true. Even worse, the components may take on different weights because of the way the answers are constructed. For example, a response with five categories may receive a score of 1 through 5, while a dichotomous answer would be 0 or 1. There is no a priori reason to suspect that a 5 on the first scale is any more important than a 1 on the second. Even when the responses are in some apparent order, a response of 5 is not necessarily five times more than a response of 1.

Deciding how to weight the components of a summary scale properly can be a serious undertaking. Ordinarily, one needs some construct to use as the basis for normalizing the values placed on each component. Techniques that vary in sophistication and ease of implementation (usually inversely) can be applied to obtaining the value weights of different constituencies. In the outcomes trade, these values are usually referred to as utility weights. Sometimes they are directly related to overt concepts; sometimes they are inferred from observed behaviors.

The science of measurement has come a long way. Before an outcomes measure can be said to have attained its pedigree, it must pass a series of tests. The criteria for a useful measure are that it is reliable (i.e., it will yield the same results consistently); it is valid (i.e., it measures what it says it does); and it is responsive (i.e., it can detect meaningful increments of change; Guyatt, Deyo, Charlson, Levine, & Mitchell, 1989).

Some measures have been extensively studied; others are more novel. Few if any can be used on all occasions. The astute outcomes researcher must weigh the measure's reputation against its actual content and the application intended. For example, some measures work well with some populations but not with others. They may cover only a limited portion of the full performance spectrum, or be better at distinguishing among some aspects of function than others.

CONCEPTUAL MODELING

There are five keys steps in outcomes research. Although they are performed sequentially, they are not as independent as they might seem. Indeed, most study design efforts involve a substantial amount of cycling back to adjust questions based on design issues and models based on data issues. Greater clarification of later steps may entail revising earlier ones. In the end, any presentation must be internally coherent. The individual steps must be shown, and they must relate to one another. The five steps are:

1. Define a researchable question.
2. Develop a conceptual model.
3. Conduct a literature review.
4. Operationalize the variables.
5. Develop a research plan.

1. *Define a researchable question.* In most cases, the research question precedes the underlying model, but not necessarily. Asking a researchable question is much harder than simply posing a question. A researchable question must be answerable by direct means. It is not a philosophic proposition. It should have a clear statement of what is done to whom, perhaps with some concerns about the context of the care. Often the test of the completeness and directness of the question will come from the conceptual model. Frequently the question will be modified after the model is refined.

2. *Develop a conceptual model.* A critical step in developing an outcomes study is the creation of a conceptual model. This need will be stressed frequently in this book, because it is so central to successful outcomes work. In essence, the conceptual model indicates what is believed to cause the outcome. It identifies the critical pathways and what other factors are likely to affect these. It should identify which variables, chosen to represent the various components of the basic outcomes equation described earlier, are pertinent to the study at hand. The variables and their relationship both to the outcomes of interest and to each other should be specified.

3. *Conduct a literature review.* The conceptual model is usually the result of a literature search, but not always. Sometimes the reverse is true; one starts with a model in mind and uses the literature review to refine it. As with all steps in this process, the actual course is typically cyclical. There are two types of literature reviews: systematic reviews and advocacy reviews. Ideally every outcomes study should be preceded by a systematic review of the literature, which identifies the current state of knowledge on the topic. Detailed methods have been developed for such systematic reviews (Agency for Healthcare Research and Quality, 2002; Juni, Altman, & Egger, 2001)

   Most research proposals (and certainly most research articles) utilize a different strategy, one that tends to lead the reader to a predetermined conclusion (i.e., the need for and feasibility of the proposed study or report). This type of review, which may be termed "advocacy" is designed with the conclusion in mind; whereas, the systematic review starts with an intellectually neutral slate and judges the results by what is unearthed—consistent and strong evidence.

Writing an advocacy review requires skill. Since you know where you want to end up, you want to shape the arguments to make the strongest case, but you cannot omit salient information (especially because the person reviewing your work may well have written it). The task then is to show what has been done and what are the limitations with that work to date. Each time you cite a limitation, you should indicate how your study will address it. You may also want to argue by analogy, suggesting that earlier work on a different topic or a different context has used methods that parallel what you propose, thereby bolstering your method, but showing it will be applied innovatively.

4. *Operationalize the variables.* Once these elements have been identified, they can be operationalized. Each one can be captured in one or more measures. The delineation of the model and the specification of variables represent two of the major components of a research design. Once again, they are reciprocal; changes in one may affect the other. The best way to lay out the variables is in a variables table, which indicates the source and form of each variable. The latter has implications for the analysis plan. Table 1-1 provides a model using elements from a congestive heart failure example.

A familiar maxim in outcomes research is that what cannot be measured does not exist. In one sense, the concept is attractive. We need to be able to reduce complex attributes to measurable representations in order to study it and to compare its presence across programs. However, one must approach measurement with respect. Measurement involves distortion; it is by nature a process of abstraction and something is inevitably lost in the process.

Likewise, the commitment to measurement should not be construed as endorsing the idea that everything that can be measured is useful. Perhaps one of the most memorable misuses of measurement was the theory behind the conduct of the Vietnam War. Body counts and arbitrary definitions of successful missions do not necessarily lead to a successful conclusion. Quantitative analysis works best when it serves conceptual thinking, not when it is a substitute for it.

5. *Develop a research plan.* The last key ingredient is the research plan, which consists of two basic components: (1) how the data will be collected (or if a secondary analysis, what data are available), and

Table 1-1   Model Variables

Element	Definition	Source	Format
Dependent variables			
Cardiac output	Ejection fraction	Medical record	Continuous
Symptoms	Shortness of breath Edema	Patient interview	Ordinal
Function	IADLs, ADLs	Patient interview	Continuous
Complications	Pneumonia	Medical record	Dichotomous
QOL	QOL score SF-36	Patient interview	Continuous
Workless/ employment	Employment status	Patient interview	Dichotomous
Independent variables			
Severity	New York Heart Classification	Medical record	Continuous
Duration	Months since onset	Medical record	Continuous
Etiology	Heart disease type	Medical record	Categorical
Comorbidity	Diagnoses	Medical record	Categorical
Age		Medical record	Continuous

ADLs, activities of daily living; IADLs, instrumental activities of daily living; QOL, quality of life.

(2) the analysis plan.[5] The conceptual model provides a general framework for the analysis, but the specifics will depend on several factors, primarily the nature of the variables. In general, there should be an analysis plan for each research question. It should provide enough detail to show that the investigator has thought about the implications of the research design. An important component of the analysis plan is the power estimate. It is important to show

---

[5]This book does not attempt to discuss the intricacies of the analytic methods for nonexperimental studies. Investigators should consult with a methodologist and/or statistician before any outcomes analysis is undertaken.

that the planned data will be sufficient to detect a real difference if one is present. Likewise, in a quasi-experimental design, one needs to address the plans for dealing with selection bias.

Most analyses, especially those that rely on an epidemiological approach will have to be multivariate. One or another variation of regression modeling will likely be employed. Although multivariate modeling can take into account the effects of intervening variables, nonrandom assignment invariably raises questions about the comparability of treatment and control groups. Even groups that seem very comparable on the basis of examined variables may vary widely along some other parameter. Some researchers have proposed statistical models to deal with this so-called selection bias. Special models are developed to identify and deal with the correlated error associated with such a bias (see Chapter 3). These corrections use factors that are related to the treatment but not to the outcome.

Interpreting the results of regression equations can be complicated. Fundamentally, the major question is whether the independent variable of greatest interest (usually treatment) is significantly related to the dependent variable (i.e., the outcome) after the effects of other factors has been considered. This relationship can be examined in two ways: (1) the extent to which a change in the risk factor affects the dependent variable (e.g., the odds ratio), and (2) the capacity of the full equation to explain the variance in the model. It is quite feasible for a variable to be very significantly related to the dependent variable in an equation that explains very little of the overall variance. Conversely, explaining the variance does not examine the relationship between the independent variables and the dependent variable. In epidemiological terms, the size and strength of a coefficient from the regression equation reflect the power of the relationship, whereas the amount of variance explained describes the power of the overall model. It is possible to have a statistically significant relationship among variables and still not explain much of the total variance in the distribution of the dependent variable. Outcomes may be influenced by many things, not all of them measurable. As a result, many outcomes equations do not account for a great proportion of the variance, although the adjusted relationship between variables of interest may be very significant. Being able to establish a clear relationship between a treatment and its purported effects is important even when that relationship does not account for all, or even most, of the effect. A clear understanding of how a treatment influences outcomes for defined subgroups of patients lays the foundation for meaningful guidelines about what constitutes appropriate care.

ORGANIZATION OF THE BOOK

The next three chapters in this introductory section address overarching design issues; two address study design issues, and one is on measurement principles. The next section of this book is organized to discuss the implications of the basic outcomes model. Each component is discussed at some length to identify the issues that must be considered and to suggest some measures that may prove useful (along with caveats about using them). The first series of chapters addresses outcomes measures including generic measures, condition-specific measures, and satisfaction. The second set of chapters covers the major components of risk adjustment, including severity of illness, comorbidity, and demographic and psychosocial characteristics. The last chapter in this section discusses treatment and proposes a taxonomy for this central component. The final three chapters address some overarching issues in conducting outcomes research. Cost-effectiveness is a growing area of related interest in outcomes research. The next chapter addresses some practical issues in implementing research studies in a clinical setting. We then offer some final thoughts for those who are anxious to launch into outcomes studies. Although these observations are intended primarily for neophytes, we hope that even more experienced outcomes researchers may gain some useful insights from them.

REFERENCES

Agency for Healthcare Research and Quality. (2002). *Systems to rate the strength of scientific evidence* (No. 47). Available at: www.ahrq .gov/clinic/epcsums/strengthsum.htm. Accessed March 31, 2010.

Angrist, J. D., Imbens, G. W., & Rubin, D. B. (1996). Identification of causal effects using instrumental variables. *Journal of the American Statistical Association*, *91*(434), 444–472.

Begg, C., Cho, M., Eastwood, S., Horton, R., Moher, D., Olkin, I., . . .Stroup, D. F. (1996). Improving the quality of reporting of randomized controlled trials: The CONSORT statement. *JAMA*, *276*, 637–649.

Berwick, D. M. (1989). Continuous improvement as an ideal in health care. *New England Journal of Medicine*, *320*(1), 53–56.

D'Agostino, R. B., Jr. (1998). Propensity score methods for bias reduction in the comparison of a treatment to a non-randomized control group. *Statistics in Medicine, 17*, 2265–2281.

Donabedian, A. (1966). Evaluating the quality of medical care. *Milbank Memorial Fund Quarterly, 44*(3), 166–206.

Donabedian, A. (1988). The quality of care: How can it be assessed? *JAMA, 260*, 1743–1748.

Field, M., & Lohr, K. (Eds.). (1992). *Guidelines for clinical practice: From development to use.* Washington, DC: National Academy Press.

Fisher, E. S., Wennberg, D. E., Stukel, T. A., Gottlieb, D. J., Lucas, F. L., & Pinder, E. L. (2003). The implications of regional variations in Medicare spending. Part 2: Health outcomes and satisfaction with care. *Annals of Internal Medicine, 138*(4), 288–298.

Glickman, S. W., Ou, F.-S., DeLong, E. R., Roe, M. T., Lytle, B. L., Mulgund, J., . . .Peterson, E. D. (2007). Pay for performance, quality of care, and outcomes in acute myocardial infarction. *JAMA, 297*(11), 2373–2380.

Guyatt, G. H., Deyo, R. A., Charlson, M., Levine, M. N., & Mitchell, A. (1989). Responsiveness and validity in health status measurement: A clarification. *Journal of Clinical Epidemiology, 42*(5), 403–408.

Heckman, J. (1979). Sample selection bias as a specification error. *Econometrica, 47*, 153–161.

Heckman, J. J. (2008). Econometric causality. *International Statistical Review, 76*(1), 1–27.

Hibbard, J. H., & Jewett, J. J. (1997). Will quality report cards help consumers? *Health Affairs, 16*(3), 218–228.

Hibbard, J. H., Peters, E., Dixon, A., & Tusler, M. (2007). Consumer competencies and the use of comparative quality information: It isn't just about literacy. *Medical Care Research Review, 64*(4), 379–394.

Juni, P., Altman, D. G., & Egger, M. (2001). Systematic reviews in health care: Assessing the quality of controlled clinical trials. *British Medical Journal, 323*, 42–46.

Kohn, L. T., Corrigan, J. M., & Donaldson, M. S. (Eds.). (2000). *To err is human: Building a safer health system.* Washington, DC: National Academy Press.

Lee, L. F. (1994). Semiparametric instrumental variable estimation of simultaneous equation sample selection models. *Journal of Econometrics, 63*(2), 341–388.

Lindenauer, P. K., Remus, D., Roman, S., Rothberg, M. B., Benjamin, E. M., Ma, A., & Bratzler, D. W. (2007). Public reporting and pay for performance in hospital quality improvement. *New England Journal of Medicine, 356*(5), 486–496.

Rosenthal, M. B., Landon, B. E., Normand, S.-L. T., Frank, R. G., & Epstein, A. M. (2006). Pay for performance in commercial HMOs. *New England Journal of Medicine, 355*(18), 1895–1902.

Sackett, D. L., Richardson, W. S., Rosenberg, W. M. C., & Haynes, R. B. (1997). *Evidence-based medicine: How to practice and teach EBM.* New York: Churchill Livingstone Press.

Shadish, W. R., Cook, T. D., & Campbell, D. T. (2002). *Experimental and quasi-experimental designs for generalized causal inference.* Boston: Houghton Mifflin.

Stukel, T. A., Fisher, E. S., Wennberg, D. E., Alter, D. A., Gottlieb, D. J., & Vermeulen, M. J. (2007). Analysis of observational studies in the presence of treatment selection bias: Effects of invasive cardiac management on AMI survival using propensity score and instrumental variable methods. *JAMA, 297*(3), 278–285.

Weed, L. L. (1968a). Medical records that guide and teach. *New England Journal of Medicine, 278*(11), 593–600.

Weed, L. L. (1968b). Medical records that guide and teach. *New England Journal of Medicine, 278*(12), 652–657.

Werner, R. M., & Asch, D. A. (2005). The unintended consequences of publicly reporting quality information. *JAMA, 293*(10), 1239–1244.

CHAPTER 2

Models and Causal Thinking

CAUSATION

One of the great challenges underlying intervention research is to determine what constitutes proof of causation. The goal of outcomes research is to isolate the effect of treatment on the patient and/or disease being treated. The underlying challenge is to demonstrate that the relationship is causal. Distinguishing cause from association is one of the great challenges of science, especially clinical science.

Much of health services research and outcomes research draws on epidemiology, which is primarily directed at identifying factors associated with illness and identifying its cause. Here we are interested in the causes of improvement that result from defined interventions. Hence, some of the principles work well, but some need extrapolations.

Principles of causation have been around for quite a while, but ironically, they have changed as scientific measurement has improved and science has become more efficient and complex. One of the early philosophers who addressed causation was David Hume (Beauchamp, 1999). He laid out a series of postulates, or criteria, for a causal relationship. For example, to say that **A** causes **B**, the following must be true:

1. **A** must be consistently associated with **B**.

2. **A** must always precede **B**.

3. There must be a theoretical connection of **A** to **B**.

This work was picked up by Jakob Henle and Robert Koch who articulated a set of principles for infection. These principles, known as Henle-Koch's postulates, are as follows:

1. The bacteria must be present in every case of the disease.

2. The bacteria must be isolated from the host with the disease and grown in pure culture.

3. The specific disease must be reproduced when a pure culture of the bacteria is inoculated into a healthy susceptible host.

4. The bacteria must be recoverable from the experimentally infected host.

However, these principles proved difficult to apply as science evolved. We came to recognize that not all persons were equally susceptible and that some agents could not be readily identified. As a result, a new approach to analyzing the chain of causation was needed, one that recognized that the effects of treatment might be mitigated by the characteristics of the patient (and even perhaps by those of the therapist). By the era of viral infection research, Henle-Koch's postulates were examples, not requirements, for causality (Evans, 1976). As knowledge of the immune process increased, the definition of a dangerous bacterium changed.

Debate on how to establish causation continues today. There is no absolute rule about causation but one of the most frequently cited descriptions comes from a famous British epidemiologist, Sir Austin Bradford-Hill. His criteria for distinguishing association from cause are shown in Table 2-1 (Hill, 1965).

Clinical science relies on the randomized clinical trial (RCT) as the highest expression of causal proof. However, the RCT is a relatively new development. Although some go back to the innovation work of James Lind in the 18th century, when he established the cause of scurvy by assigning sailors on some British Royal Navy ships to eat limes while others did not. The first reported RCT usually cited is the 1926 work of Ronald Aylmer Fisher, but it was on agriculture (Fisher, 1926). The first modern medical RCT was the 1948 report by the British Medical Research Council (Medical Research Council, 1948).

Outcomes research relies heavily on epidemiology for its methods. Whereas epidemiology is primarily interested in what causes diseases,

Table 2-1   **Bradford-Hill Criteria for Assessing Evidence of Causation**

1. Strength: Larger effect sizes provide stronger evidence for causation.
2. Consistency: Observations should be replicable by different persons at different times and places.
3. Specificity: The relationship between the putative cause and putative effect should occur only with them. It is important to distinguish the strength of the association from the clinical importance.
4. Temporality: Cause must precede effect.
5. Biological gradient: The greater the exposure the greater the effect.
6. Plausibility: A reasonable mechanism for the cause and effect relationship is desirable.
7. Coherence: Consistency between the epidemiological findings and biological findings strengthens the evidence for causation.
8. Experiment: The cause and effect relationship is supported by experimental trials.
9. Analogy: Similar effects have been observed with similar exposures.

outcomes research explores the benefits (and harms) of treatment. The modeling is basically the same; only the variables change. Epidemiology talks about risk factors and disease incidence. For outcomes research, the treatment is the risk factor of interest, the disease is the target, and other confounding factors must be considered in the design and analysis of the study (Groenwold, Hak, & Hoes, 2009).

A basic but perplexing distinction is between an association and a cause. The former reflects a consistent pattern of correlations but the latter implies a mechanism. Making the leap from association to cause means taking a big step.

There are several measures of association: odds ratio (OR), relative risk (RR), absolute risk (AR), and effect size (ES). Each conveys different information (Austin, 2010). In distinguishing among these measures, it is important to understand the difference between an odds ratio and risk ratio as measures of association. To understand the difference between these measures, it necessary to appreciate how outcomes get counted (i.e., the odds of an outcome versus the risk of an outcome).

The OR quantifies the magnitude of association between the risk factor and the outcome in terms of odds, whereas the RR quantifies the strength of the association in terms of risk. It assesses the odds of someone with the risk factor developing the outcomes as compared to someone without the risk factor. For example, the OR can be used to compare the occurrence of diabetes mellitus in a population. In the white population, there is one person with diabetes mellitus for every eight individuals without diabetes mellitus. Thus, the odds of diabetes mellitus in the white population are 1 in 8. In the African American community, the odds of diabetes mellitus are closer to 1 in 3. The OR for an association between race and diabetes mellitus is the quotient of the ratios, or 2.67 (OR = 1/3 ÷ 1/8).

Compared with the OR, the RR is based on probability estimates rather than odds. For the previous example, the probability of having diabetes mellitus, expressed as a percent, and being white is 11.1% [0.111 = 1 / (1 + 8)]. Among African Americans, the probability of having diabetes mellitus is 33.3%. For this association, the RR is the ratio of the two risks, or 3.00. This example illustrates the important distinction between the OR and RR. The two measures of association give results that are different. In fact, the OR and RR only provide comparable results when the outcome is relatively rare in the population (i.e., less than 10%). This is called the rare disease assumption. Both measures are perfectly acceptable in outcomes research, but it is important to recognize the underlying differences in how the outcomes are quantified (Schmidt & Kohlmann, 2008).

As shown in Table 2-2, the same data can be analyzed to generate an OR and a RR. Customarily, the RR is the preferred measure in prospective studies, where the group under study has been identified by the risk factor. Compared with the RR, the AR is the actual difference between the risk of the outcome with and without the exposure. For many purposes, this is the most important estimate because it speaks most directly to the ultimate impact of the intervention.

To illustrate how these differences can be used, imagine two diseases with treatments. Disease 1 Treatment A improves survival from 1 in 1 million to 2 in 1 million. Disease 2 Treatment B improves survival from 1 in 4 to 1 in 2. The relative risk (or relative benefit) is 2 in both cases. But with Disease 1, the absolute benefit of Treatment A is 1 in 1 million; whereas for Treatment B in Disease 2, it is 1 in 4.

Effect size is similar to relative benefit (or risk) but it adds some new dimensions. Essentially it reflects the distribution of the two groups (i.e., treated and not) and the distribution of outcomes associated with each. It is typically expressed as the difference in the means divided by the standard error.

Table 2-2 Outcomes Analysis Using Cross-tabulated Data

Treatment	Outcome	
	Yes	No
Exposed	a	b
Unexposed	c	d

Risk of the outcome in the exposed $= \dfrac{a}{(a + b)}$

Risk of the outcome in the unexposed $= \dfrac{c}{(c + d)}$

Relative risk $= \dfrac{\left[\frac{a}{(a + b)}\right]}{\left[\frac{c}{(c + d)}\right]}$

Odds of the outcome in the exposed $= \dfrac{a}{b}$

Odds of the outcome in the unexposed $= \dfrac{c}{d}$

Odds ratio $= \dfrac{\left[\frac{a}{b}\right]}{\left[\frac{c}{d}\right]}$ or $\dfrac{ad}{bc}$

Absolute risk $= \left[\frac{a}{b}\right] - \left[\frac{c}{d}\right]$

Another term encountered is attributable risk. It measures the proportionate excess risk of the outcome that is associated with a risk factor.

$$Attributable\ Risk = \frac{Prevalence\ of\ Risk\ Factor\ (RR - 1)}{1 + Prevalence\ of\ Risk\ Factor\ (RR - 1)}$$

where prevalence of the risk factor in the population is the proportion of those in the population with the risk factor and RR is the relative risk.

CONCEPTUAL MODELS

Developing a health outcomes project requires clearly specifying the underlying relationships and understanding what is required to establish a causal relationship. A conceptual model need not be based on disciplinary theory. It simply and clearly explicates what process the investigator believes is occurring, or at least what elements need to be controlled in the analysis. Such a model can be based on clinical experience as well as a review of prior work. Working through the model helps to think about what factors are most important.

Conceptual thinking can readily grow from insightful clinical analysis. Clinical intuition and insight is a valuable gift, which should not be discarded or devalued in the face of quantitative science. In his autobiography, Colin Powell describes an intelligence unit in Vietnam that received endless amounts of data on the enemy's shelling patterns. All this information was entered into a computer regression model, which eventually produced the result that shelling was heavier on moonless nights, an observation that any combat veteran could have provided (Powell, 1995).

Outcomes research shares some of these problems. On the one hand, if its findings do not agree with clinical wisdom, they are distrusted. On the other hand, if they support such beliefs, they are extraneous. Life is generally too complicated to attempt outcomes analysis without some sort of framework. Some analysts may believe that the data will speak for themselves, but most appreciate the value of a frame of reference. Even more important, with so much information waiting to be collected, one needs some basis for even deciding where to look for the most powerful answers.

Using outcomes wisely requires having a good feel for what question is being asked and what factors are likely to influence the answer. Outcomes research is largely still a clinical undertaking, although it has become sophisticated. At its heart is a clinical model of causation.

Before an outcomes study can be planned, the investigator needs to develop a clear model of the factors that are believed to be most salient and their relationship to the outcomes of interest. Some factors will play a direct role; others may influence events more indirectly. Each factor needs to be captured and its role defined. This model forms the basis of the analysis plan.

As noted previously, the conceptual model identifies the critical pathways and what other factors are likely to affect them. It should identify which variables, chosen to represent the various components of the basic outcomes equation, are pertinent to the study at hand. The variables themselves, and their relationship both to the outcomes of interest and to each other, should be specified. The process of creating a conceptual model is itself iterative.

A conceptual model is not necessarily the same as a theoretical model. The conceptual model lays out the expected relationship among classes of variables. It may be the result of intuition, of the literature review, or of expert judgment. A theoretical model draws upon some established set of theories that account for the observed associations among major variables.

The starting point is a set of premises based on theory and/or clinical insights. As you flesh out the model and become ever more specific about

Figure 2-1   **Basic Conceptual Model**

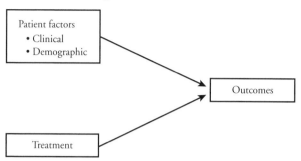

just what is involved, you can begin to think of how to operationalize this model, which may necessitate revisiting the model as it becomes further explicated and refined.

Models can vary in their complexity. Figure 2-1 offers a simple illustration of a conceptual model for looking at the outcomes of care. The two basic components of variables are those reflecting patient characteristics (both clinical and demographic) and the treatment provided. Figure 2-2 takes this model a step further by showing that the treatment may interact with the patient factors to produce an outcome. Figure 2-3 adapts the model to the case of congestive heart failure. Figure 2-4 shows the same model, but the potential relationship (exacerbated in a descriptive study) between patient clinical characteristics and the treatment is stressed. Adjusting for this selection bias will require special analyses.

Figure 2-2   **Interactive Conceptual Model**

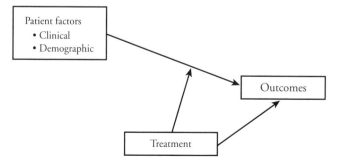

Figure 2-3 Conceptual Model of Treatment and Outcomes for Congestive Heart Failure

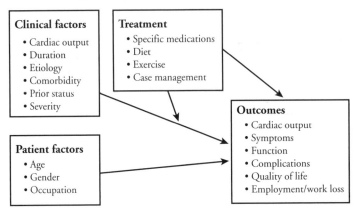

The items in the boxes are operationalized aspects of the basic elements that are addressed in the outcomes equation previously described. The arrows indicate an expected effect. In this model, the effects of treatment are expected to interact with the clinical factors to produce outcomes.

A scientific theory is a "construction of explicit explanations in accounting for empirical findings" (Bengtson, Rice, & Johnson, 1999).

Figure 2-4 Conceptual Model of Congestive Heart Failure with Selection Bias

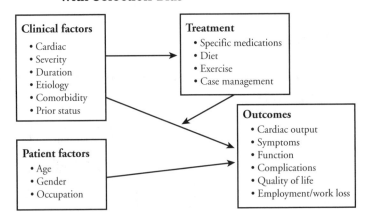

Theory is used to build knowledge and understanding in a systematic and cumulative way, so that our empirical efforts will lead to integration with what is already known, as well as a guide to what is yet to be learned (Bengtson *et al.*, 1999). Theories take time to develop and be tested. Over time they may be rejected when new evidence comes to light that is inconsistent with current beliefs (Kuhn, 1970). By contrast, a model is much simpler. It portrays a picture of how elements may be related to each other. It may be driven by an underlying theory or it may be based on clinical or other observations (some of which may come from previous studies).

EXPLANATORY MODELS

A number of explanatory models can be used in outcomes research. They may guide the actual creation of an analytically driven conceptual model or they may offer insights into how behavior can affect outcomes. Two of the most widely used are the Andersen–Aday model of utilization (Aday & Andersen, 1974; Phillips, Morrison, Andersen, & Aday, 1998) and the Health Belief Model (Stretcher & Rosenstock, 1997). The Andersen–Aday model is widely cited because it is so inclusive (Aday & Andersen, 1974). It has undergone many iterations (Andersen, 2008). The most recent version is shown in Figure 2-5. It identifies three major groups of factors that account for utilization of health resources.

1. Predisposing characteristics (demographic, social support, health beliefs)

2. Enabling resources (personal/family, community)

3. Need (perceived, evaluated)

Its strength is its weakness. It is so inclusive that almost anything can fit it. Hence, it is very attractive to people looking for a justification for their research. However, its breadth often means it explains little. Researchers may find themselves pushing variables into pigeonholes in the model to create a rationale for their inclusion when a simple, straightforward approach might work better.

The Health Belief Model (see Figure 2-6) was originally developed to explain preventive behaviors (Becker & Maiman, 1975; Stretcher &

Figure 2-5   Andersen–Aday Behavioral Model of Health Services Use

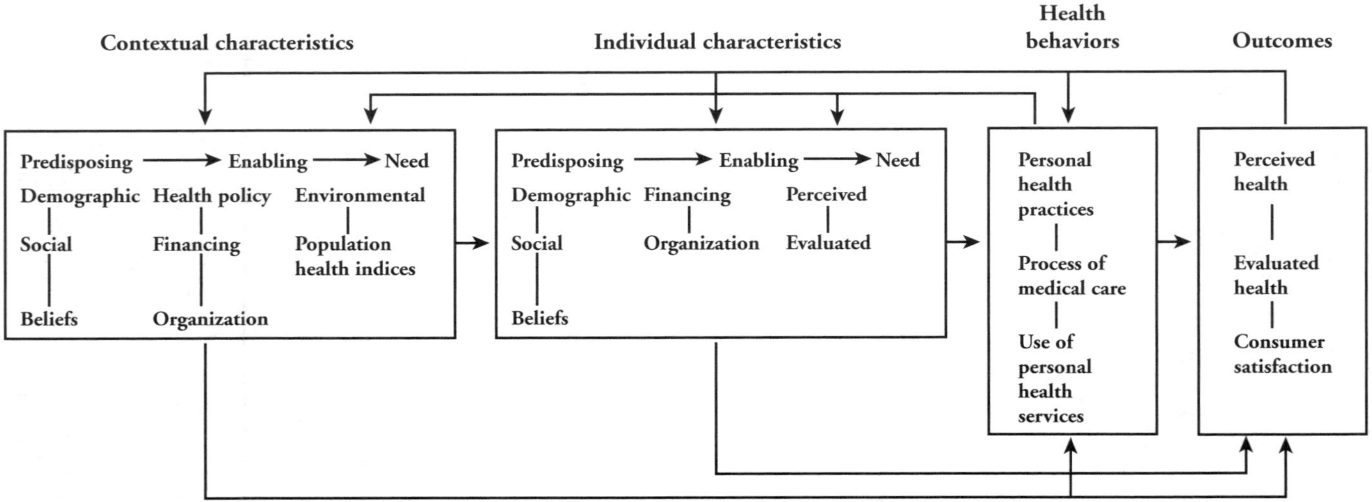

Source: (Andersen, 2008)

Figure 2-6   Health Belief Model

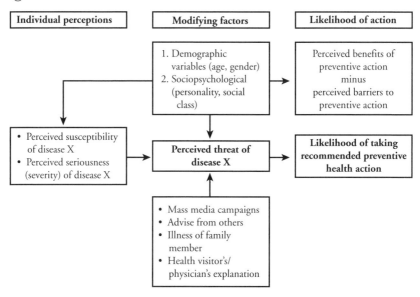

Rosenstock, 1997). Its predictive capacity has been challenged but it continues to offer a useful basic framework that suggests that people's adherence behavior is driven by their perceptions of the seriousness of a disease and their susceptibility to it. In the context of outcomes, this might be transformed into a belief in the efficacy of treatment. Thus, they conduct a crude benefit calculation that weighs the risks against the potential benefits. This calculation is susceptible to external influences.

SUMMARY

It is important but often difficult to distinguish causation from association. Various tests of association should be used deliberately and carefully. Theoretical models provide general guidance to explain phenomena, but conceptual models can offer specific details that guide the analysis of a research study. Some conceptual models are derived from theory; others may come from practice or insight. Models are simply ways of displaying what the researcher believes is happening as the basis for explicating and testing research questions.

REFERENCES

Aday, L. A., & Andersen, R. (1974). A framework for the study of access to medical care. *Health Services Research, 9*(3), 208–220.

Andersen, R. M. (2008). National health surveys and the behavioral model of health services use. *Medical Care, 46*(7), 647–653.

Austin, P. C. (2010). Absolute risk reductions, relative risks, relative risk reductions, and numbers needed to treat can be obtained from a logistic regression model. *Journal of Clinical Epidemiology, 63*(1), 2–6.

Beauchamp, T. L. (Ed.). (1999). *An enquiry concerning human understanding.* New York: Oxford University Press.

Becker, M. H., & Maiman, L. A. (1975). Sociobehavioral determinants of compliance with health and medical care recommendations. *Medical Care, 13*(1), 10–24.

Bengtson, V. L., Rice, C. J., & Johnson, M. L. (1999). Are theories of aging important? Models and explanations in gerontology at the turn of the century. In V. L. Bengtson & K. W. Schaie (Eds.), *Handbook of Theories of Aging* (pp. 3–20). New York: Springer Publishing Company.

Evans, A. S. (1976). Causation and disease: The Henle-Koch Postulates revisited. *Yale Journal of Biology and Medicine, 49*(2), 175–195.

Fisher, R. A. (1926). The arrangement of field experiments. *Journal of Ministry of Agriculture, 33,* 500–513.

Groenwold, R. H., Hak, E., & Hoes, A. W. (2009). Quantitative assessment of unobserved confounding is mandatory in nonrandomized intervention studies. *Journal of Clinical Epidemiology, 62*(1), 22–28.

Hill, A. B. (1965). The environment and disease: Association or causation. *Proceedings of the Royal Society of Medicine, 58,* 295–300.

Kuhn, T. S. (1970). *The Structure of Scientific Revolutions* (2nd ed.). Chicago: University of Chicago Press.

Medical Research Council. (1948). Streptomycin treatment of pulmonary tuberculosis: A Medical Research Council investigation. *British Medical Journal, 2,* 769.

Phillips, K. A., Morrison, K. R., Andersen, R., & Aday, L. A. (1998). Understanding the context of healthcare utilization: Assessing environmental and provider-related variables in the behavioral model of utilization. *Health Services Research, 33*(3), 571–596.

Powell, C. L. (1995). *My American journey* (1st ed.). New York: Random House.

Schmidt, C. O., & Kohlmann, T. (2008). When to use the odds ratio or the relative risk? *International Journal of Public Health, 53,* 165–167.

Stretcher, V., & Rosenstock, I. M. (1997). The health belief model. In K. Glanz, F. M. Lewis, & B. K. Rimer (Eds.), *Health behavior and health education: Theory, research, and practice* (2nd ed., pp. 41–59). San Francisco: Jossey-Bass.

Outcomes Research Study Designs

ISOLATING THE EFFECT OF THE INTERVENTION

The goal of outcomes research is to isolate the effect of treatment on the patient and/or disease being treated. The underlying challenge is to demonstrate that the relationship is causal. Distinguishing cause from association is one of the great challenges of science, especially clinical science. We discussed the principles of causation in Chapter 2.

The major threat to establishing a causal relationship is *selection bias*, by which we mean that the decision to assign a given patient to a given treatment is influenced by some set of factors that might predict the success of the treatment. The randomized clinical trial (RCT) was designed to ensure that the allocation of treatment was done in a random fashion (to all patients who qualified for the treatment). Hence, the treatment and control groups may be different, but any differences will have occurred by chance and not by prejudice. Some independent principle of assignment is used such that neither the therapist nor the patient could decide who got what treatment.[1] Obviously, the potential benefits of the treatment had to be strong (and access constrained) to induce patients to risk not getting it.

---

[1]It is important to distinguish random allocation from random sampling. The former refers to determining how patients are assigned to the treatment or control group. The latter refers to how well the persons chosen to participate in the study reflect a larger population, of which they can be called a sample. Very few studies with random allocation use random samples.

Randomized trials imply some heavy limitations. Because all patients in the trial have to be suitable and because there is great concern that the treatment should be as effective as possible, active steps are taken to assure that only extremely suitable patients who are likely to benefit are deemed eligible for the RCT. Strong inclusion and exclusion criteria were developed to facilitate targeting. As a result, the RCT could be applicable to only those who possessed the inclusion (and not the exclusion) characteristics. In other words, the stricter the selection criteria, the less generalized the RCT results. This is the inevitable trade-off. A good practical guide to trial design is *A Pragmatic–Explanatory Continuum Indicator Summary (PRECIS): A Tool to Help Trial Designers* (Thorpe *et. al.*, 2009).

Many aspects of medical care do not lend themselves easily to RCTs. Patients may be too anxious to get the treatment to tolerate a 50% chance of being a control. The greater the mortality imposed by the disease, the stronger the argument that survival is proof positive of success and randomization is not needed.

The big trade-off in clinical research is thus between potential selection bias and likely limited capacity to generalize the study findings from what is effectively a volunteer sample. Researchers from a variety of disciplines have labored long and hard to seek ways to address the impediments of selection bias. The great concern is that there may be some unmeasured factor that is linked to getting the intervention, which may affect the outcome. Perhaps the most creative work has come from economics. James Heckman, a Nobel Laureate, has been associated with some of the most creative thinking in this arena (1979; 2008). Heckman proposed a statistical approach that involves using so-called instrumental variables (IVs), variables that are related to the likelihood of getting the intervention, but not to outcomes of the intervention itself. The ideal IV should be related to the likelihood of getting treatment in question but not to the outcome (Rassen, Brookhart, Glynn, Mittleman, & Schneeweiss, 2009a; 2009b). The great challenge of these IVs (beyond the mathematics) is identifying them. It is surprisingly hard to think of factors that fit that bill of particulars. Generally, candidate variables come from access measures, which reflect the ease of getting the treatment in question, but these measures apply in only some instances and not always well.

Epidemiologists have pursued a more mundane approach. Typically, the epidemiological approach would be to statistically adjust the analysis to take cognizance of the role of any potential factors associated with getting the intervention that could affect the outcomes. A more elegant approach is called the *propensity score* (Austin & Platt, 2010a; 2010b). Basically, it models the likelihood of getting the intervention of interest using all available data, based on a conceptual model of factors that should influence such use. A logistic model is used to estimate the probability of receiving the intervention and a score is assigned to each person in the study in both the experimental and control groups. Patients are then placed into tiers based on their propensity scores and compared within each tier. This approach is easier for clinicians to follow and accept. It is less elegant than IVs and can deal with only those variables that can be measured. But adherents claim that they can predict use quite well.

Not surprisingly, the two approaches can yield different results (Stukel, Fischer, Wennberg, Alter, Gottlieb, & Vermeulen, 2007). In truth, there is no ultimate test for accuracy for either approach.

THREATS TO VALIDITY

When we talk about the validity of a study, we typically separate internal and external validity. The former refers to the extent to which the design of the study permits drawing strong (usually causal) conclusion. How strong is the study design? External validity addresses the generalizability of the findings. To whom can the findings be generalized?

According to Cook and Campbell, "external validity refers to the approximate validity with which we can infer that the presumed causal relationship can be generalized to and across alternative measures of the cause and effect and across different types of persons, settings, and times" (Cook & Campbell, 1979, p. 37). A part of that concept includes construct validity, which reflects the extent to which one can generalize the findings into a higher order construct or principle. In other words, when does a study result indicate a more general operational principle?

Threats to Internal Validity

Table 3-1 outlines a number of the most common things one should consider when planning a study. An example of the interaction between selection and maturation can be seen when children are selected on the basis of their social class (middle class and lower class) and are compared

Table 3-1 Threats to the Validity of Research Designs

Threat	Description
History	Any event that takes place outside the study and is not part of the intervention of interest
Maturation	The observed outcome may be a result of a subject growing older and wiser
Testing	Familiarity with the test when it is used repeatedly during the study
Instrumentation	Observers become experienced between a pretest and posttest or there is a shift in metric at different points in time. This may appear as a "floor" or "ceiling" effect if the intervals of measurement are narrower at the ends of the scale than they are at the midpoint.
Statistical regression	The scores for people selected as extreme (high or low) scorers regress toward the mean (average) with remeasurement.
Selection	Differences in the people in one group as opposed to the other
Mortality/Attrition	Differential drop-out between groups (treatment and control) during the project
Attention	Subjects may simply relate to the fact that they are being observed or receiving some kind of attention through the intervention, even if it has no specific benefit. This is typically countered by an attention control, whereby the control group gets an equal amount of attention.
Diffusion or imitation of treatments	Persons in the treatment group can communicate with those in the control group and learn the information that was intended for the treatment group
Interaction with selection	Any of the previously listed can interact with selection (e.g., selection–maturation, selection–history, and selection–instrumentation)

for changes in cognitive knowledge. Middle-class and lower-class children might be expected to mature at different rates.

An example of the interaction between selection and history can be seen when group differences in social class could affect members by exposing them to unique local histories such as economic hardships.

An example of the interaction between selection and instrumentation may occur when groups score at different positions on a test that has a "floor" or "ceiling." For example, evaluating change scores for physical functioning between hospitalized patients and healthy workers using a generic health status measure such as the SF-36 Health Survey.

BASIC RESEARCH DESIGNS

As we have observed, the RCT was created primarily to address selection bias. As its name implies, it has two major attributes that are both its strength and weakness: (1) allocation to study condition occurs randomly; and (2) the intervention is clearly specified and held constant. Neither of these conditions exist in nature, and hence the conceptual trade-off is always between the control of the RCT and its limited generalizability.

Feelings around RCTs run hot. Avid trialists believe that nothing can be established short of an RCT. A causal inference is impossible without such a condition. Those from the epidemiological camp suggest that much can be learned from well-designed quasi-experimental studies. Indeed some questions do not lend themselves to experiments. For those concerned about disease causation, ethical concerns would never permit deliberately exposing people to harmful substances. For disease treatment outcomes researchers, some questions may not be feasibly addressed by an RCT, or the variation in treatment would never be sufficiently captured by RCTs.

Some reserve the term "efficacy" for concepts tested by RCTs and "effectiveness" for the lessons of quasi-experimental designs.

There is a convention for diagramming research designs:

O — outcomes measures, shorthand for an observation
X — exposure, treatment, or procedure, the effects to be measures
Xs and Os in the same row are applied to the same person, unless separated by a vertical dashed line.

Temporal order is indicated by ordering the Xs and Os left to right and by subscripts.

Simultaneity is indicated by vertically ordering Xs and Os.

R — random assignment of subjects/groups to separate exposures; the subjects/groups being compared are considered equated by randomization.

The basic Pretest–Posttest Control Group Design is shown in Table 3-2. Following random assignment, one group gets the intervention and both groups are assessed at the same points in time.

Table 3-2   Pretest–Posttest Control Group Design

Group 1	R	O_1	X	O_2
Group 2	R	O_1		O_2

However, some contamination can affect even this design. The ultimate design may be the Solomon Four-Group Design, shown in Table 3-3. This design controls for the main effects of testing and the interaction of testing with the intervention. This design improves generalizability by modeling the effect of X under four different conditions. In cases where the test used is reactive with the intervention, you might well consider this design.

Table 3-3   Solomon Four-Group Design

Group 1	R	O_1	X	O_2
Group 2	R	O_1		O_2
Group 3	R		X	O_2
Group 4	R			O_2

In many instances, randomization is not feasible. A number of quasi-experimental designs are possible. A quasi-experiment is an experiment in which units (e.g., subjects, clinical areas, clinics, hospitals, health plans) are not randomly assigned to treatment conditions. Since assignment is by means of self-selection, these designs require additional measurement in order to control (through adjustment) for selection bias. The investigator lacks control of randomization and the scheduling of the intervention but does have control over the scheduling of data collection (i.e., the when and to whom of measurement), the comparison groups used, and how treatment is scheduled. These are the primary designs of outcomes research.

A quasi-experiment must meet the basic requirements for causal relationships: temporal order, an association between the putative cause and effect, and the implausibility of alternative explanations. In order to address the latter requirement, the following principles should be addressed: (1) the identification and study of plausible threats to internal validity, (2) primacy of control by design (design control over statistical control), and (3) coherent pattern matching.

A common, flawed design is the One-Group Pretest–Posttest Design (Table 3-4), which has problems that include history, maturation, testing, instrumentation, and generalizability.

Table 3-4   One-Group Pretest–Posttest Design

Group	O_1	X	O_2

This approach can be greatly strengthened by employing a time-series design (Table 3-5). Time-series experiments are possible when periodic measurement occurs. In essence, the investigator looks for discontinuities in the pattern of observations before and after the intervention. The design has limits; it fails to adequately deal with threats of history and generalizability. In addition, instrumentation changes are possible overtime. For example, over the years, the National Center for Health Statistics has modified response categories and items on their surveys in response to the science of measurement.

Table 3-5   The Time-Series Experiment

Group	O_1	O_2	O_3	O_4	X	O_5	O_6	O_7	O_8

The most common quasi-experimental design is one that incorporates a pretest and a posttest for both the group receiving the intervention and the control. Some analyses rely on so-called difference of differences tests, which compare $(O_2 - O_1)$ to $(O_4 - O_3)$, in an effort to adjust for differences in the two groups at baseline (Table 3-6). However, selection bias still remains an issue.

Table 3-6   **Untreated Control Group Design with Pretest Measures**

Group 1	NR	O_1	X	O_2
Group 2	NR	O_1		O_2

NR — Non-Random or Non-Equivalent Groups

POTENTIAL BIASES IN IMPLEMENTING A STUDY

Several potential biases should be considered when executing the experimental maneuver (or exposure).

1. *Contamination bias.* In an experiment when members of the control group inadvertently receive the experimental maneuver, the difference in outcomes between experimental and control patients may be systematically reduced.

2. *Attrition bias.* Sample loss can play havoc with a study. A well balanced sample at inception can change by differential attrition. Moreover, attrition is rarely random. Patients who withdraw from an experiment may differ systematically from those who remain. A specific case is death. It can be very misleading to simply compare survivors; the group with the better survival rate is likely to have retained more sick people.

   Even worse is *bogus control bias*, when patients who are allocated to an experimental maneuver sicken or die before or during its administration and are omitted or reallocated to the control group; the experimental maneuver will appear spuriously superior.

3. *Compliance bias.* In experiments requiring patient adherence to therapy, issues of efficacy become confounded with those of compliance.

4. *Therapeutic personality bias.* When treatment is not "blind," the therapist's convictions about efficacy may systematically influence both outcomes (positive personality) and their measurement (desire for positive results).

Rules have been established to deal with some of these concerns. One of the most widely employed is intention to treat. Basically, this step is designed to address at least some aspects of attrition, primarily differential sample loss. The operating principle is last observation forward; in other words, the last observation recorded is used as the final measure and the subject is retained. This approach provides a conservative estimate of effect if the clinical course is improvement, but it has the opposite effect if decline is anticipated (or observed). It is also important to recognize that this approach works well in the majority of circumstances where one is seeking to show a difference (because it reduces that likelihood and hence is a conservative test), but is inappropriate for studies of no different (equality).

Another aspect of attrition is mortality. As noted previously, people dying is an important event with strong implications for the outcomes of an intervention. It seems foolish to ignore them, but a surprising number of journal reviewers would have you do just that. Death is indeed an outcome—an important outcome. You have a couple of choices. Generally, the best approach is to incorporate death into the outcomes measure whenever reasonable and feasible. For example, death will usually represent the lowest level of function. In some cases it may be necessary to describe the rate of deaths in each group.

With all attrition, it is possible to model the loss of sample. While we try to estimate and account for differences in calculating propensity scores, we have even more data to estimate loss. Whereas comparability of samples usually relies on modest baseline data, we usually have a richer data source from more complete baseline data and early performance to use in contrasting those who remain and those who attrite.

REFERENCES

Austin, P. C., & Platt, R. W. (2010a). Author's response: The design of observational studies-defining baseline time. *Journal of Clinical Epidemiology, 63*(2), 141.

Austin, P. C., & Platt, R. W. (2010b). Survivor treatment bias, treatment selection bias, and propensity scores in observational research. *Journal of Clinical Epidemiology, 63*(2), 136–138.

Cook, T. D., & Campbell, D. T. (1979). *Quasi-experimentation: Design and analysis issues for field settings.* Chicago: Rand McNally.

Heckman, J. (1979). Sample selection bias as a specification error. *Econometrica, 47,* 153–161.

Heckman, J. J. (2008). Econometric causality. *International Statistical Review, 76*(1), 1–27.

Rassen, J. A., Brookhart, M. A., Glynn, R. J., Mittleman, M. A., & Schneeweiss, S. (2009a). Instrumental variables I: Instrumental variables exploit natural variation in nonexperimental data to estimate causal relationships. *Journal of Clinical Epidemiology, 62*(12), 1226–1232.

Rassen, J. A., Brookhart, M. A., Glynn, R. J., Mittleman, M. A., & Schneeweiss, S. (2009b). Instrumental variables II: Instrumental variable application—In 25 variations, the physician prescribing preference generally was strong and reduced covariate imbalance. *Journal of Clinical Epidemiology, 62*(12), 1233–1241.

Stukel, T. A., Fisher, E. S., Wennberg, D. E., Alter, D. A., Gottlieb, D. J., & Vermeulen, M. J. (2007). Analysis of observational studies in the presence of treatment selection bias: Effects of invasive cardiac management on AMI survival using propensity score and instrumental variable methods. *JAMA, 297*(3), 278–285.

Thorpe, K. E., Zwarenstein, M., Oxman, A. D., Treweek, S., Furberg, C. D., Altman, D. G., . . .Chalkidou, K. (2009). A pragmatic–explanatory continuum indicator summary (PRECIS): A tool to help trial designers. *Journal of Clinical Epidemiology, 62*(5), 464–475.

CHAPTER 4

Measurement

Measurement is fundamental to conducting health outcomes research. Poor measurement impedes health outcomes research. Measures must be recognized as imperfect. It comes at a cost. Measurement involves abstracting reality. Philosophers from Plato to Descartes (among others) have recognized that our perceptions are different from reality.

At its most basic level, measurement can be reduced to two simple concepts: scaling and classification (Nunnally & Bernstein, 1994). According to Nunnally and Bernstein, measurement "consists of rules for assigning symbols to objects so as to represent qualities of attributes numerically (scaling) or define whether the objects fall in the same or different categories with respect to a given attribute (classification)" (1994). The measurement process includes the abstraction of attributes that cannot be directly observed, the quantification of attributes in the object measured, and the standardization of rules for assigning numbers.

As discussed earlier, health outcomes research involves two critical steps: (1) conceptualization and (2) operationalization of the variables of interest. The conceptual model can be based on prior empirical work or driven by theory.

The conceptual model should display the relationships between the outcomes of interest and the factors expected to influence these outcomes. The conceptual model drives the analysis plan. The model becomes the road map for both data collection and analysis. It becomes the operating manual for the study, similar to the standard operating procedure used in clinical trials, which lays out a map of the concepts, the study hypothesis, the timing of interventions and measurements, the analysis plan, and so on.

A critical step in measurement is specifying how the model is quantified. This involves the process of *operationalization*, in which the concepts and theoretical variables are translated into empirical ones, that is, measurement. Achieving a good balance between conceptualization and measurement is a challenge in any study, but one runs the risk of focusing too heavily on one step and neglecting the other. The two steps are necessarily linked. On the one hand, an investigator may develop a complex theory on the role of psychosocial factors in achieving desirable outcomes for patients with congestive heart failure, but then rely on easily available proxy variables for psychosocial factors to test his or her hypotheses. In this scenario, if the proxy variables do not measure well what they are supposed to measure, the investigator will not be able to provide adequate evidence to test the theory. On the other hand, investigators often assume that we can measure anything that we can name without much thought to an underlying conceptual model for developing the measure (Duncan, 1984). Several different investigators might develop substantively different measures of disability but call the topic by the same name. It is easy to imagine the potential problems of comparability of results and the generalizability that could arise from the findings. The level of sophistication in measuring concepts grows as we understand them better. In practice, one may be reduced to using crude measures to first address a particular problem, such as analyzing an unanticipated insight from one's data set.

Overall, a good rule of thumb is that we should not attempt to measure something that we cannot conceptualize nor sensibly operationalize.

THE NATURE OF MEASUREMENT

Measurement is an easy concept to visualize, but a difficult one to define simply. One facet to the earlier definition of measurement (Nunnally & Bernstein, 1994) suggests that measurement defines the rules for assigning numbers to characteristics of objects, events, or people. For example, a ruler is used to measure the lengths of two boards. The ruler assigns a number to each length, say 14 in. and 28 in. Using this method, it is possible to numerically state that one board is half the length of the other. This provides a numeric description of the attribute. The ruler is the scale used for measuring what has been defined as length.

Whether using an existing measure or developing new ones, it is important to keep in mind that all measurement is imperfect for two reasons:

Anything we measure is an abstraction from reality. Anything we measure is measured with error.[1]

---

[1]This concept originally came from physics and is associated with Werner Heisenberg.

One can never measure anything directly. Instead, particular features or attributes of an object, person, or phenomenon are measured (Nunnally & Bernstein, 1994). For example, we do not measure an elderly woman, per se, but we measure her attributes, such as physical or cognitive function. Recognizing that only selected attributes are measured emphasizes that any measurement is an abstraction from the whole person in this case and from "reality." Realistically, we often end up sacrificing richness of a construct for a quantifiable measure. Other than her ability to physically function and her mental status, little information about this elderly woman is captured. In fact, even the information on functioning may be incomplete, since possible barriers and positive influences in her environment that may dramatically affect what she can and does do are unknown to us. Also, since we are constrained to using manmade instruments and protocols to measure attributes of an object or person, all of our measurements are subject to error even in the most controlled situations.

Historically, clinicians have been most confident measuring observable physical attributes of patients. However, in the current environment of outcomes research, many of the attributes of interest are not directly observable (e.g., quality of life and patient satisfaction). Phenomena such as quality of life, physical disability, depression, and even diseases like coronary artery disease, diabetes mellitus, or Alzheimer's disease, can be thought of as latent constructs. Latent constructs are abstract ideas formulated by the clinician or investigator to explain certain phenomena that are observed in a clinical setting or elsewhere. Measurement of latent constructs is even more indirect than measuring observable attributes because the clinician will never be able to absolutely confirm the former's existence. For example, a clinician has confidence in a given diagnosis only to the degree that the patient's symptoms are consistent with some past experience with the disease. Similarly, the clinician's confidence in measuring body temperature with a thermometer is based on a past experience of accurate readings with the given thermometer and competence in using the thermometer. Physical attributes are often measured as indicators of a latent construct such as disease or, in the case of the thermometer, core body temperature.

Outcomes research and clinical practice rely on many latent constructs and involve the measurement of both observable and unobservable phenomenon. Measuring the magnitude of latent constructs frequently involves constructing a scale. According to our definition of measurement, the magnitude of the latent construct in each individual causes each item in a scale to take on a given value. An individual who has trouble functioning independently should score higher on a functional disability scale than a person who has no trouble functioning. These are the rules for defining the qualities of attributes numerically; they define scaling.

SCALING

Once we identify which variables we are interested in studying, we must decide how the variable will be quantified. *Scale* is an observable expression of an underlying unobservable (latent) construct. The term scaling refers to how we assign numbers to the characteristics of the objects we are measuring. The process of scaling involves moving from a conceptual definition to an operational definition of the concept, ending with the scaling or variable definition. Table 4-1 (adapted from Aday & Cornelius, 2006) illustrates this process for the concepts of health status and physical disability.

In thinking how variables are scaled, a basic division is between those that are categorical, such as race or gender, and continuous variables like blood pressure, glucose levels, or pain ratings (Streiner & Norman, 2003). A second related feature concerns levels of measurement (see Table 4-2). It is customary to distinguish four levels of measurement: nominal, ordinal, interval, and ratio. Each defines a type of measurement scale that determines the types of statistical methods used in the outcomes analysis.

Nominal Measurement

Nominal measurement involves classification into unordered qualitative categories. In our example, individuals are classified as either healthy or disabled. Numbers are used as labels in order to classify objects into distinct categories; all objects can fit into only one category and every object must fit into a category based on our operating definition. Drawing on the earlier definition of measurement, this illustrates the fundamental importance of classification to measurement and outcomes research. Examples of nominal measures include: health status, gender, race, hospital type, and diagnosis-related groups (DRGs). Any simple yes/no question would be a nominal level measure.

Table 4-1.   Conceptual Definition, Operational Definition, and Variable Definition According to Levels of Measurement

	Levels of Measurement		
	Nominal	**Ordinal**	**Interval or Ratio**
Conceptual Definition			
Health status	Classifying subjects according to health	Ranking subjects along a continuum of health	Quantifying subjects according to their level of health
Physical disability	Classifying subjects according to disability	Ranking subjects according to their level of disability	Quantifying subjects according to their level of disability
Operational Definition			
Health status	Do you consider yourself healthy or unhealthy?	Do you consider yourself very healthy, somewhat healthy, or unhealthy?	In general, would you say your health is excellent, very good, good, fair, or poor?
Physical disability	Does your health limit you in performing any of your usual daily activities?	Which of the following activities do you have difficulty or unable to perform: bathing, dressing, feeding?	During the past month, how many days did you miss work as a result of a job-related injury? _____ number of days

(continues)

Table 4-1. *(continued)*

	Levels of Measurement		
	Nominal	**Ordinal**	**Interval or Ratio**
Variable Definition			
Health status	1 = healthy 0 = unhealthy	1 = very healthy 2 = somewhat healthy 3 = unhealthy	100 = excellent 85 = very good 60 = good 25 = fair 0 = poor
Physical disability	1 = Yes 0 = No	Count the number of activities the subject reports having difficulty or unable to perform	Number of days lost from work

Source: Adapted from Aday & Cornelius, 2006.

Ordinal Measurement

In ordinal measurement, there is an ordered categorical response set. Numbers are used to represent a rank ordering between a set of objects given a particular attribute. The magnitude of the attribute, or the distances between the objects are not equal and cannot be meaningfully interpreted. Given ordinal level of measurement, one object has more or less of the attribute than another object. In the disability example provided, disability in activities of daily living (ADL) can be quantified by counting the number of activities the individual has difficulty performing or is unable to perform. However, simply counting the number of activities is not the same in terms of the level of disability. For example, difficulty in feeding oneself reflects a greater level of disability than having difficulty dressing. Several authors have suggested approaches to quantify the magnitude of these differences (see Finch, Kane, & Philp, 1995); however, they have not found universal adoption.

Table 4-2 Levels of Measurement

Level of Measurement	Statistical Aggregation	Example
Nominal	Categorical	Gender: Female Male
Ordinal	Categorical	Can you dress and undress? Yes, without difficulty Yes, with minor difficulty Yes, with major difficulty No, not able to
Interval	Continuous	On a scale of 1 to 10 with 1 being "no difficulty dressing and undressing" and 10 being "unable to dress and undress," how much difficulty do you have dressing and undressing yourself? 1 2 3 4 5 6 7 8 9 10 No Unable to difficulty dress and undress
Ratio	Continuous	5 feet/4 feet = 60 inches/48 inches

Interval Measurement

In interval level of measurement, the response set to the variable is continuous and the distance between each response category is assumed to be equivalent. The numbers in the scale are meaningfully interpreted; for example, Fahrenheit temperature scale in degrees or blood pressure in mm of mercury (Hg). From our example, disability could be scaled in terms of the number of days missed from work. Based on interval level of measurement, the quantitative difference between 1 day and 3 days missed from work and 5 days and 7 days missed from work is 2 days. For interval measurement, 1 day is considered the same as another day. In this example, the magnitude of two differences is identical although the latter likely reflects a greater level of disability.

Ratio Measurement

When interval measures have true zeros, the level of measurement is considered ratio. Examples of ratio measurement include absolute temperature scale, such as Rankine and Kelvin temperature scales, and a person's height. There is a true zero and when the unit of measurement changes the ratio still remains fixed. A child who is 5 ft. tall is 1.25 times taller than one who is 4 ft. tall. The ratio of these two heights stays the same when converted to inches or centimeters. Except for anthropometric and biochemical measures, there are few examples of ratio measures in outcomes research.

The choice of level of measurement implies the range of acceptable statistics to use with the measure. Parametric statistics (means, least squares linear regression) are inappropriate for nominal and ordinal (categorical) measures but appropriate for interval and ratio level continuous measures. Nominal and ordinal measures should be analyzed using nonparametric statistics (Le, 1998).

A good rule of thumb is to collect continuous data or at least not dichotomous data as often as possible. You can convert variables that are continuous to categorical forms, but it is not easy to convert the other way. Such conversions to categorical data, while relying on less powerful statistics, may allow one to look for specific points of impact. For example, overall age may not show an effect, but the effect may lay in one particular subgroup, for example the oldest old or those age 85 or older. For some analyses a mean change is less meaningful than the proportion that moves from one category to the other, but it is easier to categorize or establish a cutoff point post hoc. Dichotomous measures require larger sample sizes to demonstrate an effect and are less reliable than continuous measures (Streiner & Norman, 2003). As a rule, you lose statistical power by converting continuous variables to dichotomous ones.

SCALING METHODS

Classical test theory (CTT) is the basis for most scale test construction used in outcomes research. Its appeal derives from its loose assumptions and its broad applicability to most situations. However, one of the major limitations of CTT is that the questions that make up the measure and the statistics of reliability and validity testing apply only to the group of individuals that took the test. The implication of this property is for each use of the measure, the investigator needs to test for its reliability with this group of respondents to the survey and confirm the validity of the measure for use with this group.

When measures of attributes are based on continuous variables, estimating the magnitude of the scale can be based on several techniques: rating scales, comparative methods, magnitude estimation, and econometric methods. Broadly, these represent a range of approaches to unidimensional scaling (Streiner & Norman, 2003). Each of the approaches is based on CTT.

Rating Scales

The simplest and oldest rating scales are visual analog scales (VAS; Fryed, 1923). The most frequent use for VAS is in health outcomes research is as a rating of pain. For example, the individual being evaluated for pain is asked to place a mark along a 10 cm line to indicate his or her pain, with "no pain" and "severe pain" as anchor points (see Figure 4-1 for an example of a simple VAS).

One variant of the VAS is the numerical rating scale (NRS) for pain, in which the individual responding checks one of a sequence of 11 boxes from "no pain" to "severe pain" (see Table 4-3).

Distinct from the VAS, one of the most widely used rating methods in measurement is the Likert-type scale (Guyatt & Townsend, 1987). Likert scales involve summing individual responses to a set of questions on an agree-to-disagree continuum (e.g., "strongly agree," "agree," "uncertain," "disagree," "strongly disagree") to calculate a score. The response set or response choices are symmetric. Scale values are not assigned to individual items; only the total score is scalable. While individual items in the Likert scale are ordinal, total scores are treated as interval by most investigators without introducing substantial study bias (Nunnally & Bernstein, 1994), as long as the scale is measuring only one underlying

Figure 4-1 Pain - No Pain

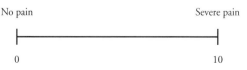

Table 4-3 **Level of Pain**

No Pain										Severe Pain
0 ☐	1 ☐	2 ☐	3 ☐	4 ☐	5 ☐	6 ☐	7 ☐	8 ☐	9 ☐	10 ☐

characteristic. Disputes over constructing the Likert scale arise around issues such as: should there be a neutral or uncertain category or the appropriate number of response choice, or whether there should be an odd or even number in the response set. The number of categories generally range from five to nine. There are no right or wrong answers in a Likert-type scale. Each question in the measure is a statement that reflects an underlying attribute. The responses to multiple items are combined by adding the response choices. This characteristic serves as the basis for referring to Likert-type scales as additive scales. Overall, their frequent use in outcomes research is based on the minimum of resources needed to design them, their comprehensibility, and their ease of administration.

Comparative Methods

Compared with rating-based techniques, comparative methods for scale construction involve significant resources, investigator time, and design effort. Items included in the measure require initial interval level scaling (usually calibrating the responses to a normal distribution). A group of judges rank a large number of statements from most favorable to least favorable, or compare each item to each other item to distinguish which one of the pairs has more of the attribute in question. After the scale has been calibrated, a respondent chooses which statements apply to him or her. Scale scores are based on the aggregation of responses to individual items through summing or averaging. The final measure is thought to have equal-appearing interval properties and guarantees interval data. As mentioned earlier, the construction of comparative scales is expensive, difficult, and does not guarantee unidimensionality of the construct or unbiased rankings by the judges (McIver & Carmines, 1981). A Thurstone-type scale is one example.

Most of the early functional disability scales relied on another comparative method, the Guttman scaling approach. This type of scale is hierarchical and deterministic in nature, and unidimensionality of the construct of interest is required (Nunnally & Bernstein, 1994). Guttman scales link response choices to an increasingly stronger expression of the attribute measured. Given the hierarchical nature of the scale, these are sometimes referred to as cumulative scales. Developmentally oriented constructs, such as ADLs and physical functioning ability work best with this method of scaling (Katz & Akpom, 1976; Spector, Katz, Murphy, & Fulton, 1987). The cumulative or hierarchical structure of the Guttman scale is illustrated for dependence in ADLs in Table 4-4. Each score on the scale indicates the exact pattern of responses to disability defined in terms of ADLs. If a respondent is dependent at functional level three, the respondent is necessarily dependent at levels one and two. In perfect Guttman scalability, individuals unable to feed themselves are dependent in the other self-care activities.

Cumulative models of scaling assume no measurement error. However, in practice, coefficients of stability and reproducibility are used to determine the degree of deviation from perfect ordering in the respondents from the sample. In reality, it is difficult to find constructs suitable for use with the Guttman method. Even the ADL construct has proven problematic. The common practice of using simple counts of activities or ADLs assumes a hierarchy, equal weighting of each ADL in the count, and interval level properties. These assumptions are somewhat tenuous.

In an effort to move beyond ordinal properties and equal weighting assumptions of standard measures, various scaling techniques have been

Table 4-4 Guttman Scaling Dependence in Activities of Daily Living

Subject	A	B	C	D
Is the individual able to				
. . . bathe without assistance?	1	1	1	1
. . . dress without assistance?	1	1	1	0
. . . toilet without assistance?	1	1	0	0
. . . feed oneself?	1	0	0	0
Scale Score	4	3	2	1

1 = Yes

0 = No

used to weight health or dependency states. For example, magnitude estimation techniques were used to obtain a weighted ratio level scale of functional dependency (Finch *et al.*, 1995). In magnitude estimation, a reference item from a given construct is chosen and given a scale value. All remaining items are rated numerically with respect to how similar or dissimilar each is from the reference item. Using bathing as the standard (500), an expert panel rated 13 function domains based on their judgment of how the need for human assistance to perform the function contributes to overall dependency. The panel then assigned weights from 0 to 100 to the level of assistance (e.g., a little assistance, a lot of assistance, complete assistance) needed to perform the functional activity. Because the scale exhibits ratio level properties, a composite score is calculated. Finch and his colleagues (1995) found that their scale was more sensitive to the nature and extent of functional losses than simple counts of ADLs and instrumental activities of daily living (IADLs), because it did not assume equal weight and did not arbitrarily dichotomize level of dependency for the ADLs and IADLs.

Econometric Methods

Econometric methods constitute the fourth unidimensional scaling technique. In studies of cost benefit analysis, the benefits of a therapy need to be numerically scaled so that there is a unitary measure of healthcare quality. Typically, this is along a continuum from worst health to best possible health. A numerical value is assigned to health states with 1 signifying a healthy state and 0 signifying death. Underlying econometric methods, the individual is forced to make choices between the benefits of the intervention and the risk that there could be a complication, the outcomes are less than desirable, or that they might die. Aggregate weights for each health state can be determined by a variety of scaling methods, including rating scales, magnitude estimation, standard gamble, or the time trade-off methods (Drummond, Sculpher, Torrance, & O'Brien, 2005; Patrick & Erickson, 1993; Torrance, Thomas, & Sackett, 1972). Economists favor the latter two methods, which are based on economic theory (Kaplan, 1995).

   Briefly, the standard gamble asks the respondent to choose between an outcome that is certain but less than ideal or gamble on an outcome that is uncertain but leads to either perfect health or death, given set probabilities. The time trade-off method discards the difficult concept of probabilities and offers respondents a choice between perfect health for a set amount of time or less than perfect health for a variable amount of time. Economists argue that aggregation is more plausible using these methods in comparison to rating scales with ordinal level properties. However, these methods assume rational decision making on the part of the respondents. Research suggests that this is not necessarily the case (Tversky & Kahneman, 1981). Moreover, people's sense of the importance of a state may change with circumstances. We refer to this as response shift (Ahmed, Schwartz, Ring, & Sprangers, 2009). Moreover, these methods are difficult for respondents to understand and time-consuming to administer (Streiner & Norman, 2003). Further, the assumptions underlying econometric methods have led to criticism by those outside economic circles.

Item Response Theory

Item response theory (IRT) is used as the basis for a new class of unidimensional models, of which the Rasch model is an example. These are widely used in psychological and educational measurement and are distinguished from other models in the information they provide about how well the questions asked measure the ability or trait of interest (Andrich, 1988). This is to be distinguished from the unidimensional models discussed earlier, in which the properties of the measures are dependent upon the subjects who took the test (Streiner & Norman, 2003). Rasch models are the simplest of the models based on IRT in which it is possible to separate parameters concerning the questions from those of the individual's taking the test. Rasch models assume unidimensionality; that is, the measure assesses only a single trait or ability and that the probability of answering any item (a single dimension) is unrelated to who takes the test. Since the psychometric properties of the measure are independent of the group taking the test, reliability and validity are established for all groups when the measure is developed.

STRATEGIC QUESTIONS IN THE SELECTION OF HEALTH OUTCOMES MEASURES

Before beginning an outcomes research study, there are six critical questions that need to be considered as part of the health outcomes measurement selection. The strategic questions in the selection of health outcomes measures are:

1. Does the use of the measure make sense? (sensibility)

2. Is the measure reliable? (reliability)

3. Can valid inferences be drawn from the use of the measure? (validity)

4. Is the measure responsive to clinically and socially relevant change? (responsiveness)

5. Does the burden for using the measure exceed available resources? (burden)

6. Does the use of the measure fit the study design and question? (design)

Following each question is a term in parenthesis that captures the essential characteristics of the question.

Sensibility

Does the use of the measure make sense? This has sometimes been referred to as "enlightened common sense," which is a mixture of common sense and reasonable knowledge of clinical reality (Feinstein, 1987). Feinstein was especially clear in terms of the constituents of sensibility. The investigator begins with knowledge of what is the study question and how this relates to the underlying conceptual model. The measure needs to be comprehensible or understandable. The outcomes researcher should have a clear understanding of what goes into the measure and what comes out. The instructions for the use of the measure are clear and replicable in order to assure reliability. The measure should be easy to use. A measure is unappealing if it is too difficult to carry out, both in terms of the burden to the investigator and to the subject. Similar to a standard operating manual for the study, the ingredients of the measure are spelled out, along with how they are combined and standardized. Finally, the scale output from the measure is well suited for its intended purpose.

Face validity and *content validity* are often considered as part of the measure of sensibility. Does the outcomes measure look reasonable? *Face validity* indicates that the measure appears to be assessing the desired qualities and underlying attributes measured. Usually this is based on the subjective judgment of experts. Considerations for face validity include: basic evidence, coherence of components, and suitable collaboration of the person to whom the index is directed (Feinstein, 1987). In the latter case, this could represent measurement of patients with the diagnosis of interest (e.g. hypertension or congestive heart failure). *Content validity* is closely related to *face validity* but is limited to whether the measure samples all the relevant content or important domains. Considerations might include: the omission of important variables from the measure, inclusion of unsuitable variables, weighting of variables, and whether the measure provides basic data of high quality. It is generally common for researchers to reject measures on the basis of face and content validity.

In the judgment of experts, the instrument measures such-and-such because the expert says it does. This is sometimes referred to as validity by assumption and it is usually a minimum prerequisite of a measure. In some cases it is inappropriate for the measure to have face validity. Examples include sensitive areas such as alcohol or spousal abuse, where direct questions are unlikely to elicit honest responses.

Reliability

An important part of selecting a measure for use in a study is establishing the usefulness of the measure. Traditionally, this process involves assessing the reliability and validity of a measure. Assessing reliability involves showing that a health outcomes measure produces reproducible results. Assessing validity, which will be discussed in detail later, means measuring what one intended to measure. Blood pressure, a measure of the internal beating and resting pressure of the cardiovascular system, is measured using a sphygmomanometer. Blood pressure that always measures the systolic, or heart beating blood pressure 10 mm Hg higher than it is in actuality is a reliable measure of pressure but not a valid measure. The measure of blood pressure is consistent but consistently high. Conversely, a sphygmomanometer might randomly read high for some patients and low for others. In the latter case, the blood pressure would be unreliable and invalid. As a rule, reliability is a necessary but not sufficient condition for validity.

Measurement error lies at the heart of reliability and validity. Measurement is always subject to error, which can be *random* and *nonrandom (bias)*. Any observed score or scale is a function of its true score, bias, and error. In the following equation, O is the observed score, T is the true score, B signifies bias, and ε is the random error component.

$$O = T + B + \varepsilon$$

Reliability is concerned with random error, whereas validity is concerned with bias.

In classical testing theory, reliability is largely a function of random error, which is completely unsystematic in nature. Random error could be caused by inconsistent responses to questionnaires, data entry errors, poor instructions or training of staff responsible for collecting data, coding and transcription errors, and so on. As random errors in the measure increase, the reliability of the measure decreases. The following formula defines reliability and illustrates this relationship (Streiner & Norman, 2003).

$$Reliability = \frac{true\ variance}{true\ variance\ +\ error\ variance}$$

Validity is largely a function of nonrandom measurement error or systematic error. This nonrandom characteristic is referred to as bias.

The relationship between reliability and validity is illustrated in Figure 4-2. In this example, core body temperature is estimated using an oral thermometer. Taking an individual's temperature by mouth is systematically biased. On average, it is 1° lower than the body's core temperature. Aside from this systematic bias, replicate measures of temperature have random, or chance, variations.

All measurement scales have inherent errors, which can be classified according to their source. As shown in Figure 4-3, the evaluation of measurement error includes testing both reliability and validity. The terms reliability and validity have very specific meanings when discussing the

Figure 4-2 Relationship Between Random Errors (Chance) and Systematic Errors (Bias) in the Measurement of Core Body Temperature Using an Oral Thermometer

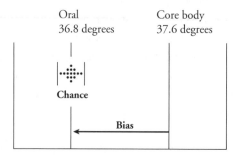

Figure 4-3   The Relationship Between Observed Scores, True Scores, and Errors in Outcomes Measurement

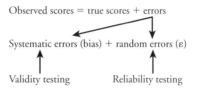

process of scale development (Streiner & Norman, 2006). Two other terms, precision and accuracy, should not be used as synonyms for reliability and validity.

A common misperception is that once the reliability and validity of a measure have been established, they are no longer an issue when the measure is used in future studies. This is false since measurement error is inherent to a particular sample and methods; thus, reliability and validity are artifacts of the given sample as well. Reliability is a function of the instrument, the user, and method employed. Comparable to using a scalpel, a scale may perform well in one set of hands and not in another. Clinicians should at least ponder whether their studies vary from previous studies along various dimensions (e.g., the population of interest, the study setting, the method of data collection, and interviewer background) that might threaten the reliability and validity of the measures.

Reliability is a measure of reproducibility and is solely an empirical issue. As such, there are five common approaches to measuring reliability: (1) interrater or interobserver reliability, (2) intrarater reliability, (3) test–retest reliability, (4) split-half reliability testing, and (5) internal consistency measures. Reliability limits the ability of a measure to detect a difference or a change. In other words, unreliable measures reduce the likelihood of finding a change in an outcomes variable when true change occurred.

Interrater or interobserver reliability is frequently used in biomedical research, in which the investigator is concerned about stable measure for a diagnosis or test result. Two radiologists are asked to independently review a series of 200 chest x-rays for evidence of lung infiltrate, which is an indicator of pneumonia or lung consolidation. Their review is recorded as either a yes or a no. The data in Table 4-5 show the results from this review.

Table 4-5 Two Radiologists Review

		Radiologist 1		Totals
		Yes	No	
Radiologist 2	Yes	60	20	80
	No	30	90	120
Totals		90	110	200

As the data show, the radiologists agree on 75% of their reviews. However, in 25% of the ratings there is a lack of agreement. Kappa (κ) is a commonly used statistic to assess *interrater agreement* in situations with dichotomous outcomes (i.e., nominal scales) such as presence or absence of a condition when more than one observer or rater is used. κ moves beyond a measure of simple agreement by taking into account the proportion of responses that are expected by chance, where p_o is the observed proportion of agreement (the addition of the diagonal elements of a 2×2 table divided by the total number of responses), p_e is the expected agreement between the two raters for the two outcomes given the marginal distributions of a 2×2 table.

$$\kappa = \frac{(p_o - p_e)}{(1.0 - p_e)} = \frac{(0.75 - 0.51)}{(1.0 - 051)} = 0.49$$

In this example, the expected agreement for presence of the condition (p_e) is calculated as

$$\left[\left(\frac{80}{200}\right) \times \left(\frac{90}{200}\right)\right] + \left[\left(\frac{120}{200}\right) \times \left(\frac{110}{200}\right)\right] = 0.51$$

The value for κ is very sensitive to the marginal frequency distributions; if the marginal frequencies are not well balanced, κ will be low even when agreement is high. However, attempts have been made to develop a weighted κ for use with ordinal data. The weighted κ focuses on disagreement, typically using quadratic weights calculated as the square of the amount of discrepancy from exact agreement (Streiner & Norman, 2003). Using Pearson's correlation, percent agreement and chi-square are not recommended for assessing interrater reliability (Streiner & Norman, 2003). Landis and Koch (1977) have provided some useful guidelines for interpreting Cohen's κ. Although there is little empirical support for their guidelines for 2×2 tables epidemiologists have found these useful. For the radiologist example, there was moderate agreement in the presence of lung infiltrate across the 200 cases.

One may be interested in the reproducibility of individual test scores across similar items in a test, of individual test scores over time, and of individual test scores by different observers. Specifically, the investigator must have repeated measures across some dimension (e.g. multiple items measuring the same construct, multiple test scores over time for the same subjects, and multiple raters scoring the same patients). This reliability coefficient, a form of an intraclass correlation coefficient (ICC), is interpreted as the percent of variance in a measure that results from true patient (or respondent) variability. The ICC provides information on the "extent to which repetition of the test yields the same values under the same conditions in the same individuals" (Guyatt, Walter, & Norman, 1987). For all reliability coefficients, a coefficient of 1 would indicate perfect reliability (i.e., no measurement error), and a coefficient of 0 represents no reliability. Since the ICC is based on analysis of variance (ANOVA) techniques, it is appropriately used only with continuous data.

The ICC is mathematically equivalent to the weighted κ mentioned earlier. Reliability for repeated measures is defined using ANOVA as follows:

$$Reliability = \frac{MS_{Subject} - MS_{Residual}}{MS_{Subject} + (k-1)MS_{Residual}}$$

where $MS_{Subject}$ is the mean square for the subject and $MS_{Residual}$ is the error variance related to subject × rater, and k is the number of raters. For example, three orthopedic surgeons grade the severity of low back pain on a 1 to 5 scale in 10 consecutive patients. Higher values indicate greater severity of low back pain. Results from this test are shown in Table 4-6.

Table 4-6 Repeated Measures ANOVA Output

Source	df	ANOVA SS	Mean Square	F Statistic	p value
Rater	2	0.887	0.433	0.22	0.835
Subject	9	29.633	3.293	1.65	0.544
Subject × Rater	18	6.467	0.390		
Total	29	36.987			

The arithmetic calculation for ICC is as follows:

$$0.713 = \frac{3.293 - 0.390}{3.293 + (3 - 1) \times 0.390}$$

The ICC value of 0.713 supports a substantial level of agreement among the physician raters in terms of the low back pain severity.

When experts use a measurement scale over time, there is a tendency to incorporate the experience gained with the measure in later uses. This proclivity leads to differences in ratings over time. This is especially troublesome in outcomes research studies involving the use of medical records. As more experience is gained by the investigator in reviewing the medical record, the reviews differ or drift from those abstracted earlier in the study. This, in essence, describes the conundrum of intrarater reliability. To evaluate this form of reliability, the raters are asked to review the same record at different stages of the study. If the within-subject ratings are similar at different stages of the project, then intrarater reliability is said to be acceptable.

Another form of reliability is *test–retest reliability*. This form of testing provides a direct measure of reliability assuming the attribute measured is relatively stable over short periods of time (e.g., physical functioning or social functioning). Pain measures, which can be quite variable over time, could not be appropriately evaluated using test–retest reliability. In order to assess test–retest reliability, the same test is given to the same individuals after a period of time elapses, say 7 to 10 days. The relationship between the scores from each test is considered the reliability of the measure. Reliability may be overestimated as a result of memory if the time interval between the tests is too short, or reliability may be underestimated if the time interval is too long and real changes within respondents occur. It is not possible to separate this form of reliability from the stability of the measure (Allen & Yen, 2002). Thus, a catch-22 exists when dealing with stability of measurement and outcomes research, since we are inherently measuring change. To paraphrase Kane and Kane, one cannot be certain about the change in a measure without reliable measurements, and one cannot readily test the measures reliability without assuming some stability over time in the characteristic measured (2004).

A common form of *internal reliability* used with scales is Cronbach's alpha coefficient (α); α is a derivation of the ICC. The Kuder–Richardson Formula 20 (K-R 20) is appropriate for dichotomous data (Cronbach, 1990).

Both Cronbach's α and K-R 20 measure reliability in terms of internal consistency (i.e., the items in the scale are homogeneous). The basic question posed is how closely each item in a scale is related to the overall scale. All variability, other than error variance and item variance, is treated as fixed since multiple observations occur due to the items in the scale rather than from multiple observers. The formula for Cronbach's α is:

$$\alpha = \frac{k}{k-1}\left[1 - \frac{\Sigma s_i^2}{s_{Total}^2}\right]$$

where k is the number of scale items, s_i is the standard deviation of each scale item, and s_{Total} is the standard deviation of the total scale score (Cronbach, 1990).

High values of coefficient α occur when the items comprising the total scale score are moderately to highly correlated with one another. If the correlation between all possible pairs of items in the scale were negligible, that is, approaching zero, the scale would have zero reliability as measured by the coefficient. In the design and development of scales, one does not want perfect correlations among the items, since this suggests that items comprising the scale are redundant. High levels of the α should be taken with a grain of salt, since they are sensitive to the number of items in the scale. By increasing the number of items in a scale, internal consistency seems to be increasing, but this may not actually be the case. It is possible that some of these scale items may be redundant or poor indicators of the attribute of interest. An adequate α level for scales used to compare groups is 0.70–0.80 (Nunnally & Bernstein, 1994), whereas values greater than 0.90 are necessary for inferences about individuals.

The classical test theory notion of reliability as a ratio of true variance to total variance is limiting, since it does not break down multiple sources of error. Essentially, each type of reliability coefficient discussed previously yields a different estimate of reliability. For some studies with multiple potential sources of error, total variability may be seen more practically as the sum of all variability in the measure, which includes both patient/respondent variability (between subject) and measurement error (within subject) and other forms of variability, such as observer, site, and training. Generalizability theory, an extension of ANOVA techniques, examines all measured sources of variance simultaneously and can address all types of reliability in a single study (Streiner & Norman, 2003). This technique has not been well utilized in the health outcomes research. This is the most appropriate approach to interrater reliability. When assessing reliability, it is important to keep in mind that it is a measure of reproducibility, not a measure of accuracy. Questions concerning the accuracy or bias associated with a measure are best answered through validity testing.

Validity

Reliability is a prerequisite for validity, but establishing validity poses significant challenges to the health outcomes investigator. Validity lies at the heart of the measurement process, since it addresses whether the scale is measuring what it was intended to measure. Validity is "not so much directed toward the integrity of tests as . . . the inferences that can be made about the attributes of the people who have produced those test scores" (Landy, 1986, p. 1186). According to Streiner and Norman, validity "is really a process whereby we determine the degree of confidence we can place on inferences we make about people based on their scores from that scale" (2003, p. 146).

One reason validity is difficult to establish is because of the number of confounding factors inherent in health outcomes research. For example, abstract ideas turned into scales are subject to the definitional whims of the individual clinician or investigator (i.e., naming a factor score from a factor analysis). Also, the interview situation may affect whether one measures what is intended. An interview of a nursing home resident on the topic of quality of life in the nursing home conducted in the presence of the nursing home administrator may produce invalid results. Results could also be affected if the interview was conducted by phone or with a proxy rather than face to face with the resident. Given all the possibilities of bias, validity becomes a matter of degree; a perfectly valid indicator is not achievable.

In practice, validity is a process of hypothesis testing that moves beyond operational definitions to demonstrate relationships between the measure of interest and other measures or observable physical properties. Although all types of validity boil down to the same consideration, a whole body of literature exists on the different types and complexities of validity. Validity is a unitary concept and types of validity are merely a useful tool for discussion. Generally, the three main types of validity discussed are content validity, criterion-related validity, and construct validity (Streiner & Norman, 2003). These are sometimes referred to as the three C's of validity. It is the responsibility of the investigator to determine the approach to assessing validity that best suits the construct of interest.

The Three C's of Validity:

- *Content validity* – refers to the comprehensiveness of the measure
  - Content
  - Face
- *Criterion validity* – correlates with a "gold standard"
  - Concurrent
  - Predictive
- *Construct validity* – scientific theory supports or refutes constructs
  - Extreme groups testing
  - Convergent and discriminant
  - Multitrait–multimethod matrix

Content validity refers to the comprehensiveness of the measure. That is, do the items in the measure cover the domain of interest? For example, how well does a specific ADL scale represent the entire range of disability? The more representative is the sample of disability, the more valid one's inferences will be. If the scale does not take into account difficulty of dressing and bathing, the picture of the extent of an individual's ability to function independently may be inaccurate. The main problem with content validity is that in the health sciences it is generally impossible to sample the entire domain due to the fuzziness of many of the concepts. For many measures, content validity reduces to a form of *face validity*, which is the judgment by the medical or research community that the measure really measures the construct and perhaps even the judgment of the respondents that the questions in the measure make sense. Sensibility is a form of content validity.

Most investigators think of validity in terms of *criterion validity*. It is assessed by correlating the measure of interest with a gold standard or an already well established measure of the characteristic (the criterion). This correlation can be assessed concurrently to establish concurrent validity or the correlation can be assessed in the future to establish predictive validity. An example of predictive validity would be the development and use of a new section on the medical school entrance exam to predict an individual's likelihood of pursuing primary care. We would not be able to know how well the section did at predicting the percentage of new primary care doctors until the class of medical school students graduated. Using the results of this exam section for admission or other type of decision prior to graduation will bias our correlation. Case mix adjusters are often validated on the basis of their ability to predict an outcome of concern such as death. In many of these cases the data on both predictors and outcomes may already have been collected. The main problem with this type of validity is that the more abstract the concept is, the less likely it will be to find a criterion for assessing a measure of it. In clinical practice, screening tests often are validated using a more comprehensive diagnosis as a criterion score.

Epidemiologists use sensitivity and specificity analysis to evaluate criterion validity. Figure 4-4 illustrates the comparison between an outcomes measure (rows) with a gold standard, or true outcome. The latter is established using some external criterion, such as physician's judgment or diagnostic test. A greater proportion of true positive and true negatives establishes the criterion validity for the outcomes measure. In practice, criterion validation is quantified in sensitivity, specificity, positive predictive value of the outcomes test, and the negative predictive value of the outcomes test. Table 4-7 provides the formal definitions for these terms. Outcomes measures with high sensitivity and high specificity discriminate between individuals with and without outcomes evaluated.

Construct validity refers to the relationship of measures to unobservable constructs. Since the constructs are unobserved and lack a criterion for validation, construct validity tests hypotheses within the context of conceptual model. The construct of interest is one of the variables. In other words, we are interested in whether the measures of the construct support our hypotheses based on the conceptual model. For example, a measure

Figure 4-4   Criterion Validation Using Sensitivity and Specificity Analysis

Outcomes measure	True outcome	
	Present	Absent
Positive	*True positives* a	*False positives* b
Negative	*False negatives* c	*True negatives* d

Table 4-7   Epidemiological Terms Used to Describe the Accuracy (Criterion Validity) of a Test

Term	Definition	Formula
Sensitivity	Proportion of persons with conditions who test positive	$\dfrac{a}{a+c}$
Specificity	Proportion of persons without conditions who test negative	$\dfrac{d}{b+d}$
Positive predictive value	Proportion of persons with positive tests who have conditions	$\dfrac{a}{a+b}$
Negative predictive value	Proportion of persons with positive tests who do not have conditions	$\dfrac{d}{c+d}$

of physical functioning should be strongly related to an individual's age, since we know that physical functioning in general declines with age. Some common methods of establishing construct validity follow.

First, we can examine group differences on the measure. If we expect two groups to differ in a predicted manner on a measure, we can directly test this difference. Often, investigators administer the scale to a group of individuals known to have the characteristic of interest and a group known not to have the characteristic. The group known to have the characteristic is expected to score higher on the measure than the other group. For example, a measure of mental health should distinguish between patients with depression and those with hypertension. However, known-groups validity testing neglects the fact that in practice the scale needs to discriminate among individuals in the middle range of the trait (Streiner & Norman, 2003).

Second, measures of similar and dissimilar constructs should be related and unrelated respectively. If two scales purport to measure physical functioning, they should be highly correlated. This is referred to as *convergent validity*. Two scales measuring different constructs, such as physical functioning and mental health, should not be highly correlated. This is called *discriminant validity*.

Campbell and Fiske (1959) proposed a third method for evaluating construct validity by interpreting traits across measurement methods. The *multitrait–multimethod matrix* presents all of the intercorrelations resulting when each of several traits is measured by each of several methods. This method is based on the concept that reliability is the agreement between two efforts to measure the same trait through similar methods. Validity is represented in the agreement between two attempts to measure the same trait using different methods.

Fourth, confirmatory factor analysis is used to determine whether or not the data are consistent with an underlying theoretical model, in other words, whether there is in fact a unique construct. This process of validation deals with the internal structure of the construct (Kim & Mueller, 1978a; 1978b), that is, can the observed correlations be explained by a small number of hypothetical constructs (i.e., the factor). Construct validity is an ongoing process. Ideally, it requires a pattern of consistent findings involving different investigators using different theoretical structures across a number of different studies (Carmines & Zeller, 1979). Unfortunately, the house of cards investigators build in trying to validate a measure can be easily toppled by a few inconsistent findings.

Responsiveness

It is the goal of medical care to produce a positive change in health through appropriate treatment of disease. A principal goal of outcomes research is to assess the effectiveness of that medical treatment. Outcomes measures must be reliable and valid but measures that evaluate the effectiveness of treatment must also be responsive to change (Guyatt *et al.*, 1987; Guyatt, Deyo, Charlson, Levine, & Mitchell, 1989; Kirshner & Guyatt, 1985). This property of outcomes measures is often called *responsiveness*. In the literature, responsiveness is sometimes referred to as sensitivity to change; however, the use of the term sensitivity should be reserved for evaluating the accuracy of tests discussed earlier.

Responsiveness should be evaluated in terms of what is relevant to the patient and the illness being studied (Fischer *et al.*, 1999). Death is usually quite reliable and has validity as an outcomes measure, but it is unresponsive as an outcomes measure for detecting change associated with arthritis treatment. Taken at face value, responsiveness should be relatively easy to assess. However, few measures are systematically evaluated for their responsiveness.

Responsiveness can be measured using either serial measures of an outcome or retrospectively by asking whether the individual's condition has changed. Asking patients about their levels of pain at the beginning and end of therapy sessions is considered serial outcomes measurement, whereas asking patients at the conclusion of their therapy sessions whether their pain level has changed for better or worse is considered a retrospective approach. The assumption is that the serial outcomes measures are somehow more accurate than retrospective measures. However, there is some evidence that retrospective measures might hold greater relevance to the patient (Fischer *et al.*, 1999). In addition, the results from serial and retrospective approaches to measuring responsiveness appear to be moderately correlated and strongly related for the more extensive treatment procedures. As a rule of thumb, in the design of health outcomes studies, serial measures should be supplemented by retrospective measures.

Responsiveness describes the ability of an instrument to detect small but important clinical changes. There is a multiplicity of statistical measures for measuring responsiveness, but the majority of these measures have a fundamental form (Norman, 1989). The following formula provides a theoretical definition of the responsiveness.

$$Responsiveness = \frac{variance\ to\ change}{variance\ to\ change + error\ variance}$$

The easiest method for assessing responsiveness is to compare outcomes measures at the beginning and end of a study using paired t statistics. This approach has some limitations, since it fails to account for variability in the outcomes scale, learning with readministration of the test, and improvement in the subject's score with retesting. The principal limitation to using a change score is the possibility of a regression effect (Nunnally & Bernstein, 1994). A second, more common, approach to measuring responsiveness is the use of effect size. One simple version calculates the difference between the baseline and follow-up score divided by the standard deviation of the baseline score. Much of the criticism concerning the use of the effect size centers on the source of variation (standard deviation) used in the denominator. In response to this criticism, Guyatt devised the responsiveness statistic, which divides the change by the standard deviation among subjects that show no change (Guyatt *et al.*, 1987). This has the advantage of accounting for nonspecific score changes. For an instrument to be responsive, it must account for change above and beyond this nonspecific component or the variability among stable subjects who do not show any clinical change. This has the effect of inflating the statistic over the standard method for computing the effect size. There are disadvantages to each method because even stable subjects are likely to improve as a result of the regression effect.

In response to criticisms of the *t* statistic, Liang, Larson, Cullen, and Schwartz (1985) recommended the *F* statistic and the relative precision of an outcomes measure as an alternative. In measuring the precision of an outcomes measure (its usefulness in making clinical comparisons) the *F* statistic takes two sources of variation into account, the groups being compared and within-group variance. In this regard, Liang and colleagues' approach more closely approximates the theoretical formula presented earlier. The relative precision indicates how much more or less precise a measure is in proportional terms than the standard measure.

The receiver operating characteristic (ROC) analysis is another method for measuring responsiveness. This approach works especially well when the results can be expressed in terms of subjects who improve and those who do not (i.e., nominal measures). The ROC curve is constructed by plotting the sensitivity (expressed as a proportion) against one minus the specificity of the measure. Alternatively, subjects that truly changed according to the measure are compared with subjects that truly changed but were undetected by the measure. In addition to evaluating patient change, ROC analysis is used in evaluating the effectiveness of screening tests. A simple illustration of the latter is shown in Figure 4-5.

Figure 4-5   **Receiver Operating Characteristic Curve for the CAGE Questionnaire Compared with Alcohol Dependency or Abuse by Extensive Clinical Evaluation**

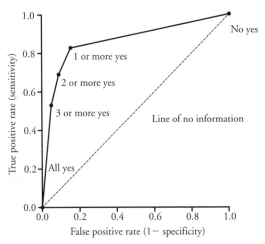

The ROC curve shows the effectiveness of the CAGE questionnaire in identifying individuals with alcohol dependency as confirmed by clinical investigation. The CAGE is a four-item yes or no questionnaire that asks about drinking habits (Ewing, 1984). Deviations of the ROC curve toward the upper left-hand corner support the strength of discrimination of the measure. The area beneath this curve, called the area under the curve (AUC), can be empirically measured and reflects the test of the measure. Values greater than 0.7 are necessary to accept a measure as responsive or discriminative (Iezzoni, 2003).

Burden

No outcomes study can be conducted without sufficient resources and the adherence of subjects to treatment protocols. A fifth strategic question in selecting a measure is: Does the burden for using the measure exceeds available resource? Burden takes on multiple forms and can be viewed from various vantage points in relation to the investigator, the treatment, and the study subject.

From the perspective of the subject, measurement burden can be in terms of the time spent completing forms, uncomfortable or intrusive tests, and so on. In cases where the burden of completing measures exceeds benefits of participating, subjects can choose to withdraw from studies, fail to complete questionnaires, become inattentive when completing surveys, and provide erroneous information. For any of these reasons, significant biases can be introduced into the measurement process. The investigator might be faced with the need to compensate subjects for completing forms or participating in the health outcomes research study. Subject compensation can take the form of monetary incentives for completing forms, gift cards, and trinkets such as pens, cards, and so on. There is extensive literature evaluating the effectiveness of various forms of incentives and approaches taken to measurement that reduces respondent burden and increases participation (Dillman, 2006).

From the vantage point of the investigator, measurement burden takes on several forms. First, the study might have inadequate resources for collecting the data necessary for the study or may collect too much data. As a general rule, most studies collect more data that they can realistically analyze and report. The skill set of the investigator is deficient for collecting the data or technically scoring the measure.

Design

Health outcomes studies are undertaken for any number of reasons. The proverbial cookie-cutter approach for selecting measures by pulling the next and greatest measure off the shelf is likely to lead to failure. The final question you need to address before embarking on an outcomes research study is: Does the use of the measure fit the study design and question? In some ways this is an extension of the notion of sensibility discussed earlier. Health outcomes measurement can be undertaken for a variety of reasons, characterizing the health of a population, predicting health outcomes, and evaluating the effectiveness of treatment interventions (Kirshner & Guyatt, 1985). The wrong outcomes measures can be placed in the appropriate study design and fail to answer the underlying study question. Alternatively, the right measure for answering the study question can be incorporated into a study design that fails to address the purpose of the study. A single item measure of health might be appropriate for assessing the overall health of a population of study patients, but is likely to be a poor choice for outcomes studies, because these measures have poor reliability and are more susceptible to regress toward the population mean. Design and analytical questions need to be weighed in the context of each of the properties discussed earlier.

FINAL THOUGHTS ABOUT OUTCOMES MEASURES

Advantages of Multiple-Item Versus Single-Item Measures

Frequently, the outcomes researcher is faced with the choice of using a multiple-item measure or a single-item measure for an outcome. There are three good reasons to choose multiple-item scales over single questions: improved reliability, scope, and precision (Haley, McHorney, & Ware, 1994; Nunnally & Bernstein, 1994; Spector, 1992). Single-item scales are not as reliable as multiple-item scales, since multiple-item scales average out measurement error when they are summed to obtain a total score. Generally, individual items have considerable measurement error, but it is not typically assessed. An implication of a loss in reliability with single-item measures is a tendency for high and low values for the baseline measure to regress toward the population mean at follow-up (Nunnally & Bernstein, 1994). Regression toward the mean is a particularly thorny problem in health outcomes research that select study subjects on the basis of extreme scores (i.e., high and low scores at baseline) and use unreliable single-item measures (Campbell & Stanley, 1963; Cook & Campbell, 1979; Shadish, Cook, & Campbell, 2002).

A second problem with using single-item scales to measure an outcome is that in many clinical instances, a single item is inadequate to capture the complexity of a construct. For example, complex constructs such as quality of life or mental health are necessarily measured along multiple dimensions. Finally, multi-item scales make it possible to discriminate more finely between the degrees of an attribute. Categorical response sets allow more discrimination than a simple yes or no question. For example, asking whether individuals can dress independently, with response options being: limited help from assistive devices or taking excessive time, with help from another person, or unable to perform, provides more information on the level of disability than simply asking whether the individual dresses without assistance and expecting a yes or no response. Several aggregated multiple category questions measuring a single construct provide many times the precision.

Other Useful Terms to Describe Measures

Some of the differences between multiple-item and single-item measures are best illustrated by defining other terms to describe measures. Outcomes measures for an attribute show varying levels of gradations, or *calibration*. For example, in the Medical Outcomes Study (MOS), mental health was measured using a single question with five response choices, the five-item Mental Health Inventory (MHI-5), a subscale from the 36-item health survey (SF-36) and the 18-item health survey (MHI-18). Each of the three approaches to measuring mental health have different levels of calibration, 5 levels, 26 levels, and 91 levels, respectively (McHorney, 1999). As a rule, increased calibration is associated with increased likelihood of detecting true differences in outcomes. This is referred to as increased statistical power. Multiple-item measures have better calibration compared with single-item measures.

Measures can be described in terms of *floor effects* and *ceiling effects*, and summarized as the percent of lowest and highest possible values on the scale. As a rule, single-item measures are more prone to floor and ceiling effects. A three-item measure of physical functioning, which is a component the 12-item Health Status Questionnaire (HSQ-12), found 63.8% of scale scores at the ceiling compared with 41.9% at the ceiling from the 10-item Physical Functioning Scale (PF-10) score from the SF-36 (Radosevich & Pruitt, 1996).

Measurement scales can also be described in terms of their *fidelity* and *bandwidth*. The term fidelity has a more general meaning and concerns accurate reproduction. It is intended to assess the thoroughness of the measure, its depth, and its quality. Bandwidth refers to the breadth of attributes assessed and the dimensionality. Multidimensional measures and multiple-item scales have greater bandwidth than unidimensional and single-item measures.

For subject reported outcomes, multiple-item measures are preferable to single-item measures.

SUMMARY

Measurement is a critical component to health outcomes research. Its intuitive appeal and accessibility lead many researchers to underestimate its importance and minimize its underlying complexities. Essential steps in measurement involve the abstraction of qualities or attributes that cannot be directly observed and the quantification of these qualities into scales. The process of measurement has become increasingly complex and empirically grounded. This is often unrecognized by new outcomes researchers. In many cases, technical assistance is needed from experts familiar with measurement and its subtle complexities.

REFERENCES

Aday, L. A., & Cornelius, L. J. (2006). *Designing and conducting health surveys: A comprehensive guide.* San Francisco: Jossey-Bass.

Ahmed, S., Schwartz, C., Ring, L., & Sprangers, M. A. (2009). Applications of health-related quality of life for guiding health care: Advances in response shift research. *Journal of Clinical Epidemiology, 62*(11), 1115–1117.

Allen, M. J., & Yen, W. M. (2002). *Introduction to measurement theory.* Long Grove, IL: Waveland Press.

Andrich, D. (1988). *Rasch models for measurement.* Beverly Hills, CA: Sage Publications.

Campbell, D. T., & Fiske, D. W. (1959). Convergent and discriminant validation by the multitrait–multimethod matrix. *Psychological Bulletin, 56,* 81–105.

Campbell, D. T., & Stanley, J. (1963). *Experimental and quasi-experimental designs for research.* Boston: Houghton Mifflin.

Carmines, E. G., & Zeller, R. A. (1979). *Reliability and validity assessment.* Beverly Hills, CA: Sage Publications.

Cook, T. D., & Campbell, D. T. (1979). *Quasi-experimentation: Design and analysis issues for field settings.* Boston: Houghton Mifflin.

Cronbach, L. J. (1990). *Essentials of psychological testing* (5th ed.). New York: Harper Collins.

Dillman, D. A. (2006). *Mail and Internet surveys: The tailored design method: 2007 update with new Internet, visual, and mixed-mode guide* (2nd ed.). New York: John Wiley and Sons.

Drummond, M. F., Sculpher, M. J., Torrance, G. W., & O'Brien, B. J. (2005). *Methods for the economic evaluation of health care programmes.* New York: Oxford University Press.

Duncan, O. D. (1984). *Notes on social measurement: Historical and critical.* New York: Russell Sage.

Ewing, J. A. (1984). Detecting alcoholism: The CAGE Questionnaire. *JAMA, 252,* 1905–1907.

Feinstein, A. R. (1987). *Clinimetrics.* New Haven, CT: Yale University Press.

Finch, M., Kane, R. L., & Philp, I. (1995). Developing a new metric for ADLs. *Journal of the American Geriatrics Society, 43*(8), 877–884.

Fischer, D., Stewart, A. L., Bloch, D. A., Lorig, K., Laurent, D., & Holman, H. (1999). Capturing the patient's view of change as a clinical outcome measure. *JAMA, 282*(12), 1157–1162.

Fryed, M. (1923). The graphic rating scale. *Journal of Educational Psychology, 43,* 83–102.

Guyatt, G., Walter, S., & Norman, G. R. (1987). Measuring change over time: Assessing the usefulness of evaluative instruments. *Journal of Chronic Diseases, 40*(2), 171–178.

Guyatt, G. H., Deyo, R. A., Charlson, M., Levine, M. N., & Mitchell, A. (1989). Responsiveness and validity in health status measurement: A clarification. *Journal of Clinical Epidemiology, 42*(5), 403–408.

Guyatt, G. H., & Townsend, M. B. (1987). A comparison of Likert and visual analogue scales: A critical review. *Journal of Chronic Diseases, 40*, 1129–1133.

Haley, S. M., McHorney, C. A., & Ware, J. E. (1994). Unidimensionality and reproducibility of the Rasch item scale. *Journal of Clinical Epidemiology, 47*(6), 671–684.

Iezzoni, L. I. (2003). *Risk adjustment for measuring health care outcomes* (3rd ed.). Chicago: Health Administration Press.

Kane, R. L., & Kane, R. A. (2004). *Assessing older persons: Measures meaning and practical applications.* New York: Oxford University Press.

Kaplan, R. M. (1995). Utility assessment for estimating quality adjusted life years. In F. A. Sloan (Ed.), *Valuing health care* (pp. 31–60). New York: Cambridge University Press.

Katz, S., & Akpom, C. A. (1976). A measure of primary socio-biological functions. *International Journal of Health Services, 6*, 493–507.

Kim, J.-O., & Mueller, C. W. (1978a). *Factor analysis: Statistical methods and practical issues.* Beverly Hills, CA: Sage Publications.

Kim, J.-O., & Mueller, C. W. (1978b). *Introduction to factor analysis: What it is and how to do it.* Beverly Hills, CA: Sage Publications.

Kirshner, B., & Guyatt, G. H. (1985). A methodological framework for assessing health indices. *Journal of Chronic Diseases, 27*(3), S178–S189.

Landis, J. R., & Koch, G. G. (1977). The measurement of observer agreement for categorical data. *Biometrics, 33*, 159–174.

Landy, F. J. (1986). Stamp collecting versus science. *American Psychologist, 41,* 1183–1192.

Le, C. T. (1998). *Applied categorical data analysis.* New York: John Wiley and Sons.

Liang, M. H., Larson, M. G., Cullen, K. E., & Schwartz, J. A. (1985). Comparative measurement efficiency and sensitivity of five health status instruments for arthritis research. *Arthritis and Rheumatism, 25*(5), 542–547.

McHorney, C. A. (1999). Health status assessment methods for adults: Past accomplishments and future challenges. *Annual Review of Public Health, 20,* 309–335.

McIver, J. P., & Carmines, E. G. (1981). *Unidimensional scaling.* Newbury Park: Sage Publications.

Norman, G. R. (1989). Issues in the use of change scores in randomized trials. *Journal of Clinical Epidemiology, 42*(11), 1097–1105.

Nunnally, J. C., & Bernstein, I. H. (1994). *Psychometric theory.* New York: McGraw-Hill.

Patrick, D. L., & Erickson, P. (1993). *Health status and health policy: Quality of life in health care evaluation and resource allocation.* New York: Oxford University Press.

Radosevich, D. M., & Pruitt, M. (1996). Twelve-item Health Status Questionnaire (HSQ-12) cooperative validation project: Comparability study. *AHSR FHSR Annual Meeting Abstract Book, 13,* 59.

Shadish, W. R., Cook, T. D., & Campbell, D. T. (2002). *Experimental and quasi-experimental designs for generalized causal inference.* Boston: Houghton Mifflin.

Spector, P. E. (1992). *Summated rating scale construction: An introduction.* Newbury Park, CA: Sage Publications.

Spector, W. D., Katz, S., Murphy, J. B., & Fulton, J. P. (1987). The hierarchical relationship between activities of daily living and instrumental activities of daily living. *Journal of Chronic Diseases, 40*(6), 481–489.

Streiner, D. L., & Norman, G. R. (2003). *Health measurement scales: A practical guide to their development and use* (3rd ed.). Oxford: Oxford University Press.

Streiner, D. L., & Norman, G. R. (2006). "Precision" and "accuracy": Two terms that are neither. *Journal of Clinical Epidemiology, 59,* 327–330.

Torrance, G. W., Thomas, W. H., & Sackett, D. L. (1972). A utility maximization model for evaluation of health care programs. *Health Services Research, 7,* 118–133.

Tversky, A., & Kahneman, D. (1981). The framing of decisions and the psychology of choice. *Science, 211,* 453–458.

Generic Health Outcomes Measures

Two classes of measures can be used to assess outcomes: condition-specific measures and generic measures.[1] *Condition-specific measures* (discussed in Chapter 7) focus on symptoms and signs that reflect the status of a given medical condition. They may also assess the direct sequelae of a disease on a person's life. As a result, they are likely to be sensitive to subtle changes in health. *Generic measures*, on the other hand, are comprehensive, broadly applicable across diseases, treatments (or interventions), and demographic groups that assess a single aspect or multiple aspects of health-related functioning in daily life. These measures summarize a wide spectrum of health concepts that apply to individuals and populations in different health states (Patrick & Erickson, 1993). The strength of the generic measures is their ability to compare across different conditions. For example, the Sickness Impact Profile (SIP; Bergner, Bobbitt, Carter, & Gilson, 1981) has been used to evaluate physical and social health in rheumatoid arthritis (Deyo, Inui, Leininger, & Overman, 1982), low back pain (Deyo, 1988; Deyo & Diehl, 1983), and myocardial infarction patients (Ott *et al.*, 1983). The 36-item Short-Form Health Survey (SF-36; Ware, Kosinski, & Keller, 1994; Ware & Sherbourne, 1992; Ware, Snow, Kosinski, & Gandek, 1993) was used to

---

[1]Generic measures may also be used as independent variables to control for health status differences between patients or groups. Usually, generic measures used as independent variables are collected at baseline to adjust for patient differences without confounding outcomes through the contemporaneous measurement of the outcome of interest and health status. Contemporaneous measurement of outcomes and health status can lead to differences affecting how a person reports outcomes. For example, being depressed may influence how a person reports his or her overall health status.

compare the several chronic conditions studied in the Medical Outcomes Study (MOS; Kravitz *et al.*, 1992; Safran, Tarlov, & Rogers, 1994). The SF-36 has become the most widely used generic measure today and has been translated into more than 120 different languages (QualityMetric, 2009). In effect, you are trading the broad coverage of a generic measure against the greater responsiveness and discrimination of a condition-specific measure. Thus the choice should reflect the purpose of the measurement.

WHY USE GENERIC MEASURES?

Generic measures capture elements that transcend single diseases. They can thus be used to compare the effects of treatments across diseases and disparate populations. Compared to condition-specific measures, they trade responsiveness for breadth of measurement.

Generic measures are designed to capture the physical, psychological, and social aspects of health first captured when the World Health Organization (1948) defined health as "a state of complete physical, mental and social well-being and not merely the absence of disease or infirmity" (p. 100).

Generic health has been evaluated in terms of both quantity and quality of health. Many of the traditional outcomes measures used in epidemiological and clinical research are based on counts of the frequency of occurrence of specific events (usually bad events that reflect some level of dysfunction). These traditional measures tend to have face validity for clinicians and can be applied across populations. Many of these quantitative health measures, such as mortality, morbidity, and average life expectancy, can be aggregated as easily understandable summary figures. Statistics derived from vital records, such as census counts, birth, and death, are the basis of traditional quantity of health measures.

The breadth of generic measures extends beyond these traditional health measures to reflect the importance of, or value attributed to, overall health and functioning. Generic measures are useful for clinical assessment and research. In clinical practice, providers interested in broadly assessing patient health can find generic measures useful as bottom-line indicators of the effects of treatments. Generic measures can be used to measure health along the entire range of health from well-being to disability. These measures can augment other types of clinical data and provider perceptions of patient health that focus on symptoms and signs of disease. Generic health measures, such as the Cooperative Information Project (COOP) Charts (Nelson,

Landgraf, Hays, Wasson, & Kirk, 1990; Nelson, Wasson, Johnson, & Hays, 1996) or the SF-36 (Ware & Sherbourne, 1992), have been used to track the "natural history" of a patient's perceived health status and quality of life. Patients' perceptions of physical, emotional, and social health cannot be obtained except by their direct assessment. Clinicians and patient proxies may be able to make statements about a patient's experience, but the proxy responses can both overestimate or underestimate patient health in ways that vary by domain and type of proxy (Boyer, Novella, Morrone, Jully, & Blanchard, 2004; Essen, 2004). While such potential biases do not threaten the validity of generic measures, they do raise caution flags.

Generic measures often include the concept of health-related quality of life (HRQL) addressed in Chapter 6. Such measures are useful for research applications. In randomized clinical trials and clinical research, the inclusion of generic (and condition-specific) outcomes measures can complement the analysis of morbidity and mortality by providing information from the patient's perspective of the impact of treatment on relevant aspects of patient experience. In addition, generic measures that assign relative values to different health states, such as the Health Utilities Index Mark 3 (Feeny *et al.*, 2002; Feeny, Torrance, & Furlong, 1996), the EuroQol or EQ-5D (EuroQol Group, 1990; Johnson, Coons, Ergo, & Szava-Kovats, 1998), or the Quality of Well-Being Scale (Kaplan & Anderson, 1988), enable the construction of quality-adjusted life years that are the typical denominator in a cost-effectiveness ratio. These types of generic measures, called health utility or health preference measures, assign values to health states that reflect patient preferences for being in a given health state (e.g., death; Patrick & Erickson, 1993). For example, the EQ-5D is able to identify 243 possible health states with five questions (EuroQol Group, 1990), while the Health Utilities Index Mark 3 can identify 972,000 possible health statuses with eight questions (Feeny *et al.*, 2002). In general, these measures can: (1) assess treatment effects in terms most relevant to patients, and (2) measure the effectiveness of treatments for cost-effectiveness analyses.

There are two other potential uses for generic measures: risk adjustment and profiling. Generic measures have proven to be useful predictors in cost estimation compared to diagnosis- or pharmacy-based measures of patient risk (Pope, Adamache, Walsh, & Khandker, 1998). The Duke Health Profile was more predictive of primary care charges than diagnoses or provider severity measures (Parkerson, Hammond, Michener, Yarnall, & Johnson, 2005). In this type of risk adjustment, generic measures potentially explain variation in costs. Finally, generic measures may also be useful in profiling healthcare organizations, such as hospitals or nursing homes. Researchers profiled 40 nursing homes using a generic quality of life measure and found that it was possible to differentiate nursing homes using a quality of life measure that was completed by the nursing homes' residents (Kane *et al.*, 2004). Profiling is typically done using health outcomes or costs, but this novel approach to profiling via quality of life measures is likely to increase in the future.

ADVANTAGES AND DISADVANTAGES OF USING A GENERIC HEALTH OUTCOMES MEASURES

There are advantages and disadvantages in using generic health outcomes measures. On the positive side, generic measures tap domains that are relevant to the patient and permit comparisons across patient groups that are different in terms of their personal characteristics or underlying diagnoses. Since generic measures have a wider use, they have tended to be more standardized. That is, the breadth of use promotes more consistent use and valid application. On the negative side, generic health outcomes measures tend to be less responsive to change and lack specificity when treatment effects are measured. Table 5-1 summarizes advantages and disadvantages of generic health outcomes measures.

The criteria for selecting a generic health outcomes measure are summarized in Table 5-2.

Table 5-1 **Advantages and Disadvantages of Generic Health Outcomes Measures**

Advantages	Disadvantages
Ability to make comparison across studies and patient groups	Lack specificity with respect to treatment effects
Widespread use of generic health outcomes measures permits greater standardization and more thorough psychometric evaluation	Floor and ceiling effects
Understood and used by nonprofessionals	Lack responsiveness to small but clinically important changes
Tap domains that hold relevance to the patient	May fail to tap dimensions that hold relevance to the clinician

Table 5-2   Criteria for Choosing a Generic Measure

Criterion	Impact on Measure
Domains of health	Choice of domains affects the treatment effects observed
Range of health	Range of measure affects the coverage of the spectrum of performance and change in health status
Clinical relevance	The degree to which the measure taps into health domains relevant to the population
Level of emphasis	The emphasis determines the relative weight of each domain in the measure
Sensitivity	The ability of the measure to detect subtle but meaningful variations in health status without significant floor or ceiling effects that might limit its usefulness in the population of interest
Responsiveness	The ability of the measure to detect important changes over time
Reliability	Reliable measures yield consistent, interpretable results
Validity	Valid measures provide information about the dysfunction of interest and measures the domains that it was designed to measure
Practical concerns	The burden of administration influences the response rates and rate of item completion from patients

HEALTH OUTCOME DOMAINS

Generic health outcomes measures assess either a single health domain or multiple health domains. Single domain measures are referred to as unidimensional, whereas measures of multiple domains are multidimensional. HRQL are multidimensional measures that assess function, social activity, cognitive function, emotional well-being, sleep and rest patterns, energy and vitality, perceived health, and general life satisfaction. These measures are also known as health status and quality of life, although the distinctions between the two are unclear. HRQL is discussed in greater detail in Chapter 6.

What health domains characterize the scope of generic health outcomes measures? Beyond mortality and morbidity, a core set of dimensions defines the scope of generic measurement. Within academic medical centers and large hospitals, mortality and morbidity reviews serve as the backbone of the peer review process. Physicians and surgeons meet as part of a peer review process to discuss mistakes made (i.e., poor outcomes) during the care of patients and to learn from complications and errors to prevent their reoccurrence. These M&M (mortality and morbidity) conferences serve as a forum for clinical education. Coming from this academic preparation, it is little wonder physicians are inclined to emphasize death and disease as core generic outcomes measures.

The traditional medical view of generic health outcomes as limited to mortality and morbidity has, however, been expanded (Fries, Spitz, Kraines, & Holman, 1980). Used predominantly for patients with arthritis, the Stanford Health Assessment Questionnaire (HAQ) expanded the scope of generic health measurement to include domains that hold importance to the patient, such as functioning and pain (Bruce & Fries, 2003; Fries & Spitz, 1990).

The scope of generic outcomes measures are easily remembered as the 6 Ds of generic outcomes:

- Death
- Disease
- Disability
- Discomfort
- Dissatisfaction
- Destitution or Dollars Expended for Health Services

The mnemonic lays out the broad scope of measures considered generic. The scope of generic outcomes measures includes the traditional end points, such as death and disease, along with other domains that provide a door into the individual's health within a social environment.

Table 5-3 lists the seven generic domains of health. Table 5-4 provides some examples of unidimensional scales. A comprehensive review is beyond the scope of this book; however, excellent reviews of generic measures are available in print (Kane & Kane, 2000; McDowell, 2006) and through online databases (MAPI Research Trust, 2009).

Table 5-3   **Seven Generic Domains of Health**

Domain	Definition
Physical functioning	Mobility and independence in physical abilities, self-care activities, and advanced, integrated independent living activities
Psychological well-being	Range of positive and negative emotions; anxiety and depressive symptoms
Social functioning	Social interaction and interdependence of the individual with the social environment
Pain	Self-reported degrees of physical discomfort
Cognitive functioning	Range of intellectual ability, specifically memory, reasoning, and orientation
Vitality	Energy, fatigue, sleep, and rest quality
Overall well-being	Global assessment of contentment and health

Physical Functioning

Compared with the other domains of generic health, there has been a proliferation of scales measuring physical functioning. In general, physical functioning refers to the range of an individual's mobility and independence in three types of physical ability:

1. Fitness or physiological health

2. Basic self-care activities (activities of daily living [ADLs])

3. Advanced, integrated independent living activities (instrumental activities of daily living [IADLs])

Fitness or physiological health refers to an individual's capacity to engage in varying levels of physical activity. For example, can the individual perform moderate-to-vigorous physical activities such as walking several miles or playing tennis? The ability to carry out basic self-care activities, such as bathing, dressing, and feeding oneself is fundamental to assessing physical health. Referred to as ADLs, there is a hierarchical relationship among the activities that gives these scales Guttman-type characteristics (see Chapter 4). As the physical activities become more complex and integrated within the individual's social fabric, physical activity becomes more critical in supporting independent living. Activities such as shopping, doing

Table 5-4 Selected Unidimensional Measures

Measure	Domain of Health	Number of Questions	Focus of Questions
Katz Index of ADLs (Katz, Ford, Moskowitz, Jackson, & Jaffee, 1963)	Physical functioning	Six dichotomous questions to create a scale of dependency	Bathing, dressing, toileting, transfer, continence, feeding
Barthel Index of ADLs (Mahoney & Barthel, 1965)	Physical functioning	Ten questions on performance based on 100-point scale	Feeding, grooming, toileting, walking, climbing stairs, continence
Profile of Mood States (McNair & Lorr, 1964)	Emotional functioning	Sixty-five questions	Affective mood states of anxiety, depression, anger, vigor, fatigue, and bewilderment
Beck Depression Inventory (Beck, Ward, Mendelson, Mock, & Erbaugh, 1961)	Emotional functioning	Twenty-one questions	Body image, sadness, feeling of failure, dissatisfaction, social withdrawal, low energy
Mental Status Questionnaire (Kahn *et al.*, 1960)	Cognitive functioning	Ten questions that sum to 10	Orientation based on current date, location, birthday
RAND Social Health Battery (Donald & Ware, 1984)	Social functioning	Eleven questions	Social resources and contacts in family and community
MOS Social Support Survey (Sherbourne & Stewart, 1991)	Social functioning	Twenty questions	Emotional support, informational support, tangible support, positive social interaction, affection

ADLs, activities of daily living; MOS, Medical Outcomes Study.

chores, and cleaning are examples of these IADLs. The choice of a physical functioning measure depends on the population measured and its underlying characteristics. For physically disabled populations, for whom basic self-care activities are critical, ADLs might be a better focus of physical functioning; whereas populations with greater physical ability would be better measured using physical ability or instrumental activity measures.

Psychological Well-Being

Psychological well-being refers to an individual's range of positive and negative emotions. Much of the assessment in this area focuses on anxiety and depression. In fact, next to physical functioning, depression is one of the more frequently measured generic health domains. Frequently used measures such as the SF-36 (Ware *et al.*, 1993; Ware *et al.*, 1994; Ware & Sherbourne, 1992), include psychological health measurement scales as one component of the multidimensional instrument. The 5-item mental screener, referred to as the MHI-5 assesses depressive symptoms, anxiety, and mood (Berwick *et al.*, 1991). This simple set of items has been shown to be effective in identifying individuals at risk of major mental illness.

Social Functioning

Social health is less frequently discussed and assessed as a part of health outcomes research. Social functioning, which is a key facet of social health (Donald & Ware, 1984; Sherbourne & Stewart, 1991), describes social interaction and interdependence of the individual within the social environment in the following ways:

1. Social roles;

2. Engagement in the community or neighborhood;

3. Closeness of interpersonal relationships; and

4. Social support.

Social roles define the ability of the individual to perform a social responsibility that has been prescribed by society, for example, a job role or parenting role. A health problem can directly impair the ability to perform these prescribed social roles. A second facet of social functioning involves the connectedness of the individual with the community or neighborhood of which he or she is a member. Stated in another way, this refers to the degree of integration one has with his or her social environment.

The final two facets are interrelated. The closeness of interpersonal relationships refers to the quality of the individual's social network. One dimension of social support is emotional. This concerns the comfort provided by family, friends, and others. More tangible support that involves physical aid (e.g., financial aid, shelter) is referred to as instrumental support. The physical assistance and emotional support provided through our interpersonal relationships are critical to coping with the impact health has on our lives.

Pain

In addition to mental health problems, pain is the most frequently cited reason for physician visits (the reason for physician visit is referred to as the chief complaint; Agency for Healthcare Research and Quality, 2008). Generic measures of pain assess the degree of debilitating physical discomfort. This can be in the form of bodily pain and sensations that are bothersome to the individual. Pain is individually and personally defined and can be uniquely described in terms of uncomfortable sensations, like aches and cramps. Pain is assessed in terms of its intensity, duration, frequency, timing, and participating and alleviating factors. These characteristics are critical to developing a history of present illness.

Cognitive Functioning

The assessment of cognitive functioning serves as the basis for neurological testing routinely performed at the bedside by clinicians. Cognitive functioning refers to an individual's range of intellectual ability in three ways: (1) memory, (2) reasoning abilities, and (3) orientation. The ability to remember significant dates and events in the past or future is a common measure of cognitive functioning, but thinking is a much more complex process. Several different generic measures test memory, including the Mental Status Questionnaire (Kahn, Goldfarb, Pollack, & Peck, 1960). *Reasoning ability* refers to an individual's ability to do simple reasoning or computational tasks. Although these are best tested directly, it is possible to ask respondents to note problems they are experiencing in these areas. Multidimensional measures, like the SIP, has a question asking the individual about difficulties making plans or decisions, or learning new things (Bergner *et al.*, 1981). *Orientation* captures an individual's awareness of current surroundings and is a common aspect of cognitive functioning queried in older adult patients. A note such as "orientation times 3" is often recorded in the patient record signifying orientation to person, place, and time.

Vitality

The degree of vitality that an individual feels is captured by two constructs: (1) energy and (2) sleep and rest. Besides food and shelter, sleep and rest are basic human needs. The Pittsburgh Sleep Quality Index (PSQI) provides a useful paradigm for thinking about the assessment of sleep and rest in health outcomes studies (Buysse, Reynolds, Monk, Berman, & Kupfer, 1989; Buysse *et al.*, 1991). Sleep is viewed as a highly complex phenomenon characterized by sleep quality, bedtime routine, wake-up time, sleep latency, and sleep duration. In addition to these facets of sleep and rest, the PSQI asks the bed partner or roommate about the individual's sleep. In health outcomes research studies where sleep is affected by an underlying medical condition, measures of sleep and rest could prove useful. Several conditions likely to impact on sleep are management of hot flashes, nocturia (going to the bathroom at night), and gastroesophageal reflux disease (GERD).

Energy and fatigue characterize the positive and negative ranges of vitality. For example, four questions on the SF-36 comprise the Vitality or Energy/Fatigue Scale. In the instrument, individuals are asked about their level of pep and if they feel tired. Similar to the SF-36, the SIP asks patients if they sit during much of the day and if they sleep or nap during the day.

Overall Well-Being

Overall life satisfaction, or overall well-being, is a global evaluation of an individual's sense of contentment. This domain provides a comprehensive assessment of the patient's sense of his or her health status and happiness. In essence, overall well-being implicitly incorporates the physical, psychological, and social dimensions and their interactions. This domain is commonly assessed with broad questions asking patients about their overall health and well-being. The best known question used to assess overall health is, "In general, would you say your health is excellent, very good, good, fair, or poor?" Overall well-being is a useful domain to include in most studies because this deceptively simple question has been found to be a good predictor of mortality (Idler & Kasl, 1991; Mossey & Shapiro, 1982). Combined with the other domains of health, assessment of overall well-being can provide a complete conception of HRQL.

PRACTICAL CONSIDERATIONS

If a generic measure is used as an outcome, it should be collected at baseline as well as follow-up. This permits tracking the individual's health trajectory. Based on years of experience of health outcomes investigators, the baseline measure will serve as the best predictor of follow-up outcomes. The measurement of health status to indicate improving or worsening health is only meaningful if a before and after comparison can be made.

The serial assessment of generic outcomes is the core for health outcomes research. With few exceptions, a simple health transition item should be included with the generic health outcomes used. These retrospective measures ask individuals to compare their present health state against their previous states of health (Feinstein, 1987). Practically, this strategy enhances the interpretation of the measurement and provides other useful information about perceived changes in health status (Fischer *et al.*, 1999). This latter retrospective approach has been employed to assess a range of generic health status domains, such as health in general, physical functioning, and pain, to name a few.

In almost all cases, investigators are advised to use an extant generic health status measure (or portions of it) instead of trying to create one de novo. (The development work involved is extensive and would dwarf most applied studies.) Several practical considerations must be addressed when choosing a generic health status measure. These practical issues should be considered once the conceptual model and psychometric issues are dealt with, not the other way around. These considerations include:

- The length of time required to administer and complete the questionnaire;
- The appropriate format for the survey (telephone, face-to-face, or self-administered);
- The use of proxy respondents;
- The cost of administration (data collection and data entry);
- The complexity of the measurement and scoring methods;
- The acceptability of the survey to patients/respondents and clinicians; and
- The expected format for presenting the results.

Policy makers and clinicians generally find single, comprehensive values of health or quality of life more palatable than a set of scale values associated with different domains. (The simplicity of traditional generic measures, such as infant mortality or life expectancy, may partly explain their persistence in public policy analysis.) However, scores may not be meaningful per se. To get someone's attention, the score has to be understood in a context that is significant to the audience. Moreover, the same score may mean different things to different people. For those working actively with a scale, score values may become rectified as facts, but, for most people, they are not. Treating score values as indisputable, objective indicators of underlying health should be avoided.

Investigators must balance the burden of survey administration on interviewers and respondents with the breadth of health domains covered. Respondent attention will vary with the underlying nature of the respondents and the situation. Long questionnaires cannot be completed in a busy clinic while people are waiting to see the physician. There is a trade-off between the length of a questionnaire and the response rate for the overall measure and for particular items in the measure that have to be balanced. Older adults or chronically ill populations may have problems of comprehension and/or fatigue.

The time frame of a question can be important. There is often a trade-off between the time needed to generate enough events and the accuracy of recall. Different types of information can be reliably remembered for various times. Questionnaires must be designed to minimize the difficulty in answering them. Pilot testing to ensure that the questions are interpreted as they were intended can prevent disastrous mistakes.

In many cases, the cost of survey administration will influence the choice of generic measure. As a general rule, complicated, high-quality data on patient quality of life will be expensive to collect. They usually require interviewers to administer the questions and interpret them or probe for further responses. New forms of interactive computerized interviews may reduce the need for interviewers, but several logistical issues must be resolved before this approach is widely available.

The acceptability of the survey to patients and clinicians is important to ensure reasonable response rates. The COOP Charts (Nelson *et al.*, 1990) are unique among multidimensional generic measures in accompanying survey questions by pictures associated with Likert-type responses. For example, a question about physical functioning has answers ranging from "very little work," with an associated picture of someone doing dishes to "very heavy work," with a picture of someone running (Nelson *et al.*, 1990). This intuitive format was highly acceptable to patients and clinicians. The results were also easily interpreted because the COOP Charts have only one question for each health construct. Investigators have to balance presentation of results and the psychometric properties of their measure. Surveys that use single measures may have deficiencies in validity and reliability. By contrast, the results from complex, multidimensional measures may provide results that require careful interpretation.

Each of these criteria should be considered for all measures, but all do not need to be satisfied before a generic measure can be considered useful. Often, it is a trade-off between the ideal characteristics for a measure and the practicalities of application.

CHOOSING A MEASURE

In recent years, improved psychometric work has fostered the development of more sophisticated measures of generic health. Clinical investigators now have a variety of alternative generic measures that can be used as substitutes or complements to these traditional indicators of health.

The most commonly used measures—mortality, morbidity, and utilization are frequently used because they are the most accessible from medical records, vital records, and hospital charts. Mortality is a valuable endpoint when there is a reasonable expectation that the problem being studied has a chance of leading to premature death. Solid organ transplant is an exemplar. Mortality is most meaningful if expressed as the proportion of deaths from a particular cause over a defined time interval. These are expressed in terms of survival percentages. However, mortality suffers from both floor and ceiling effects.[2] On the one hand, a living status says little about any other point on the continuum of dysfunction.

Morbidity can be assessed in several ways. It may reflect the incidence or prevalence of a disease, or it may be expressed as days of work missed or bed disability days. Evaluations relying solely on morbidity measures may exclude important extremes in outcomes, such as excellent health or death. These types of floor and ceiling effects are a frequent concern in any generic status measure. Morbidity usually focuses only on physical health, but it can also capture the consequences of mental health and work-related limitations. If a broader range of dysfunction and other domains of health

---

[2]A floor effect is a value that observations cannot fall below. A ceiling effect is a value that observations cannot exceed (Nunnally & Bernstein, 1994).

is relevant, then morbidity is not as useful as other, more comprehensive measures (Kaplan, Anderson, Wu, Mathews, Kozin, & Orenstein, 1989).

Utilization of health services measures has been used as a proxy of health status. Utilization is difficult to interpret as a measure of health because of differences in access to services and other factors related to a population's utilization. Cultural and economic factors in the patient population of interest may distort the relationship between health and utilization data (Johnson *et al.*, 1995; Meredith & Siu, 1995).

CONCLUSION

The evaluation of generic health status deserves greater consideration than may seem indicated at first. Careful attention to conceptualization of health domains and their components is critical. Four main points can serve as guidelines for selecting these measures:

1. It is best to determine which of the generic health domains are salient to your problem and then choose the generic measure that captures those domains. Each measure will have one or more questions that focus on a specific aspect of functioning, and different measures incorporate different combinations of domains. No single measure will work best in all possible patient populations and medical conditions. Choosing the measure appropriate for one's study is a critical first step in effective outcomes research.

2. Generic measures are the best way to capture multidimensional aspects of health. These types of measures are designed to assess patient health across several domains (physical/social/emotional/cognitive functioning, pain, vitality, and overall well-being). In any case, generic measures are the ones to use if overall patient health is the desired outcome.

3. Generic measures should be collected at baseline (as well as follow up) to indicate where the individual's health course began. The measurement of health status to indicate improving or worsening health is only meaningful if a before and after comparison can be made. With few exceptions, a simple health transition item should be included as a measure. This strategy enhances the interpretation of the replicate measurement and provides other useful information about changes in health status.

4. The more easily understood the measure, the more useful it is. Generic measures generally have life anchors to relate a numeric value to a state or condition of health. In other words, results based on scale scores need to be placed in the context of daily life to be easily interpreted. The values obtained from a generic measure must have a clinical context to be useful sources of information.

REFERENCES

Agency for Healthcare Research and Quality. (2008). Mental health woes remain one of the top reasons for doctor visits. *AHRQ News and Numbers.* Available at: http://www.ahrq.gov/news/nn/nn030608.htm. Accessed April 6, 2010.

Beck, A. T., Ward, C. H., Mendelson, M., Mock, J., & Erbaugh, J. (1961). An inventory for measuring depression. *Archives of General Psychiatry, 4*, 561–571.

Bergner, M. B., Bobbitt, R. A., Carter, W. B., & Gilson, B. S. (1981). The Sickness Impact Profile: Development and final revision of a health status measure. *Medical Care, 19*(8), 787–805.

Berwick, D. M., Murphy, J. M., Goldman, P. A., Ware, J. E., Barsky, A. J., & Weinstein, M. C. (1991). Performance of a five-item mental health screening test. *Medical Care, 29*(2), 169–176.

Boyer, F., Novella, J. L., Morrone, I., Jully, D., & Blanchard, F. (2004). Agreement between dementia patient report and proxy reports using the Nottingham Health Profile. *International Journal of Geriatric Psychiatry, 19*(11), 1026–1034.

Bruce, B., & Fries, J. F. (2003). The Stanford Health Assessment Questionnaire: A review of its history, issues, progress and documentation. *Journal of Rheumatology, 30*(1), 167–178

Buysse, D. J., Reynolds, C. F. I., Monk, T. H., Berman, S. R., & Kupfer, D. J. (1989). The Pittsburgh Sleep Quality Index: A new instrument for psychiatric practice and research. *Psychiatry Research, 28*(2), 193–213.

Buysse, D. J., Reynolds, C. F. I., Monk, T. H., Hoch, C. C., Yaeger, A. L., & Kupfer, D. J. (1991). Quantification of subjective sleep quality in healthy elderly men and women using the Pittsburgh Sleep Quality Index (PSQI). *Sleep*, *14*(4), 331–338.

Deyo, R. A. (1988). Measuring the functional status of patients with low back pain (Review). *Archives of Physical Medicine and Rehabilitation*, *69* (12), 1044–1053.

Deyo, R. A., & Diehl, A. K. (1983). Measuring physical and psychosocial function in patients with low-back pain. *Spine*, *8*(6), 635–642.

Deyo, R. A., Inui, T. S., Leininger, J., & Overman, S. (1982). Physical and psychosocial function in rheumatoid arthritis: Clinical use of a self-administered health status instrument. *Archives of Internal Medicine*, *142*(5), 879–882.

Donald, C. A., & Ware, J. E. J. (1984). The measurement of social support. *Research in Community & Mental Health*, *4*, 325–370.

Essen L. von (2004). Proxy ratings of patient quality of life—factors related to patient-proxy agreement. *Acta Oncologica*, *43*(3), 229–234.

EuroQol Group. (1990). EuroQoL—A new facility for the measurement of health-related quality of life. *Health Policy*, *16*(3), 199–208.

Feeny, D., Furlong, W., Torrance, G. W., Goldsmith, C. H., Zhu, Z., DePauw, S., . . . Boyle, M. (2002). Multiattribute and single-attribute utility functions for the health utilities index mark 3 system. *Medical Care*, *40*(2), 113–128.

Feeny, D. H., Torrance, G. W., & Furlong, W. J. (1996). Health utilities index. In B. Spilker (Ed.), *Quality of life and pharmacoeconomics in clinical trials* (2nd ed., pp. 239–252). Philadelphia: Lippincott-Raven.

Feinstein, A. R. (1987). *Clinimetrics*. New Haven, CT: Yale University Press.

Fischer, D., Stewart, A. L., Bloch, D. A., Lorig, K., Laurent, D., & Holman, H. (1999). Capturing the patient's view of change as a clinical outcome measure. *JAMA*, *282*(12), 1157–1162.

Fries, J. F., & Spitz, P. W. (1990). The hierarchy of patient outcomes. In B. Spilker (Ed.), *Quality of life assessments in clinical trials* (pp. 25–35). New York: Raven Press.

Fries, J. F., Spitz, P. W., Kraines, R. G., & Holman, H. R. (1980). Measurement of patient outcomes in arthritis. *Arthritis and Rheumatism, 23*(2), 137–145.

Idler, E. L., & Kasl, S. (1991). Health perceptions and survival: Do global evaluations of health status really predict mortality? *Journal of Gerontology, 46*(2), S55–S65.

Johnson, J. A., Coons, S. J., Ergo, A., & Szava-Kovats, G. (1998). Valuation of EuroQOL (EQ-5D) health states in an adult US sample. *PharmacoEconomics, 13*(4), 421–433.

Johnson, P. A., Goldman, L., Orav, E. J., Garcia, T., Pearson, S. D., & Lee, T. H. (1995). Comparison of the Medical Outcomes Study Short-Form 36-item health survey in black patients and white patients with acute chest pain. *Medical Care, 33*(2), 145–160.

Kahn, R. L., Goldfarb, A. I., Pollack, M., & Peck, A. (1960). Brief objective measures for the determination of mental status in the aged. *American Journal of Psychiatry, 117*(4), 326–328.

Kane, R. L., Bershadsky, B., Kane, R. A., Degenholtz, H. B., Liu, J., Giles, K., & Kling, K. C. (2004). Using resident reports of quality of life to distinguish among nursing homes. *The Gerontologist, 44*(5), 624–632.

Kane, R. L., & Kane, R. A. (Eds.). (2000). *Assessing older persons: Measures, meaning, and practical applications.* New York: Oxford University Press.

Kaplan, R. M., & Anderson, J. P. (1988). A general health policy model: Update and applications. *Health Services Research, 23*(2), 203–235.

Kaplan, R. M., Anderson, J. P., Wu, A. W., Mathews, W. C., Kozin, F., & Orenstein, D. (1989). The quality of well-being scale: Applications in AIDS, cystic fibrosis, and arthritis. *Medical Care, 27*(3), S27–S43.

Katz, S., Ford, A. B., Moskowitz, R. W., Jackson, B. A., & Jaffee, M. W. (1963). Studies of illness in the aged. The index of ADL: A standardized measure of biological and psychosocial function. *JAMA, 185*(12), 914–919.

Kravitz, R. L., Greenfield, S., Rogers, W., Manning, W. G., Zubkoff, M., Nelson, E. C., . . .Ware, J. E. (1992). Differences in the mix of patients among medical specialties and systems of care: Results from the Medical Outcomes Study. *JAMA, 267*(12), 1617–1623.

Mahoney, F. I., & Barthel, D. W. (1965). Functional evaluation: The Barthel Index. *Maryland State Medical Journal, 14*, 61–65.

MAPI Research Trust. (2009). Patient-reported outcome and quality of life instruments database (PROQOLID). Available at: http://www.proqolid.org/. Accessed April 16, 2010.

McDowell, I. (2006). *Measuring health: A guide to rating scales and questionnaires* (3rd ed.). New York: Oxford University Press.

McNair, D. M., & Lorr, M. (1964). An analysis of mood in neurotics. *The Journal of Abnormal and Social Psychology, 69*(6), 620–627.

Meredith, L. S., & Siu, A. L. (1995). Variation and quality of self-report health data: Asian and Pacific Islanders compared with other ethnic groups. *Medical Care, 33*(11), 1120–1131.

Mossey, J. M., & Shapiro, E. (1982). Self-rated health: A prediction of mortality among the elderly. *American Journal of Public Health, 72*(8), 800–808.

Nelson, E. C., Landgraf, J. M., Hays, R. D., Wasson, J. H., & Kirk, J. W. (1990). The functional status of patients: How can it be measured in physicians' offices? *Medical Care, 28*(12), 1111–1126.

Nelson, E. C., Wasson, J. H., Johnson, D. J., & Hays, R. D. (1996). Dartmouth COOP Functional Health Assessment Charts: Brief measures for clinical practice. In B. Spilker (Ed.), *Quality of life and pharmacoeconomics in clinical trials* (2nd ed.). Philadelphia: Lippincott-Raven Publishers.

Nunnally, J. C., & Bernstein, I. H. (1994). *Psychometric theory*. New York: McGraw-Hill.

Ott, C. R., Sivarajan, E. S., Newton, K. M., Almes, M. J., Bruce, R. A., Bergner, M. B., & Gilson, B. S. (1983). A controlled randomized study of early cardiac rehabilitation: The Sickness Impact Profile as an assessment tool. *Heart & Lung: The Journal of Critical Care, 12*(2), 162–170.

Parkerson, G. R., Jr., Hammond, W. E., Michener, J. L., Yarnall, K. S. H., & Johnson, J. L. (2005). Risk classification of adult primary care patients by self-reported quality of life. *Medical Care*, *43*(2), 189–193.

Patrick, D. L., & Erickson, P. (1993). *Health status and health policy: Quality of life in health care evaluation and resource allocation.* New York: Oxford University Press.

Pope, G., C., Adamache, K. W., Walsh, E. G., & Khandker, R. K. (1998). Evaluating alternative risk adjusters for Medicare. *Health Care Financing Review*, *20*(2), 109–129.

QualityMetric. (2009). Generic health surveys. Available at: http://www.qualitymetric.com/WhatWeDo/GenericHealthSurveys/tabid/184/Default.aspx?gclid=CMa7lfHBn54CFQ_xDAodOUiFlg. Accessed April 16, 2010.

Safran, D. G., Tarlov, A. R., & Rogers, W. H. (1994). Primary care performance in fee-for-service and prepaid health care systems: Results from the Medical Outcomes Study. *JAMA*, *271*(20), 1579–1586.

Sherbourne, C. D., & Stewart, A. L. (1991). The MOS social support survey. *Social Science and Medicine*, *32*(6), 705–714.

Ware, J. E., Jr., Kosinski, M., & Keller, S. D. (1994). *SF-36 physical and mental health summary scales: A user's manual.* Boston: The Health Institute.

Ware, J. E., Jr., & Sherbourne, C. D. (1992). The MOS 36-item Short-Form health survey (SF-36). *Medical Care*, *30*(6), 473–483.

Ware, J. E., Jr., Snow, K., K, Kosinski, M., & Gandek, B. (1993). *SF-36 health survey: Manual and interpretation guide.* Boston: The Health Institute, New England Medical Center.

World Health Organization. (1948). *World Health Organization constitution.* Geneva: World Health Organization.

CHAPTER 6

Health-Related Quality of Life

Increasingly, the central role that quality of life (QOL) plays as part of the outcomes of care is being recognized. QOL is obviously a subjective concept. It addresses the elements of life that give our lives meaning and, in effect, define who we are. Even a few moments of thought make it clear that, while being in good shape would undoubtedly add to one's QOL, it is possible to enjoy a high QOL even while suffering severe disease. Stephen Hawking, the well-known theoretical physics professor, is often used as a model, but other examples closer to home abound. In your everyday life you undoubtedly have met someone who is enjoying a high QOL despite severe handicaps.

In some ways the World Health Organization (WHO) definition of health opened the door to an excessively grandiose conception of how medical care can affect QOL when it defined health as not simply the absence of illness but a positive state of physical, emotional, and social well-being[1] (World Health Organization, 1948). In truth, aspects of QOL are not generally within the influence of medical care. For instance, although heavy medical expenses can pauperize a person, in general, medical care does not contribute to one's financial well-being.

Just because the bounds of QOL can extend so far, health care has opted to manage its liability by taking responsibility for only those aspects of QOL it might hope to influence. Hence, the bounded concept of health-related quality of life (HRQL) was created. HRQL refers to the

---

[1]You are unlikely, however, to get your health insurance company to buy you a Mercedes-Benz because it is necessary for your social well-being.

various aspects of a person's life that are strongly affected by changes in health status (health related) and that are important to the person (quality of life; Cleary, Wilson, & Fowler, 1994).

Most conceptualizations include multiple dimensions: physical functioning, social functioning, role functioning, mental health, general health, vitality, pain, and cognitive functioning. Recent iterations (specifically the WHO's Quality of Life Assessment) include spiritual dimensions. In essence, one might ask what aspects of life medical care be expected to influence. Table 6-1 shows some elements that might be considered in assessing HRQL.

Figure 6-1 shows a model that links elements of care to HRQL. In effect, biological and systems factors create symptoms (which are actually the body's responses to insults like infection), which in turn affect function, which leads to global health status. This progression is influenced at each stage by feelings and other psychosocial factors.

HRQL can be thought of as a summation measurement, wherein a host of factors contribute. Measuring health status is a summative process. Perhaps the easiest example lies with rheumatoid arthritis. The common way to measure the effectiveness of acute joint inflammation treatment is with a joint count (a count of the number of target joints that are inflamed and painful) or a sedimentation rate (or a C-reactive protein) test of inflammatory activity. The next stage of measure for arthritis would be to examine function. One might use a timed walk to assess the lower body, or grip strength

Table 6-1   **Components of Health-Related Quality of Life**

Components
Physical functioning
Social functioning
Emotional functioning
Cognitive functioning
Pain
Vitality
Overall well-being
Spirituality
Mortality

Figure 6-1   Conceptual Model Depicting the Relationships
Among Measures of Patients Outcome
in Health-Related Quality of Life

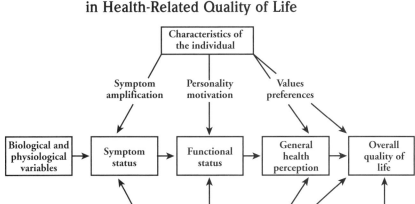

Source: (Wilson & Cleary, 1995)

for the upper body. These functional measures would be affected by the
acute state addressed previously; but they would also be sensitive to other
factors, like joint deformity. Even in the absence of an acute flare up, function would be influenced by joint deformity. A more comprehensive level of
functioning might come from examining activities of daily living (ADLs).
ADLs require everything already addressed, but also may be influenced
by motivation, depression, or even cognitive ability (Spiegel *et al.*, 1988).
HRQL is similarly affected by an accumulation of factors.

One can view this progression as a distal–proximal continuum. Essentially,
the nearer the event to the outcome of interest, the easier it is to detect the
effect. As factors cumulate, the relationships become more complex. The
implications of this proximal–distal continuum for measuring HRQL are:

   a. Distal outcomes are influenced more heavily by nontreatment factors.
   b. Larger effects are seen when proximal outcomes are assessed, initial
       illness is more severe, and pretreatment distal outcomes show high
       impairment.
   c. You should include disease-specific measures.

    d. If the disease is severe, any outcome measure selected is useful.

    e. Any previous experience with measurement in the population informs decisions regarding measurement selection.

    f. The strongest predictors of generic health are baseline health status and demographics.

    g. The timing of the outcome of interest is a primary determinant of whether to emphasize generic or condition-specific measures.

    h. Systematic assessment of treatment processes is of critical importance. (Brenner, Curbow, & Legro, 1995)

APPLICATIONS FOR HEALTH-RELATED QUALITY OF LIFE MEASURES

HRQL measures are used in a variety of settings. They have become a mainstay in clinical trials that evaluate new pharmacological agents and biomedical devices, where some measure of the ultimate benefit of the intervention is increasingly demanded. They are likewise important to consider in tests of clinical effectiveness. They are a central part of health needs assessments and associated resource allocation efforts, which measure health status and health deficits. Perhaps the best example of how they have been used in a policy context around such assessments was the attempt to allocate health care based on effectiveness in the state of Oregon (Kitzhaber, 1993).

    Clinical applications of HRQL face several major obstacles: (1) clinicians are uncertain about how to use these measures as part of their practices; (2) many clinicians see these as "soft data"; (3) clinicians are reluctant to use HRQL as an outcome because they believe that many of the factors that affect HRQL are outside the influence of medical care; and (4) the validity of using HRQL scales to make clinical decisions has not yet been well established. However, the growing popularity of patients and clinicians sharing decisions make a strong case for HRQL, which is a critical part of any thoughtful decisions about health treatments.

Condition-Specific HRQL

Although HRQL is generally considered a generic measure used across health conditions, it can also be used for specific conditions. The Functional Assessment of Chronic Illness Therapy (FACIT) Measurement System is a collection of QOL questionnaires targeted to the management of chronic illness. FACIT (Functional Assessment of Chronic Illness Therapy) was adopted as the formal name of the measurement system in 1997 to portray the expansion of the more familiar Functional Assessment of Cancer Therapy (FACT) series of questionnaires into other chronic illnesses and conditions. Thus, FACIT is a broader, more encompassing term that includes the FACT questionnaires under its umbrella.

The measurement system, under development since 1987, began with the creation of a generic CORE questionnaire called the Functional Assessment of Cancer Therapy–General (FACT-G). The FACT-G (now in its fourth version) is a 27-item compilation of general questions divided into four primary QOL domains: Physical Well-Being, Social/Family Well-Being, Emotional Well-Being, and Functional Well-Being. The fifth component allows for additional items that relate to the condition of specific interest. It is considered appropriate for use with patients with any form of cancer, and has also been used and validated in other chronic illness conditions (e.g., HIV/AIDS and multiple sclerosis) and in the general population (using a slightly modified version).

David Cella and his colleagues have developed 40 different FACIT scales and nine symptom indices (Bruner *et al.*, 2007; Cella *et al.*, 2007; Garcia *et al.*, 2007; Hahn *et al.*, 2007; Hahn, Rao, Cella, & Choi, 2008; Rao, Debb, Blitz, Choi, & Cella, 2008; Sloan *et al.*, 2006). Tables 6-2 and 6-3 show the range of the scales that have been created from this basic template. Another example of a condition-specific HRQL scale is the Minnesota Living with Heart Failure Questionnaire (MLHFQ; Rector, Kubo, & Cohn, 1987). For this measure, the patient is asked to grade the extent to which his or her heart failure prevented them from doing various tasks or engaging in activities. Table 6-4 gives an example of the items that comprise the MLHFQ.

Examples of HRQL Measures

Karnofsky Scale

One of the earliest efforts to address HRQL (before the concept was even defined) was created to assess the status of cancer patients, where QOL was recognized as a major component of clinical outcomes (Karnofsky, Abelmann, Craver, & Burchenal, 1948). Despite its limitations, the Karnofsky Scale has persisted, perhaps because it was introduced so early. Among its several limitations is the large problem that it is designed to reflect a clinician's judgment of a patient's condition rather than ask the

Table 6-2   **FACT Measures of Health-Related Quality of Life for Various Conditions**

Measure	Description
FACT-G	Functional Assessment of Cancer Therapy–General version of the scale constitutes the core of all subscales. FACT-G can be used with patients of any tumor type.
FACT-GP	Functional Assessment of Cancer Therapy–General Population includes 21 FACT-G items.
FANLTC	Functional Assessment of Non-Life Threatening Conditions (The FANLTC is the FACT-G less one item.)
FACT-B	For patients with breast cancer
FACT-Bl	For patients with bladder cancer
FACT-Br	For patients with brain cancer
FACT-C	For patients with colorectal cancer
FACT-CNS	For patients with cancer in the central nervous system
FACT-Cx	For patients with cancer of the cervix
FACT-E	For patients with esophageal cancer
FACT-En	For patients with endometrial cancer
FACT-Ga	For patients with gastric cancer
FACT-H&N	For patients with head and neck cancer
FACT-Hep	For patients with hepatobiliary cancer (liver, bile duct, and pancreas)
FACT-L	For patients with lung cancer
FACT-Leu	For patients with leukemia
FACT-Lym	For patients with lymphoma (non-Hodgkin's lymphoma)
FACT-M	For patients with melanoma
FACT-O	For patients with ovarian cancer
FACT-P	For patients with prostate cancer
FACT-V	For patients with vulva cancer
FKSI 19	For patients with kidney cancer
Peds-FACT-BrS	Pediatric Functional Assessment of Cancer Therapy–Brain tumor Survivors

Table 6-3   **FACIT Measures of Health-Related Quality of Life for Cancer-Specific Symptom Indices, Treatment Measures, and Noncancer-Specific Measures**

Measure	Description
Symptom Indices	
FAACT	Functional Assessment of Anorexia/Cachexia Treatment
FACIT-D	For patients with diarrhea
FACIT-F	Functional Assessment of Chronic Illness Therapy–Fatigue
FACIT-Fatigue	Functional Assessment of Chronic Illness Therapy–Fatigue, a 13-item FACIT Fatigue scale.
FACT-An	For patients with anemia/fatigue
FACT-B+4	For patients with lymphedema (to be used with FACT-B)
FACT-Bone Pain	For patients with bone pain
FACT-Cog	For patients with cognitive function issues
FACT-ES	For patients with endocrine symptoms
FACT-N	For patients with neutropenia
FACT-Th	For patients with thrombocytopenia
Treatment Measures	
FAIT-F	Functional Assessment of Incontinence Therapy–Fecal
FAIT-U	Functional Assessment of Incontinence Therapy–Urinary
Peds-FAACT	Pediatric–Functional Assessment of Anorexia Cachexia
FACT-AD	Functional Assessment of Cancer Therapy–Abdominal Discomfort
FACT-Liver Transplant	For patients of liver transplants
Non-Cancer Specific Measures	
FACIT-Pal	Functional Assessment of Chronic Illness Therapy–Palliative Care
FACIT-Sp	Functional Assessment of Chronic Illness Therapy–Spiritual Well-Being
FACIT-Sp-12	Functional Assessment of Chronic Illness Therapy–Spiritual Well-Being (the 12-item Spiritual Well-Being Scale)

(continues)

Table 6-3   *(continued)*

Measure	Description
Non-Cancer Specific Measures	
FACIT-Sp-Ex	Functional Assessment of Chronic Illness Therapy–Spiritual Well-Being, Expanded version
FACIT-SWiP	Satisfaction with pharmacist scale
FACIT-TS-G	Functional Assessment of Chronic Illness Therapy–Treatment Satisfaction–General
FACIT-TS-PS	Functional Assessment of Chronic Illness Therapy–Treatment Satisfaction–Patient Satisfaction
FAHI	Functional Assessment of HIV Infection
FAMS	Functional Assessment of Multiple Sclerosis

patient individually, a clear and flagrant violation of a subjective concept like HRQL. The scoring system, shown in Table 6-5, was developed intuitively rather than psychometrically.

COOP Charts for Primary Care Practices

The Dartmouth Primary Care Cooperative Information Project (COOP) was looking for a simple method to measure health status in physicians' offices. They created response charts that used simple pictures of facial expressions to indicate agreement or disagreement with a series of statements. They

Table 6-4   **Example of Questions from the Minnesota Living with Heart Failure Questionnaire**

Did your heart failure prevent you from living as you wanted during the last month by: (selected items, graded very little to very much on a 5-point scale, plus "No")
• Causing swelling in your ankles, legs, etc.?
• Making going places away from home difficult?
• Costing you money?
• Making you feel you are a burden to your family or friends?
• Making you feel a loss of self-control in your life?
• Making you feel depressed?

Table 6-5 **Scoring the Karnofsky Performance Index by a Healthcare Professional**

Definition	Index	Criteria
Able to carry on normal activity and to work. No special care is needed.	100	Normal; no complaints; no evidence of disease
	90	Able to carry on normal activity; minor signs or symptoms of disease
	80	Normal activity with effort; some signs or symptoms of disease
Unable to work. Able to live at home, care for most personal needs.	70	Cares for self. Unable to carry on normal activity or to do active work
	60	Requires occasional assistance but is able to care for most of his or her needs
	50	Requires considerable assistance and frequent medical care
Unable to care for self. Requires equivalent of institutional or hospital care. Disease may be progressing rapidly.	40	Disabled; requires special care and assistance
	30	Severely disabled; hospitalization is indicated although death not imminent
	20	Very sick; hospitalization necessary; active supportive treatment necessary
	10	Moribund; fatal processes progressing rapidly
	0	Dead

were designed to provide a quick assessment of health and functioning in routine clinical practice. The charts represent a unique approach to measuring the health status of patients since they are built on simple visual pictures to represent response categories. Single items are used to measure each of nine distinct health status domains. The charts assess function, health perception, symptoms, and social support. The COOP charts should be thought of more as a screener than a research tool suitable for outcomes research.

The charts are either self-administered or administered by personal interview. They have been used internationally and have been adapted for use in adolescents. The developers report that the charts can be completed in less than 5 minutes. Studies report generally good interrater reliability (physician vs nurse administered; kappa above 0.65) and retest reliability (1 week apart; correlation coefficients of 0.42 to 0.88; Nelson, Landgraf, Hays, Wasson, & Kirk, 1990; Nelson, Wasson, Johnson, & Hays, 1996). Results indicate adequate discrimination and poorer relative efficiency than comparable scales from the Medical Outcomes Study (MOS) instruments and the Sickness Impact Profile (SIP; McHorney, Ware, Rogers, Raczek, & Lu, 1992). The COOP charts offer a useful metric for current health status and screening but are inadequate for measuring changes in health.

Medical Outcomes Studies Short-Form Measures

This generic indicator of health status was originally developed as part of the RAND Corporation's Health Insurance Experiment (HIE) in the 1970s. The instruments used in the HIE were refined and became part of the MOS Questionnaire, which was designed to study the outcomes of treating series of chronic illnesses (Reisenberg & Glass, 1989; Stewart *et al.*, 1989; Tarlov *et al.*, 1989). The 36-item Short-Form Health Survey (SF-36) measure was derived from the 245-item MOS Questionnaire. It has since been widely applied and adapted for use in several versions: self-administered, personal interviews, and even a voice response system.

The SF-36 includes measures for eight dimensions of health and two component summary scales (Ware *et al.*, 1995; Ware, Kosinski, & Keller, 1995; Ware & Sherbourne, 1992). Each of the scales is based on multiple items. Table 6-6 lists the eight SF-36 scales, a brief description, and the items that comprise each scale. Scores for each of the eight health dimensions vary from 0 to 100. Higher scores indicate the more positive health attributes. Each component of the SF-36 is designed to be reported on a scale of 0–100. For each of the health dimensions, there are US population norms. The total scale was not designed to create a single score; however, two aggregate subscales that have been widely used were empirically derived using factor analytic techniques. Separate aggregate scales for a physical component summary (PCS) and a mental component summary (MCS) can be calculated based on either the full SF-36 or a shorter, 12-item version called the SF-12.

The SF-36 has been widely used and has been translated into many languages. It was carefully constructed and psychometrically tested. It is now available in a new computerized version based on item response theory (IRT). Computer-based testing builds assessments using the least

Table 6-6 The 36-Item Short-Form Health Survey
(SF-36)*—Eight Scales, Brief Description,
and Items Comprising the Scale

Scale	Description and Items
Physical functioning	Limitations with varying levels of physical activities, walking, climbing stairs, bending, carrying objects, and self-care activities (10 items)
Role limitations– physical	Physical health forced a reduction in activities and accomplishing less than normal (4 items)
Bodily pain	Severity of bodily pain and the interference of pain with normal daily activities (2 items)
General health	Health perception and health constitution (5 items)
Social functioning	Extent to which health interferes with normal social activities (2 items)
Vitality	Energy and fatigue level (4 items)
Role limitations– emotional	Emotional problems forced a reduction in activities and accomplishing less than normal (3 items)
Mental health	Anxiety, depression, happiness, and well-being (5 items)

*The 36th item found on the SF-36 is a health transition question. The question asks about how the patient's health is compared with 12 months previously. This item does not contribute directly to any of the eight scales.

number of questions that can locate a person on each health dimension, thereby dramatically reducing the response burden. Despite its wide use, the SF-36 has been criticized for having a ceiling effect, which renders it less useful with older and sicker patients. In effect, it is good for distinguishing the well from the sick but not nearly as useful in distinguishing the sick from the very sick and disabled. Although the SF-36 was not initially designed to include utility weights, recent work has developed a method to assign utility weights to each SF-36 score (Fryback, Lawrence, Martin, Klein, & Klein, 1997).

Sickness Impact Profile

The Sickness Impact Profile (SIP) was developed to be a versatile tool that was both comprehensive and flexible. It consists of 12 subscales that could be aggregated using a utility-based weighting scheme or could be used individually. Table 6-7 shows the basic dimensions and categories of the SIP. Because all scales were weighted from the same base, they can be combined as needed and still provide meaningful aggregated scores. The SIP focuses on behaviors and performance rather than feelings and capacities. It reflects changes in a person's behavior attributed to sickness.

The SIP is broadly applicable and intended to measure the outcomes of care in health surveys, in program planning and policy formation, and in monitoring patient progress. The SIP has been described as the gold standard against which other HRQL measures are compared. The SIP provides a comprehensive assessment of health, where the ultimate aim of health care is to reduce sickness (i.e., the individual's experience of illness) or modify its effects on everyday life. This approach clearly differs from disease, which denotes the professional definition of illness based on clinical observations made by a medical professional.

The SIP takes a behavioral approach to assessment. It focuses on activities and behaviors that are observable and accessible to external validation over feelings that are culturally biased. In addition, behaviors can be verified externally by observation and can be obtained whether or not the patient is receiving care, whereas clinical reports are obviously limited to those receiving care. The SIP focuses on changes in performance rather than capacity. The behaviors are considered significant from the individual, social, and healthcare points of view. These are intended to represent universal patterns of limitations regardless of the specific condition, treatment, individual characteristics, or prognosis.

The original version of the SIP included 136 items in 12 categories. It was designed as a self-administered questionnaire where people check statements that describe them on a given day. Item weights indicate the relative severity of limitations implied by each statement. Scores can be calculated for the overall SIP and for each of the categories. The SIP can be administered by an interviewer in 20 to 30 minutes, or it can be self-administered.

The SIP is based on Thurstone Scaling methods. Approximately 100 judges from various backgrounds were used to assign weights to each item on the instrument. These items from the SIP closely approximate an equal-appearing interval scale. The test–retest reliability for the 136-item version has been consistently high (0.88–0.92). Reliability was slightly higher for the interviewer version than the self-administered. Internal consistency for the overall score was greater than 0.97 but lower for the

Table 6-7 Sickness Impact Profile: Dimensions, Category, and Items Describing Behavior

Dimension	Category	Items Describing Behavior Related to	Selected Items
Independent categories	SR	Sleep and Rest	I sit during much of the day.
	E	Eating	I am eating special or different food.
	W	Work	I am not working at all.
	HM	Home management	I am not doing heavy work around the house.
	RP	Recreation and pastimes	I am going out for entertainment.
Physical	A	Ambulation	I walk shorter distances or stop to rest often.
	M	Mobility	I stay within one room.
	BCM	Body care and movement	I do not bathe myself at all, but am bathed by someone else.
Psychosocial	SI	Social interaction	I am doing fewer social activities with groups of people.
	AB	Alertness behavior	I have difficulty reasoning and solving problems; for example, making decisions, learning new things.
	EB	Emotional behavior	I laugh and cry suddenly.
	C	Communication	I am having trouble writing or typing.

Adapted from: McDowell, I., & Newell, C. (1996). *Measuring health: a guide to rating scales and questionnaires* (2nd ed.). New York: Oxford University Press.

mail-out mail-back versions. Validation studies have compared the SIP with other subjective ratings and with clinical assessments. It has been mostly compared to the leading health indicators. The SIP has been more widely tested for responsiveness to change than other measures of health. Conclusions were that the SIP is relatively insensitive to small changes but may mirror changes over a longer period of time.

The SIP has been adapted for use in different countries. A short, 64-item version was designed for use among arthritics; a 66-item version was developed for nursing home use. Neither of the shorter versions are recognized or supported by The Johns Hopkins University, which owns the rights to the SIP. Roland adapted the SIP for use among low back pain patients (Roland & Morris, 1983). In summary, the SIP was carefully developed and tested. It is applicable to a wide range of age groups, countries, and conditions. A major drawback is its length. Its emphasis on behaviors may limit its ability to detect changes.

Quality of Well-Being Index

The Quality of Well-being (QWB) Index scale is a utility assessment measure that summarizes a person's current symptoms and disability in a single number that represents the social undesirability of the problems and expresses it in terms of quality-adjusted life years (QALYs). The value can be adjusted to reflect the likely prognosis of any existing medical condition. It can be used with any population or disease. It was developed specifically to support economic models that utilize utility weights as a common metric to assess QOL (Kaplan & Anderson, 1988; Kaplan *et al.*, 1989).

QWB is part of a General Health Policy Model that defines an approach to quantifying the output of the healthcare system. The model quantifies the health output in terms of years of life, adjusted for their diminished quality. Thus, a person living a whole year free of disability and symptoms has the equivalent of one, whereas a person whose QOL is reduced by one half will have only 0.500 QWB years. Dividing the cost of the program by the number of well years gives the relative efficiency or cost-effectiveness. (The concept of utilities follows.)

The QWB is based on a three-component model of health (symptoms, functioning, and prognosis).

- Functional status is based on performance.
- A value or utility reflecting the relative desirability associated with each functional level. Death is an anchor and is assigned zero.

- Health implies a consideration not only of present health but also the future prognosis of any illness present. This permits distinguishing between people with the same functional state but markedly different prognosis. The prognosis may reflect either positive health (health promotion and rehabilitation) or negative health (malignancy).

Classifying the person occurs in stages. First, functional status is assessed by a structured interview that asks about symptoms and medical problems in the previous 8 days. The symptoms or problems (CPX) have a corresponding weight. Next, screening questions lead to a more detailed set of questions. The questions cover performance rather than capacity in three areas: mobility and confinement (Mobility scale, or MOB), physical activity (Physical Activity Scale, or PAC), and social activity (Social Activity Scale, or SAC). The interview also records the presence of each of 27 symptoms or problems complexes.

Preference weights were derived from an equal appearing interval scale. These reflect the relative importance of social preferences associated with each function. Studies have indicated stability of preference weights. Correlations between weights (W), populations, and on subsequent days were in excess of 0.93 (Balaban, Sagi, Goldfarb, & Nettler, 1986). Content validation has been studied extensively. Criterion and construct validation were extensively tested. QWB responsiveness to change was found as intermediate compared with other health measures.

$$QWB\ Score = 1 - (MOB\ Step \times MOB\ Weight) - (PAC\ Step \times PAC\ Weight) - (SAC\ Step \times SAC\ Weight) - (Symptoms\ or\ Problems \times CPX\ Weight)$$

W represents a person's well-being at a point in time. To indicate QALYs, W is multiplied by the time spent in that state. For example, assume that a person lives well for 65 years (W = 1.00); lives for 5 years disabled (W = 0.59); and has 3 years of bed disability (W = 0.34). At age 73, that person's QWB score would be 68.9 well years (65 × 1.00) + (5 × 0.59) + (3 × 0.34).

The QWB was one of the earliest HRQL measures to confront conceptual and methodological issues of combining length and quality of life in a single score. There are QWB norms for the general population. It has been widely used in cost-effectiveness studies. This technique was used as part of the ill-fated Oregon medical coverage redistribution project (Kaplan, 1994).

Criticism of the QWB focuses on two areas: the items included and the scoring method. The QWB is strongly oriented toward physical problems. It has been criticized for under representing mental health problems. Inclusion of symptoms appears to improve the sensitivity of the QWB. Major criticism has focused on the scale weights because of the inconsistencies of certain disabled states over another. Another concern addresses the complexity of interviewer training required. Typically, it takes 1 to 2 weeks. A self-administered version may rectify this concern but it is lengthy and not suitable for all populations.

EuroQol

The EuroQol (EQ-5D) measure was developed to create a simple summary score that could be used across cultures (largely in Europe) to capture HRQL (EuroQol Group, 1990; see Table 6-8). It addresses five domains (mobility, self-care, usual activities, pain/discomfort, and anxiety/depression); and each domain has three levels (no problem, moderate, extreme; see Table 6-8). An aggregate score of 0 to 100 is derived

Table 6-8 EuroQol Domains and Levels

Domain	Level
Mobility	I have no problems in walking about.
	I have some problems in walking about.
	I am confined to bed.
Self-care	I have no problems with self–care.
	I have some problems washing or dressing myself.
	I am unable to wash or dress myself.
Usual activities (e.g., work, study, housework, family, or leisure activities)	I have no problems with performing my usual activities.
	I have some problems with performing my usual activities.
	I am unable to perform my usual activities.
Pain/discomfort	I have no pain or discomfort.
	I have moderate pain or discomfort.
	I have extreme pain or discomfort.
Anxiety/depression	I am not anxious or depressed.
	I am moderately anxious or depressed.
	I am extremely anxious or depressed.

from a pattern of responses to levels within each of the five domains. As an alternative to the recommended weights based on the pattern of responses, responses can be weighted using a visual analog scale (VAS). There are norms for many populations. The copyright is held by the EuroQol Foundation, and it is necessary to register to use the system (Brooks, Rabin, & Charro, 2003).[2]

World Health Organization Quality of Life-BREF

The World Health Organization Quality of Life-BREF (WHOQOL-BREF) was developed by the WHO to assess QOL. The WHOQOL-BREF is a shorter version of the original WHOQOL, which measured a range of areas, including self-rated health, satisfaction with health and self, feelings about life, pain, concentration, safety, physical environment, energy, appearance, finances, leisure, mobility and transportation, sleep, ADLs, work capacity, relationships, sex, access to care, and mood. For large research and clinical trials, the longer version is recommended, assuming these are the concepts of study interest.

The WHOQOL-BREF has 26 items that cover 4 broad domains: (1) physical health, (2) psychological health, (2) social relationships, and (4) environment. Table 6-9 gives the 26 items and corresponding domains (Murphy, Herrman, Hawthorne, Pinzone, & Evert, 2000). Most of the questions are rated in reference to the past 4 weeks. The scoring algorithm is based on a Likert-type model.

Health Utilities Index

The Health Utilities Index (HUI) is a family of generic health status and HRQL measures developed by a team of Canadian researchers (Feeny, Furlong, Boyle, & Torrance, 1995; Feeny, 2005). The family of measures includes the Health Utilities Index Mark 1 (HUI1), Mark 2 (HUI2), and Mark 3 (HUI3) systems. Each HUI measure includes a health-status classification system and a preference-based scoring formula. Although HUI1 is still used, HUI2 and HUI3 are much more frequently used, both in clinical and population health studies. HUI3, which was originally developed for the 1990 Statistics Canada Ontario Health Survey, has

---

[2]Instructions on how to register are available at: www.euroqol.org/eq-5d/how-to-obtain-eq-5d.html). Accessed April 17, 2010.

Table 6-9   Domains and Questions for the World Health Organization Quality of Life–BREF

Domain	Question
Physical health	To what extent do you feel that physical pain prevents you from doing what you need to do?
	How much do you need any medical treatment to function in your daily life?
	Do you have enough energy for everyday life?
	How well are you able to get around?
	How satisfied are you with you sleep?
	How satisfied are you with your ability to perform your daily living activities?
	How satisfied are you with your capacity for work?
Psychological health	How much do you enjoy life?
	To what extent do you feel your life to be meaningful?
	How well are you able to concentrate?
	Are you able to accept your bodily appearance?
	How satisfied are you with yourself?
	How often do you have negative feelings such as blue mood, despair, anxiety, depression?
Social relationships	How satisfied are you with your personal relationships?
	How satisfied are you with your sex life?
	How satisfied are you with the support you get from your friends?
Environment	How safe do you feel in your daily life?
	How healthy is your physical environment?
	Have you enough money to meet your needs?
	How available to you is the information that you need in your day-to-day life?
	To what extent do you have the opportunity for leisure activities?

Environment *(continued)*	How satisfied are you with the conditions of your living place?
	How satisfied are you with your access to health services?
	How satisfied are you with your transport?
General questions that aid with interpretation	How would you rate your quality of life?
	How satisfied are you with your health?

eight attributes (vision, hearing, speech, ambulation, dexterity, emotion, cognition, and pain) with five to six levels per attribute. A multiplicative, multiattribute utility function and single-attribute utility functions for HUI3 have been released (Furlong *et al.*, 1998).

QOL Coverage

Table 6-10 contrasts coverage of health domain for each of the HRQL instruments. The extent that various QOL domains from the SIP are captured by each HRQL score is reviewed here. As can be seen, several measures cover only a few domains. The WHOQOL has the broadest coverage.

Utility Assessment

Economic analysis seeks to compare the return on various levels of investment. In the context of health, such analyses are greatly simplified if the health outcome can be reduced to a single number that can be applied across conditions and populations. The technique for converting health status to this ultimate summary number is utility weighting. Cost-utility studies require a standard metric for outcomes studies. In cost-utility studies, the cost of a medical intervention is related to the number of QALYs. In general, one QALY is equivalent to a year life spent (alive) and free of disability and functional limitations. The notion of QALY incorporates its approaches to assessing outcomes: mortality and morbidity. The latter is usually assessed by measuring general health and physical disability.

This procedure is essentially the economist's variation on transubstantiation. It converts subjective information into analyzable data. To accomplish this end, a set of weights are determined for a whole variety of health states. Because every combination cannot be tested, various rules of addition and interpolation are created.

Table 6-10 Health Domains Covered by Each of the Health-Related Quality of Life Instruments

Health Domain	Karnofsky	COOP	SF-36	EQ-5D	SIP	QWB	WHOQOL	HUI3
Physical function	X	X	X	X	X	X	X	X
Impairment		X	X	X	X	X	X	X
Psychological function		X	X	X	X	X	X	X
Cognitive function					X		X	X
Social support		X			X		X	
Social activity		X	X		X	X	X	X
Role function			X	X	X	X	X	X
Sexual function					X	X	X	X
Pain		X	X	X	X	X	X	X
Energy/fatigue			X		X	X	X	X

COOP; EQ-5D, EuroQol; HUI3, Health Utility Index 3rd version; SF-36, Short Form-36; SIP, Sickness Impact Profile; QWB, Quality of Well-being scale; WHOQOL, World Health Organization Quality of Life.

The two most familiar ways of creating these utility weights are the standard gamble and the time trade-off. Basically the first approach asks you to choose between your own health status and a gamble that you might die immediately or achieve full health status for the remainder of your life. Time trade-off asks you to consider your health state to last for a fixed period of time. The specific treatment will allow you to live for a shorter period of time but you will die or be disabled at the end of that time. You are asked to trade off the time with reduced capacity for living with normal health for a shorter period of time. The spent in normal health is varied until the point of indifference is found. Another variation is willingness to pay, which asks how much one would be willing to pay to avoid a given state.

Utility weighting has been criticized as relying on invalidated value judgments that often lack a conceptual basis and lack data to support their reliability and validity. They use nonrepresentative samples for their development. There are fundamental issues about who should provide the data.

Using QALYs has major implications. If you accept its premise, then the life of someone with a disability or a shorter life expectancy is always going to be worth less than someone who is healthy. It is important to appreciate that respondents have generally never experienced the state they are rating. In some cases it is even hard to imagine it (Ubel, Loewenstein, Schwarz, & Smith, 2005). Thus, much of this exercise relies on hypothetical situations. Evidence suggests that most people place a much more negative value on a hypothetical level of disability than they do on the actual state. Proponents argue that this may create error but not necessarily bias; if all hypotheticals are equivalent, it may not matter if the analyses are relative. Historically, the collection of these data has been burdensome. They have required skilled interviewers and complex scoring algorithms, but newer approaches use computerized methods that make collecting the data easier, although respondents must still respond to large numbers of situations. Participating can be very time consuming.

Other approaches have been used as well. One more direct approach is magnitude estimation, whereby the rater is asked to place a numerical value on each of various states in relation to each other. The rating scale approach developed by George Torrance specifies six attributes that are important in health: physical function, emotional function, sensory function, cognitive function, self-care, and pain. The patient is asked to rate the desirability of varying levels of each attribute on a 0 to 100 scale. Multiple attribute theory is used to derive a utility value for each health state. Table 6-11 provides an example of how values can be assigned to health states that combine perceived health status and activity limitation.

The QALY approach has broadened to include various approaches to assessing health-adjusted life expectancy. The choice of measures often reflects the data available. QALYs morphed into two types of disability adjusted life expectancy (DALYs). One uses disability measures derived from the Katz ADL scale to create disability-adjusted life expectancy. It is sometimes broadened to include IADLs as well and labeled years of healthy life expectancy. Instrumental activities of daily living are higher level, complex tasks that are necessary for living in the community. They include tasks such as doing housework, taking medications, shopping for groceries, using the telephone, and balancing a checkbook.

Table 6-12 offers an illustration of how the value of a health state can be combined with survival data to create a life table based on years of expected healthy life expectancy. The second type of DALY uses diagnoses to create a system that can be used across many countries including developing nations with weak vital statistics; it is call the disease-adjusted QOL score.

Table 6-11   **Values for Health States Defined in Terms of Activity Limitation and Perceived Health Status**

	Perceived Health Status				
Activity Limitation	Excellent	Very Good	Good	Fair	Poor
Not limited	1.00	0.92	0.84	0.63	0.47
Limited–other	0.87	0.79	0.72	0.58	0.38
Limited–major	0.81	0.74	0.67	0.46	0.34
Unable–major	0.68	0.62	0.55	0.38	0.25
Limited in IADL	0.57	0.51	0.45	0.29	0.17
Limited in ADL	0.47	0.41	0.36	0.21	0.10

ADL, activities of daily living; IADL, instrumental activities of daily living.

Source: Erickson, P., Wilson, R., & Shannon, I. (1995, April). Years of healthy life. *Healthy People 2000.* DHHS Publication No. (PHS) 95-12374-1484 (4/95).

Table 6-12   Calculation of Years of Healthy Life for the US Population

Age interval	Number living at beginning of age interval of 100,000 born live (I_x)	Stationary population in the age interval ($_nL_x$)	Average health-related quality of life of persons in the age interval (Q_x)	Quality-adjusted stationary population — In the age interval ($Q_x \cdot {}_nL_x$)	Quality-adjusted stationary population — In this and all subsequent age intervals T'_x	Years of healthy life remaining	Life years remaining
Period of life between two exact ages stated in years x to x + n (1)	(2)	(3)	(4)	(5)	(6)	(7)	(8)
0–5 years	100,000	495,073	0.94	465,369	6,403,748	64.0	75.4
5–10 years	98,890	494,150	0.93	459,560	5,938,379	60.1	75.1
10–15 years	98,780	493,654	0.93	459,098	5,478,819	55.1	71.2
15–20 years	98,653	492,290	0.92	452,907	5,019,721	50.9	66.3
20–25 years	98,223	489,794	0.91	455,713	4,566,814	46.5	61.3
25–30 years	97,684	486,901	0.91	443,080	4,121,101	42.2	56.6
30–35 years	97,077	483,571	0.90	435,214	3,678,021	37.9	51.9
35–40 years	96,334	479,425	0.89	426,688	3,242,807	33.7	47.2
40–45 years	95,382	474,117	0.88	417,223	2,816,119	29.5	42.6

(continues)

Table 6-12　*(continued)*

Age interval — Period of life between two exact ages stated in years x to x + n (1)	Number living at beginning of age interval of 100,000 born live (l_x) (2)	Stationary population in the age interval ($_nL_x$) (3)	Average health-related quality of life of persons in the age interval (Q_x) (4)	Quality-adjusted stationary population — In the age interval ($Q_x \cdot {}_nL_x$) (5)	Quality-adjusted stationary population — In this and all subsequent age intervals T'_x (6)	Years of healthy life remaining (7)	Life years remaining (8)
45–50 years	94,179	456,820	0.86	401,465	2,398,896	25.5	38.0
50–55 years	92,420	455,809	0.83	378,321	1,997,431	21.6	33.4
55–60 years	89,735	439,012	0.81	355,600	1,619,110	18.0	29.0
60–65 years	85,634	143,879	0.77	318,687	1,263,510	14.8	24.8
65–70 years	79,590	378,369	0.76	287,560	944,823	11.9	20.8
70–75 years	71,404	330,846	0.74	244,826	657,263	9.2	17.2
75–80 years	50,557	270,129	0.70	189,090	412,437	6.8	13.9
80–85 years	47,168	197,857	0.63	124,650	223,347	4.7	10.9
85 years and over	31,892	193,523	0.61	98,697	98,697	3.1	8.3

Source: Erickson, P., Wilson, R., & Shannon, I. (1995, April). Years of healthy life. *Healthy People 2000.* DHHS Publication No. (PHS) 95-12374-1484 (4/95).

REFERENCES

Balaban, D. J., Sagi, P. C., Goldfarb, N. I., & Nettler, S. (1986). Weights for scoring the Quality of Well-Being instrument among rheumatoid arthritics: A comparison to general population weights. *Medical Care, 24*(11), 973–980.

Brenner, M. H., Curbow, B., & Legro, M. W. (1995). The proximal-distal continuum of multiple health outcome measures: The case of cataract surgery. *Medical Care, 33*(4), AS236–AS244.

Brooks, R., Rabin, R., & Charro, F. (Eds.). (2003). *The measurement and valuation of health status using EQ-5D: A European perspective: Evidence from the EuroQol BIO MED Research Programme.* New York: Springer.

Bruner, D. W., Bryan, C. J., Aaronson, N., Blackmore, C. C., Brundage, M., Cella, C., . . . Whalen, G. (2007). Issues and challenges with integrating patient-reported outcomes in clinical trials supported by the National Cancer Institute-sponsored clinical trials networks. *Journal of Clinical Oncology, 25*(32), 5051–5057.

Cella, C., Wagner, L., Cashy, J., Hensing, T. A., Yount, S., & Lilenbaum, R. C. (2007). Should health-related quality of life be measured in cancer symptom management clinical trials? Lessons learned using the functional assessment of cancer therapy. *Journal of the National Cancer Institute. Monographs, 37,* 53–60.

Cleary, P. D., Wilson, I. B., & Fowler, F. J. (1994). A theoretical framework for assessing and analyzing health-related quality of life. In G. L. Albrecht & F. Ray (Eds.), *Advances in medical sociology: Quality of life in health care* (p. 311). Greenwich, CT: JAI Press.

EuroQol Group. (1990). EuroQoL—A new facility for the measurement of health-related quality of life. *Health Policy, 16,* 199–208.

Feeny, D. (2005, Spring). The Health Utilities Index: A Tool for Assessing Health Benefits. *PRO Newsletter, 34,* 2–6.

Feeny, D., Furlong, W., Boyle, M., & Torrance, G. W. (1995). Multi-attribute health status classification systems: Health Utilities Index. *PharmacoEconomics, 7*(6), 490–502.

DROPFryback, D. G., Lawrence, W. F., Martin, P. A., Klein, R., & Klein, B. E. K. (1997). Predicting quality of well-being scores from the SF-36: Results from the Beaver Dam Health Outcomes Study. *Medical Decision Making, 17*(1), 1–9.

Furlong, W., Feeny, D., Torrance, G. W., Goldsmith, C., DePauw, S., Zhu, Z., . . . Boyle, M. (1998). *Multiplicative multi-attribute utility function for the Health Utilities Index Mark 3 (HUI3) system: A technical report.* London, Ontario: McMaster University Centre for Health Economics and Policy Analysis.

Garcia, S. F., Cella, C., Clauser, S. B., Flynn, K. E., Lad, T., Lai, J.-S., . . . Weinfurt, K. (2007). Standardizing patient-reported outcomes assessment in cancer clinical trials: A patient-reported outcomes measurement information system initiative. *Journal of Clinical Oncology, 25*(32), 5106–5112.

Hahn, E. A., Cella, C., Chassany, O., Fairclough, D. L., Wong, G. Y., & Hays, R. D. (2007). Precision of health-related quality-of-life data compared with other clinical measures. *Mayo Clinical Proceedings, 82*(10), 1244–1254.

Hahn, E. A., Rao, D., Cella, C., & Choi, S. W. (2008). Comparability of interview- and self-administration of the Functional Assessment of Cancer Therapy-General (FACT-G) in English- and Spanish-speaking ambulatory cancer patients. *Medical Care, 46*(4), 423–431.

Kaplan, R. M. (1994). Value judgment in the Oregon Medicaid experiment. *Medical Care, 32*(10), 975–988.

Kaplan, R. M., & Anderson, J. P. (1988). A general health policy model: Update and applications. *Health Services Research, 23*(2), 203–235.

Kaplan, R. M., Anderson, J. P., Wu, A. W., Mathews, W. C., Kozin, F., & Orenstein, D. (1989). The quality of well-being scale: Applications in AIDS, cystic fibrosis, and arthritis. *Medical Care, 27*(3), S27–S43.

Karnofsky, D. A., Abelmann, W., Craver, L. F., & Burchenal, J. H. (1948). The use of the nitrogen mustards in the palliative treatment of carcinoma. *Cancer, 1*(4), 634–638.

Kitzhaber, J. A. (1993). Prioritising health services in an era of limits: The Oregon experience. *British Medical Journal, 307*(6900), 373–377.

McHorney, C. A., Ware, J. E. Jr., Rogers, W., Raczek, A. E., & Lu, J. F. (1992). The validity and relative precision of MOS short- and long-form health status scales and Dartmouth COOP charts. Results from the Medical Outcomes Study. *Medical Care, 30*(5 Suppl), MS253–MS265.

Murphy, B., Herrman, H., Hawthorne, G., Pinzone, T., & Evert, H. (2000). *Australian WHOQoL instruments: User's manual and interpretation guide.* Melbourne, Australia: Australian WHOQoL Field Study Centre.

Nelson, E. C., Landgraf, J. M., Hays, R. D., Wasson, J. H., & Kirk, J. W. (1990). The functional status of patients: How can it be measured in physicians' offices? *Medical Care, 28*(12), 1111–1126.

Nelson, E. C., Wasson, J. H., Johnson, D. J., & Hays, R. D. (1996). Dartmouth COOP Functional Health Assessment Charts: Brief measures for clinical practice. In B. Spilker (Ed.), *Quality of life and pharmacoeconomics in clinical trials* (2nd ed., pp. 161–168). Philadelphia: Lippincott-Raven.

Rao, D., Debb, S., Blitz, D., Choi, S. W., & Cella, C. (2008). Racial/ethnic differences in the health-related quality of life of cancer patients. *Journal of Pain & Symptom Management, 36*(5), 488–496.

Rector, T. S., Kubo, S. H., & Cohn, J. N. (1987). Patients' self-assessment of their congestive heart failure, part 2: Reliability and validity of a new measure, The Minnesota Living with Heart Failure Questionnaire. *Heart Failure, 3*(5), 198–209.

Reisenberg, D., & Glass, R. M. (1989). The Medical Outcomes Study. *JAMA, 262*(7), 943.

Roland, M., & Morris, R. (1983). A study of the natural history of back pain, part I: Development of a reliable and sensitive measure of disability in low-back pain. *Spine, 8*(2), 141–150.

Sloan, J. A., Frost, M. H., Berzon, R., Dueck, A., Guyatt, G., Moinpour, C., . . . Cella, D. (2006). The clinical significance of quality of life assessments in oncology: A summary for clinicians. *Supportive Care in Cancer, 14*(10), 988–998.

Spiegel, J. S., Leake, B., Spiegel, T. M., Paulus, H. E., Kane, R. L., Ward, N. B., & Ware, J. E., Jr. (1986). What are we measuring? An examination of self-reported functional status measures. *Arthritis and Rheumatism, 31*(6), 721–728.

Stewart, A., Greenfield, S., Hays, R. D., Wells, K. B., Rogers, W. H., Berry, S., . . . Ware, J. E., Jr. (1989). Functional status and well-being of patients with chronic conditions: Results from the Medical Outcomes Study. *JAMA, 262*(7), 907–913.

Tarlov, A. R., Ware, J. E., Jr., Greenfield, S., Nelson, E. C., Perrin, E., & Zubkoff, M. (1989). The Medical Outcomes Study: An application of methods for monitoring the results of medical care. *JAMA, 262*(7), 925–930.

The WHOQOL Group (1993). Study protocol for the World Health Organization project to develop a Quality of Life assessment instrument (WHOQOL). *Quality of Life Research, 2*(2), 153–159.

Ubel, P. A., Loewenstein, G., Schwarz, N., & Smith, D. (2005). Misimagining the unimaginable: The disability paradox and health care decision making. *Health Psycholology, 24*(2), S57–S62.

Ware, J. E., Jr., Kosinski, M., Bayliss, M. S., McHorney, C. A., Rogers, W. H., & Raczek, A. (1995). Comparison of methods for the scoring and statistical analysis of the SF-36 Health Profile and Summary Measures: Summary of results from the Medical Outcomes Study. *Medical Care, 33*(4), AS264–AS279.

Ware, J. E., Jr., Kosinski, M., & Keller, S. D. (1995). *SF-12: How to score the SF-12 Physical and Mental Health Summary Scales.* Boston: The Health Institute, New England Medical Center.

Ware, J. E., Jr., & Sherbourne, C. D. (1992). The MOS 36-Item Short-Form Health Survey (SF-36). *Medical Care, 30*(6), 473–483.

Wilson, I. B., & Cleary, P. D. (1995). Linking clinical variables with health-related quality of life. *JAMA, 273*(1), 59–65.

World Health Organization. (1948). *Constitution of the World Health Organization.* Geneva, Switzerland: Author.

CHAPTER 7

Condition-Specific Measures

Earlier chapters discussed the use of generic health status measures in the measurement of outcomes. Although generic health status measures can successfully measure outcomes in a wide variety of settings, they generally trade depth for breadth. Condition-specific health status measures are more likely to show responsiveness to changes in health status because they are more sensitive.

CONDITION-SPECIFIC MEASURES VERSUS GENERIC HEALTH STATUS MEASURES

"Condition-specific measures are available for many different diseases and afflictions. Condition-specific health status measures are measures designed to assess specific diagnostic groups or patient populations, often with the goal of measuring responsiveness or 'clinically important' changes" (Patrick & Deyo, 1989, p. S217). They are designed to measure changes in the most salient aspects of a specific condition, reflecting aspects of functioning that are closely tied to the condition. There are essentially two types of condition-specific measures: (1) clinical and (2) experiential. The clinical type primarily measures signs, symptoms, and tests, whereas the experiential type captures the impact of the disease or problem on the patient. The experiential type of measure evaluates health in ways similar to those used in generic measures but is more fine tuned to the specifics of the underlying condition.

Condition-specific measures are designed to be extremely responsive to small treatment effects. Generic measures, however, could fail to detect small changes associated with treatment. Condition-specific measures are designed to tap the domains of greatest salience to a particular condition.

WHY NOT GENERIC HEALTH STATUS MEASURES?

"Generic health status measures purport to be broadly applicable across types and severities of disease, across different medical treatments or health interventions and across demographic and cultural subgroups" (Patrick & Deyo, 1989, p. S217).

Generic health status measures, in contrast, cast a broad net across different facets of health. For example, the SF-36 health survey described in Chapter 6 measures health across a broad spectrum. As a generic health status measure, it attempts to tap eight conceptually separate aspects of functioning and mental well-being (Ware, Kosinski, & Keller, 1994; Ware & Sherbourne, 1992; Ware, Snow, Kosinski, & Gandek, 1993), as well as component summaries that measure physical and mental health (Ware *et al.*, 1994; Ware, Kosinski, & Keller, 1996). Differences across the SF-36 scales illustrate both the strengths and weaknesses of a broad health status measure. The SF-36 taps different dimensions of an intervention in different ways. For example, certain drugs could improve physical functioning while causing fatigue as an untoward side effect. A generic health status measure could incorporate the sum of both of these effects in the form of a component summary; however, the resulting outcome measure could miss clinically important changes (Patrick & Deyo, 1989). In this instance, the breadth and flexibility belies the weakness of the generic health status measure. By not isolating the dimensions of greatest interest, a true treatment effect could be masked. In contrast, a condition-specific measure specifically designed to assess pain focuses directly on the precise area of interest, for instance, low back pain, hip pain, and so on. In effect, one is trading depth for breadth. The breadth of a measure involves both the range of the domains addressed and the response range within each domain. Whereas generic measures are typically designed to cover a wide range, condition-specific measures hone in on what is especially salient for that condition.

This focus is important not just to enable measures to be concise, but also to ensure that the health status measure is sensitive to clinically important differences or changes in health states. Determining whether or not a given treatment had an effect requires that the estimated effect is both statistically and clinically significant. Statistical significance, which refers to the likelihood that a result occurred by chance, is determined by such factors as sample size and variance. The clinical significance of the treatment effect must be determined by the investigator and may involve decisions regarding the effectiveness of the treatment vis-à-vis alternative treatments (Fletcher & Fletcher, 2005; Haynes, Sackett, Guyatt, & Tugwell, 2006).

A generic health status measure may miss clinically significant treatment effects for several reasons. First, there may be a floor or ceiling effect. A scale is considered to have a ceiling effect if individuals rated by the scale as perfectly healthy can be found to have health problems on other scales (Bombardier *et al.*, 1995); the converse is a floor effect. For example, the SF-36 is designed to be used to distinguish the health status of reasonably healthy populations from those who are ill, but it is not as useful in distinguishing between the ill and the very ill. If the SF-36 was used to assess the effect of an intervention on a population of frail elderly, the scale might miss a true treatment effect because the entire sample would be bunched at the lower end of the scale *both before and after* the intervention. The condition-specific measure can be aimed at the proper segment of the distribution (i.e., avoid ceiling and floor effects).

Moreover, generic health status measures lack responsiveness (Kessler & Mroczek, 1995). A successful treatment should result in an increase in the scores of a health status measure. Generic measures may not meet this challenge. For example, generic health status measures were unresponsive to positive health changes resulting from successful treatment of benign prostatic hyperplasia, changes successfully captured by condition-specific measures (Barry *et al.*, 1995).

More importantly, generic health status measures might simply fail to tap the necessary dimensions of health. For example, the effects of successful treatment for hypertension would not be reflected using a self-administered generic health status measure such as the SF-36. Improved blood pressure control is imperceptible to patients despite its profound influence on the long-term health of the individual.

CONDITION-SPECIFIC HEALTH STATUS MEASURES

Although condition-specific measure can successfully tap the domains of greatest interest, they come with a cost and have inherent drawbacks. In order to measure a given condition more precisely, condition-specific measures cast a far narrower net than do generic measures. As a result, some unanticipated (or anticipated in a separate domain) effects from an intervention could be missed (Bombardier *et al.*, 1995).

A second drawback associated with condition-specific health status measures is the difficulty comparing the results of one study with those of another study. For example, improvements in diabetes care cannot be readily compared to a decrease in arthritis symptoms.

In many settings, the investigator is not merely interested in finding a treatment effect, but also in estimating the magnitude or importance of the treatment effect relative to treatment alternatives. Most readers prefer some clinical translation of a numerical scale. What does a 3-point increase in the Arthritis Impact Measurement Scales (AIMS) mean clinically (Kazis, Anderson, & Meenan, 1989)? How does a 3-point AIMS increase compare to an improvement on another scale? One possibility is to compare the findings to previous studies. However, for most health conditions a plethora of scales is available. If the investigator is concerned not merely with finding the presence of a treatment effect but also with comparing the treatment with other similar studies, a condition-specific measure may complicate that comparison. One approach to quantifying differences in treatment effects is using statistical techniques such as "effect sizes" (Guyatt, Feeny, & Patrick, 1993). Often effect-size estimates are unavailable for the condition-specific measure. But some generic health status measures, such as the SF-36 and EuroQual 5D, have become sufficiently widely used that comparisons across different treatments, conditions, or populations are possible.

Condition-specific outcome measures have strength; they are often intuitively appealing to clinicians. If one wishes to investigate the impact of a treatment for arthritis, a common sense approach is to use a scale that specifically taps the dimensions of health affected by arthritis. The ultimate goal of outcomes research is to provide insights that lead to greater efficiency and higher quality of care. To actually have an impact on the delivery of care, the researcher must be able to persuade the medical care community that the findings truly reflect clinical reality, rather than simply a theoretical construct.

An excellent example of the strengths and limitations of the two types of measures was provided in a study of patients who underwent cataract surgery (Damiano *et al.*, 1995). This study used both a generic health status measure (the Sickness Impact Profile [SIP]) and a vision specific measure (the VF-14) to evaluate the impact of the surgery. The study found postoperative improvement in visual acuity unrelated to the SIP score; conversely, the VF-14 was highly responsive to changes in visual acuity. The authors concluded that the SIP is simply not sensitive or responsive enough to measure changes such as those caused by cataract surgery. However, the SIP did provide interesting insights that would have been missed using only the VF-14. Several behaviors measured by the SIP that were not expected to be related to vision, such as "I act irritable and impatient," were found to be highly correlated with presurgery better eye-visual acuity. This suggests that vision may impact health in ways not detected by a vision-specific measure or clinical measures of visual acuity.

Almost all measures of complications are condition specific. By definition, a complication of treatment is an untoward outcome associated with the treatment of a condition. Therefore, a complication is necessarily condition specific. (The definition of complications is discussed in more detail in Chapter 11 on risk adjustment).

PHYSIOLOGICAL MEASURES

One type of condition-specific measures is the physiological measure. Physiological outcomes are clinimetric measures of the organic function or state of an individual. Broadly, these measures fall into the following six domains: (1) physical findings, (2) laboratory results, (3) physiological tests, (4) diagnostic procedures, (5) the presence of disease, and (6) mortality. Table 7-1 gives examples of these types of outcomes.

In Chapter 4, psychometrics was described as the study of psychological measures such as those for measuring health status and health-related quality of life (HRQL). The complementary science for the study of physiological outcomes is clinimetrics. As described by Feinstein, clinimetrics concerns the measurement of clinical phenomena (Feinstein, 1987). It includes the process of assessing symptoms, signs, and laboratory tests creating scales, indexes, or metrics for summarizing.

Table 7-1 **Physiological Outcomes According to Domain**

Domain	Example
Physical findings	Blood pressure: systolic and diastolic blood pressure Lung sounds: rales, rhonchi, wheezes Edema: pitting edema Heart sounds: S1 and S2, extra heart sounds S3 and S4, murmurs Skin: erythema, petechiae, nodules, bullae
Laboratory results	Hemoglobin A1C Chest radiograph Degree of stenosis
Physiological tests	Exercise treadmill Pulmonary function test
Diagnostic procedures	Ejection fraction Colonoscopy
Presence of disease	Medical diagnosis Diagnostic code
Mortality	Condition-specific mortality All-cause mortality

Physiological measures serve as the primary end points in many randomized controlled trials (RCTs) and epidemiological studies. These measures tend to be more responsive as study end points and are considered by clinicians to be important for evaluating medical effectiveness, on par with (or, for some, surpassing) HRQL. For diabetes mellitus, long-term serum glucose management and diabetes-related complications (such as retinopathy, nephropathy, and macrovascular disease) are of primary interest. The challenge is selecting the appropriate physiological outcomes.

There are three types of physiological measures: (1) intermediate or surrogate measures, (2) in vitro measures, and (3) disease state. Intermediate or surrogate measures correlate with the outcomes of interest. For example, blood pressure is correlated with stroke and, as a consequence, with physical functioning and HRQL. In studies of diabetes mellitus, hemoglobin A1C is associated with glucose control during the patient's last 120 days. It is an intermediate measure associated with the complications of diabetes, which is the true interest.

Intermediate or surrogate measures offer advantages over other physiological measures. These measures are easier to collect and they are readily available. A major drawback of these measures is that their reliability cannot be assured. This is especially true in the case of physical findings. There is nothing objective about physical findings. Clinicians' examinations are carried out inconsistently, and the lack of standardization makes them difficult to use in outcomes studies. In addition, the validity of many measures remains unclear. New laboratory tests are developed and become part of routine practice before testing for their validity. The prostate specific antigen (PSA) test is a prime example of one that yields a high proportion of false positives.

In vitro measures, on the other hand, are measured in a way different or in different settings from "the real world." The treadmill is a frequently used in vitro measure. The examiner might measure the functional status of a patient with claudication (i.e., pain in the calf of the leg with exertion) by measuring exercise tolerance on a treadmill, although we may really be interested in the patient's ability to walk in "the real world." Many clinical trials that collect physiological outcomes measures are conducted in a clinical research center (CRC) or a general clinical research center (GCRC). These are in vitro settings, usually within academic research centers, that provide a controlled setting for conducting the clinical trial and collecting physiological measures.

Much like other physiological measures, in vitro measures are acceptable to clinicians and, in many cases, responsive to small clinical changes in patients. The major drawbacks to these measures are the validity, costs, and burden associated with collecting data. The cost of data collection within a CRC is driven by the overhead associated with the cost of the test and the professional staff necessary to carry out the test.

Finally, disease state refers to the most distal end point for many outcomes studies. This encompasses all-cause mortality, disease-specific mortality, and the incidence of new disease. For clinicians, measures of disease state have significant face validity and can frequently be obtained using secondary data, such as medical records and administrative data. The time and resources required to collect these data might be a disadvantage; and, except in the case of conditions with a high prevalence, inadequate statistical power might be a threat. The validity of disease state measures might be questioned because of the lack of a standardized case definition. Epidemiologists have long known that imprecision in the case definition of a disease state attenuates the relationship between the factors of interest and the outcome. Case definitions define the case of disease in terms of person, place, and time. Administrative data sets, like billing data and death certificates, use diagnoses as listed by clinicians with no specific criteria as a basis for inclusion or definition.

CASE DEFINITION DISEASE DOES NOT EQUAL DISEASE

The definition of a case may vary with the circumstances. In ordinary practice, diagnoses depend on the skill and precision of the treating clinician. In research contexts, the criteria can vary with the study. This difference may explain inconsistencies with findings across studies. For example, the case definition for ischemic coronary heart disease (CHD) in a major study included symptoms, signs, laboratory tests or biomarkers, and EKGs (Luepker *et al.*, 2003). For the laboratory tests, at least two tests of myocardial ischemia were taken 6 hours apart.

OTHER ALTERNATIVES

Although a discussion of the use of condition-specific health status measures versus the use of generic health status measures is useful, often the best alternative is to employ a combination of the two approaches. The generality of the generic measures is both a strength and a weakness; the generic measures exhibit breadth, but not depth. The generic measures are able to find treatment affects across many domains, but they may fail to focus intently enough on the domains of most interest. Conversely, the condition-specific measures exhibit great depth, but little breadth.

As resources permit, the combined strategy is probably the best alternative and is a relatively common approach (Fitzpatrick, Davey, Buxton, & Jones, 1998; Guyatt Feeny, & Patrick, 1991; Patrick & Deyo, 1989). This was the course followed by Bombardier and colleagues in a study of pain and physical function after knee surgery (Bombardier *et al.*, 1995). Among patients who reported knee pain, a generic measure (the SF-36) was unable to distinguish patients in need of knee surgery; but the knee pain-specific measure (the Western Ontario and McMaster Universities Osteoarthritis Index [WOMAC]) was able to do so (Bellamy, Buchanan, Goldsmith,

Campbell, & Stitt, 1988). After surgery, patients often recovered enough that the WOMAC was unable to distinguish among patients, although some were extremely disabled, while the SF-36 was able to do so.

Some people worry that responses to surveys may be altered by the order in which the questionnaires are administered (i.e., whether the generic or condition-specific survey is given first). Previous research has found that the order in which questions are asked can alter responses to the questions based on factors such as interviewee fatigue, relevance of the question or topic, and learning effects (Sudman & Bradburn, 1974). However, the little work that has been done examining the effect of generic versus condition-specific survey ordering suggests that this is not a major issue and that responses do not vary based on order (McColl *et al.*, 2003).

If it is necessary to use a single instrument, two approaches are available. First, a generic instrument can be modified for a specific condition. For example, an (unsuccessful) attempt was made to modify the SIP to make it more sensitive to head injury (Temkin, Dikmen, Machamer, & McLean, 1989). Items deemed nonapplicable to head injury were removed and items believed particularly applicable were added. The scale was then reweighted. In this case, the modified SIP was no more effective than the unmodified SIP, so it was discarded. One drawback of this approach is that the strength of generic measures is the ability to compare to other studies that have used the same measure. Once a scale has been modified and reweighted, it is no more comparable to the original than a completely unrelated condition-specific measure. The Roland–Morris Low Back Pain Disability Questionnaire represents a successful adaptation of the SIP for a specific condition (Roland & Morris, 1983; Stroud, McKnight, & Jensen, 2004).

Second, a generic instrument can have an attached condition-specific supplement. The goal of this approach is to have the condition-specific supplement not overlap measurement of the domains covered by the generic measurement, but instead expand it into domains of particular interest (Patrick & Deyo, 1989). Since the measures are retained, this approach retains the comparability of the generic measurement and taps the domains of greatest interest in the supplement.

A final alternative is to use a battery of condition-specific measures. Since one of the major shortcomings of condition-specific measures is their narrowness and specificity (Kessler & Mroczek, 1995), the use of several different condition-specific tests may be an option. This approach expands the domains measured. For example, Kjerulff and Langenberg (1995), in a study examining fatigue among patients having a hysterectomy, used four different fatigue measures (Symptom Fatigue Scale, Profile of Mood States, and two scales from the Medical Outcome Study Short-Form General Health Survey). Although each of the four scales ostensibly measured the latent construct "fatigue," each provided slightly different insights into how hysterectomy affected fatigue. Using this strategy, fatigue was broken down into three separate components: frequency of fatigue, the extent to which fatigue is problematic for the individual, and the extent to which fatigue causes limitations in activities. Although the correlation of the components was high, each predicted different events. For example, the extent to which fatigue is problematic was the best predictor of the number of physician contacts. Each scale contained unique information, and the authors of this study suggest that measurement of all three components is necessary for a complete analysis of fatigue. Table 7-2 summarizes the four options for using condition-specific measures, either alone or in combination.

Table 7-2   Approaches to Using Condition Specific Measures

Approach	Discussion
Use a condition-specific and a generic measure	Administer two different measures. This is potentially costly, but, this is the best option.
Modify generic measure	A modified measure is not truly comparable with an unmodified measure; lose main advantage of generic measure.
Attach a condition-specific supplement to a generic measure	This is a solid option. It retains comparability gained by using a generic measure. The investigator is required to find or develop supplement.
Use battery of condition-specific measures	Pick condition-specific measures that tap all domains of research interest. It may be easier, cheaper, and more thorough to use generic and condition-specific measures. A battery of condition-specific measures does not retain the easy comparability of generic measures.

THE CHOICE OF A CONDITION-SPECIFIC MEASURE

The Conceptual Model

Simply choosing the "best" measure available for a given condition from a statistical perspective is inadequate. The choice of a particular condition-specific measure should be guided more strongly by the investigator's conceptualization of what the condition-specific measure *ought* to measure than by narrow statistical guidelines. *The first step in picking a measure is to understand the natural history of the disease and to construct a theory regarding precisely how the intervention will impact the condition and when, during the course of the natural history, the measurement occurs.* With that model in place, available condition-specific measures can be evaluated to find one that taps the exact domain, along with when and where the intervention is expected to have an impact.

Diseases can affect the life of an individual in many ways, and a *single* disease can impact *multiple* domains of the individual's life. Although the selection of domains is a difficult task, choosing appropriate domains is key to selecting the appropriate condition-specific health status measure.

> The first issue that has to be confronted in selecting outcome measures concerns the appropriate domains. This is an easy issue to address in the abstract, because the researcher usually wants to measure all domains that might be importantly affected by the medical intervention under investigation. It is much more difficult to determine what these domains are in practice, however, because the intervention effects can be complex. (Kessler & Mroczek, 1995, p. AS109)

One way to conceptualize this issue is to consider the types of information that can be drawn from study participants regarding the nature of their ailments. A health status measure can be thought of as evaluating symptoms, signs, tests, or function (see Table 7-3). A *symptom* would be something reported by the patient but not confirmed by other "scientific" means. Symptoms are typically the easiest and least costly event to measure—you simply need to ask the patient (Sherbourne & Meredith, 1992). Some domains, like pain, are very difficult (but possible) to measure in any other way.

Table 7-3 Types of Condition-Specific Measures

	Definition	Example
Symptoms	Reported, but not confirmed by other means	Pain, shortness of breath
Signs	Result reported by medical profession	Heart murmur
Test	Objective, reproducible finding by medical professional	Blood pressure, blood glucose level
Function test	Measurement of item related to condition, but not condition itself	Test of patient's ability to walk up stairs

Symptoms are inherently subjective since they reflect the individual's perception of how one feels. There is a prejudice against using subjective patient opinions; patient opinions are not considered as scientific as opinions rendered by trained medical professionals. The major difficulty with symptoms is establishing their validity. For example, many different health questionnaires ask patients to rate their own level of pain. What precisely does this measure? Is it compared to the worst pain imaginable? The worst pain the individual has ever felt? The worst pain felt recently? The level of pain the individual typically feels? The level of pain the individual fears they might feel? Self-reported health measures are strongly influenced by such factors as ethnicity (Meredith & Siu, 1995) and social class (Koos, 1954). One example of this is the classic study of the relationship between culture and pain, which showed that individual responses to pain depend on social, family, and culturally patterned responses (Zborowski, 1952). Methods to standardize pain reporting to permit comparisons across patients have been developed (Kane *et al.*, 2005).

But, it is not clear that symptoms reported by patients are, in fact, less reliable than other types of measures. Symptoms have inherent face validity and hold relevance to the patient. Moreover, patient feelings can provide unique insights. For example, studies of self-reported health have found that it is one of the best available predictors of mortality (Idler & Kasl, 1991). The problem may be less one of lower actual validity than one of lower perceived validity.

A *sign* is a result reported by a medical professional after a direct examination of the patient. Signs are opinions or reports expressed by medical professionals. For example, a physician listening to a patient's heart may report hearing a heart murmur. Signs are typically considered more valid than symptoms, although that may be affected by professional prejudice rather than empirical truth. The validity and reliability of a professional opinion is dependent on such factors as the training of the professional, the focus and quality of the instrument, and the level of ambiguity of the topic (Feinstein, 1987). Although clinicians place much faith in clinical observation, the accuracy of such observations is well worth testing for reliability and validity.

A *test* is an objective finding by a medical professional, such as a laboratory test. A test is typically considered to be superior to symptoms and signs because of better validity. When a population is tested for a disease, for example, the exact same procedure and exact same criteria can be used for every single member of the population. Every member of the population can give a blood sample of the same size. Every blood sample can be treated in the same way. The exact same antibody threshold can be used every time. With tests, extreme precision and standardization can be established.

With most tests, interpretation of the results by a clinician is necessary. For example, in an echocardiogram, after the test is complete, a physician or technician needs to interpret the ultrasonic record, which is shown as shadows on a monitor. The rater must make a judgment about the presence of potential anomalies. The quality, reliability, and validity of the test therefore depend entirely on the quality of the image and the reliability and validity of the interpretation by the rater.

Radiologists do not agree to the presence of abnormal findings. In a study of the accuracy of radiological findings, the rate of correct interpretations of mammograms of patients with cancer was 74–96% (Elmore *et al.*, 1994). The correct interpretation rate for patients without cancer ranged from 11–65%. The results of such studies strongly suggest that tests can be just as fallible as symptoms or signs.

Although one may feel confident in using a direct physiological measure as an outcome, even the simplest measure can produce unforeseen problems and potential for measurement bias. For example, blood pressure seems like a straightforward parameter, but however simple a measure it is, the results can be presented in different ways and not standardized as a measure (Pickering *et al.*, 2005). The way the variable is defined can affect the result and even dramatically alter the interpretation. One analysis showed that depending on how blood pressure was used (e.g., last diastolic blood pressure [DBP] determination $\geq$ 90, mean DBP over 1 year) the relative performance of clinical sites changed (Berlowitz *et al.*, 1997). If the measurement of blood pressure is not standardized in an outcomes study, the researcher runs the risk of an attenuated relationship with treatments of interest (Pickering *et al.*, 2005).

Finally, a *function test* does not attempt to measure aspects of the condition directly, as do symptoms, signs, and tests, but rather measures the impact of the condition on day-to-day life. Many generic health status measures operate on the functional level, but most of them use reported function rather than direct testing of performance. A function test may be directed at a single joint (e.g., range of motion) or at the lower or upper extremities (e.g., walking or grip strength).

Care needs to be exercised with measures that utilize function tests. For example, a test which measures a patient's ability to walk a specified distance measures just that: the ability of a patient to walk a specified distance. This point may seem quite obvious, but it is often overlooked. Investigators often use function tests to measure some underlying disease state. For example, if arthritis limits the ability to walk, does a test of a person's ability to walk measure arthritis? To answer yes involves a leap of faith (and is also a logical fallacy). This leap can be made, but should be made only in the presence of a strong conceptual model. Consider the following as an example of the type of mistake that this approach could allow: An investigator attempts to measure the relationship between an intervention and arthritis, using walking distance as a test of function. The intervention is exercise. Although the arthritis is unchanged, the experimental group increases their fitness level as a result of the exercise, and therefore, patients walk further. Increased scores on the function test, driven by changes in fitness levels, are then falsely interpreted as improvements in arthritis.

Hierarchy of Measurement

Each type of test has inherent shortcomings and tap different domains measuring the impact of the condition on the patient. Many domains can be measured by each of the different methods. For example, a measure of health could be a function test (like performance ADL) or a symptom reported by a patient (self-reported health).

Rheumatoid arthritis can provide an example of the hierarchy of measure. Spiegel and her colleagues (1986) examined some of the available condition-specific tests for rheumatoid arthritis to explore which domains each measure covered. First, symptoms are reported by the patient: morning stiffness and pain. Next, signs can be discovered upon physical examination: tenderness, swelling of joints, and joint deformity. Tests are available, such as x-rays and laboratory tests, for the presence of an inflammatory disorder. A series of performance tests are available, notably a grip test and a walk time test. Finally, generic health status measures such as activities of daily living can measure functional status. Which is the correct test to use?

Rheumatoid arthritis is a chronic, symmetrical arthritis affecting synovial lining of joints. Initially, the patient typically experiences swelling and tenderness of affected joints, followed by pain and stiffness. Eventually, the range of motion of the joints may become limited, joints may become deformed, and cysts may form. Other problems associated with rheumatoid arthritis include malaise and anemia. Although other complications are much less common, rheumatoid arthritis can affect almost every organ system, including the heart and lungs. This is an example of a disease primarily associated with the musculoskeletal system having complications in many different systems (which argue for the inclusion of a generic health status measure along with a condition-specific measure).

There is no cure for rheumatoid arthritis. Interventions include exercises and splints for sleeping to increase range of motion (also surgery in extreme cases). Symptomatic pharmacologic therapy can reduce inflammation and pain. Rheumatoid arthritis is rarely fatal, but pain, suffering, and impairment can be extreme. Up to 15% of patients become fully incapacitated (Fishman, 1985).

With this background, the question of which test to use can be asked again. Which measure is appropriate depends entirely on the research question. Measures that address treatment for an acute exacerbation may be very different from those that address performance. Acute measures concentrate on evidence or effects of inflammatory response, such as joint counts and sedimentation rates. Using performance measures like walk time and grip strength to detect acute events must consider that they are strongly related to joint deformity. Regardless of a person's acute status, extensive joint deformity may dramatically impair performance. In contrast, clinical estimates of disease activity and pain by physicians and patients appear to be strongly related to disease activity, but not as strongly to functional status. Global functioning may be affected by a person's mental state. Depressed or discouraged patients may find themselves less able to cope with social roles at the same level of disease activity as those unimpaired by such feelings. The choice of an appropriate outcome measure for rheumatoid arthritis depends entirely on the expected impact of the intervention and knowledge of the relationship of the measure to other clinically significant factors.

When selecting a particular condition-specific measure, the investigator should have built a conceptual model to facilitate the identification of important domains. In this rheumatoid arthritis example, it is necessary to understand the natural history of the disease and the expected impact of the intervention prior to the selection of the condition-specific measure. The bottom line is that in order to select an appropriate condition-specific measure, investigators must know what they wish to measure.

THE ROLE OF CONDITION-SPECIFIC VERSUS GENERIC MEASURES

Generic and condition-specific measures can complement each other. The domains measured by condition-specific measures may resemble those addressed by generic measures, but they are treated differently. When an investigator selects a condition-specific measure, the reason is typically to measure domains more deeply than they are measured by generic measures. The cataract eye surgery study mentioned earlier provides an example of this goal (Damiano *et al.*, 1995). If it is decided to use both condition-specific and generic measures, investigators should be clear as to why both are being included in the study. Often, generic measures are used as a safety net; they are designed to capture unexpected results of the intervention. This strategy is associated with statistical trolling, casting a wide net without an underlying model in the hopes that something will prove interesting in retrospect. This strategy is often used early on in the research of a new treatment. As noted in the first chapter, hypothesis-driven investigations will lead to stronger conclusions and avoid misleading observations based on chance findings.

Typical statistical measures, such as t tests, are designed to test hypotheses. If a 95% significance level is used to test hypotheses, then Type I errors (rejecting the null hypothesis when the null hypothesis is true) will occur 5% of the time. Therefore, in 20 tests, one would be expected to be statistically significant simply due to chance. Simply throwing a battery of tests at a problem, without any underlying conceptual model, can lead to false conclusions.

Instead, generic measures should be incorporated to test specific hypotheses. An intervention's primary impact may be in one domain, but the intervention may also be expected to have secondary impacts in several different domains. For example, knee surgery might affect not just mobility, but could potentially also affect other domains such as mental health (if increased mobility reduced depression caused by isolation). Bear in mind that more generic effects are usually the result of more complex interactions.

Another reason for incorporating generic measures into a study is that overall health, as measured by generic health measures, may differentially affect the intervention's impact on the main (condition-specific) outcome measure. Consider, for example, back surgery as an intervention for patients with back pain. The purpose of the intervention is to decrease pain. A condition-specific outcome, such as the Roland–Morris Low Back Pain and Disability Rating Scale (Roland & Morris, 1983), could be used to measure the levels of pain both before and after the intervention. The success of the intervention may depend on overall health status. People suffering from a multitude of ailments may not gain much relief from the surgery, even if the surgery worked perfectly. Such a result does not mean the intervention was a failure. Rather, it means that the success of the surgery depends on overall health status. A condition-specific measure can convey the result that the surgery worked, which is necessary information for the narrow evaluation of the surgery. A generic measure could reveal that for some patients the surgery had no positive impact on the overall well-being of the patient. The latter information is necessary for evaluating, for example, the cost-effectiveness of a treatment, or it could be used in targeting a treatment toward populations likely to gain benefit from the treatment.

The notion that generic and condition-specific measures should be used in tandem has been criticized by Dowie (2002) as being inconsistent with the goal of making decisions on the allocation of scarce healthcare resources in a transparent and explicitly coherent, preference and evidence-based process. Dowie argues that in situations when the generic and condition-specific measures disagree, there must be a transparent prespecified decision rule for selecting which measure to accept as definitive (2002). However, if the decision maker has already decided that one or the other measure (generic or condition-specific) will be disregarded if it disagrees with the preferred measure, what is the purpose in using both? Further, the argument that a condition-specific measure can find small but important differences is also criticized; if a change is too small to impact overall health, what is the purpose in inflating the change to make it seem larger? This is likened to selecting a larger map to make two cities seem further apart—the distance between the cities is the same regardless of the scale of the map. Similarly, if a change in health status is too small to impact overall health, what is the purpose of administrating a measure sensitive enough to detect irrelevant differences?

But this argument presupposes that there is agreement on the definition of a meaningful difference. Generic measures typically find changes in HRQL. In contrast, condition-specific measures are often more akin to clinical measures and can more easily find clinically relevant differences. But what is the purpose in making a clinically relevant change in a person's health that has no effect on his or her HRQL? Clinicians and decision analysts often disagree about this question. Decision analysts argue that treatment should be focused on the person, not the condition, which leads to the conclusion that a generic measure—examining the impact on the entire person—is preferable to a condition-specific measure, which focuses only on the condition. But most measures have a set of patient preferences implicitly built in, which determine the relative value of different health states. Generic measures often reflect community preferences, while condition-specific measures may reflect the preferences of the particular population with the condition (Guyatt, 2002). Many condition-specific measures cover multiple domains, as do the generic measures, and may measure HRQL, as do the generic measure, with the key difference being that the preference weights built into the measures for condition-specific measures more accurately reflect the preferences of the target population.

The argument that differences that are important to the individual's HRQL will be found by a generic measure also assumes that the generic measure is the final arbitrator of meaningful differences. But this is a difficult argument given the dramatic differences in widely accepted generic measures in the number of questions, number of possible levels of responses, and included domains, as detailed in the previous chapter. For example, on a 0–1 scale, the difference between perfect health and any level of illness in the EQ-5D is 0.12 points (from a score of 1 to 0.88; Brazier & Fitzpatrick, 2002). So, for example, a decline in health from full health to 0.95 health units is undetectable by the EQ-5D, although a different measure, such as the SF-36, might be able to demonstrate such a change. If different generic measures disagree on the effect of a treatment or condition on an individual's HRQL, how can a particular generic measure be considered definitive?

CHOOSING A MEASURE

Selecting the best condition-specific health status measure for a study can be difficult. Investigators can either create a new measure or use an already developed measure. Despite the appeal of a customized measure, the work involved is substantial. Moreover, the acceptance of the results of the study may hinge on the acceptance of the measure. Pioneering investigators must first provide strong and convincing evidence that their measure is reliable, internally consistent, and valid before even beginning to discuss the substantive results of the study. Further, the results of the study with the new measure will be hard to compare with those from any previous study. These drawbacks, combined with the time and cost associated with the development of a new measure, argue strongly against developing a new measure unless no available measures are acceptable.

The better option is to choose a condition-specific measure developed and validated by other investigators. For many conditions there are a multitude of condition-specific measures (for example, for the measurement of arthritis, at least five standard condition-specific outcome measures are available; Patrick & Deyo, 1989). The book *Measuring*

Health: A Guide to Rating Scales and Questionnaires (McDowell, 2006) presents nearly 100 measures for common conditions, such as pain, mental status, depression, and physical disability. *Measuring Disease: A Review of Disease-Specific Quality of Life Measurement Scales* provides a comprehensive but less exhaustive discussion of condition-specific measures (Bowling, 2001). The Ovid database interface provides access to the Health and Psychosocial Instruments database, which contains more than 15,000 references to articles and measures. The MAPI Research Trust has an extensive battery of self-reported condition-specific measures in their Patient Reported Outcome and Quality of Life Instruments Database (PROQLID; MAPI Research Trust, 2009). Much of the work of MAPI has centered on the cross-cultural use and translation of measures (Acquadro, Joyce, Patrick, Ware, & Wu, 2004). Unless there is a royalty associated with the measure, the condition-specific measures are free to use.

The selection of a particular condition-specific measure from the measures available should be guided by statistical, theoretical, and practical criteria. Statistically, the investigator should seek measures that are reliable, valid, responsive, unbiased, precise in the range where effects are expected, and easy to implement (Kessler & Mroczek, 1995). Theoretically, the measure should cover the domains of greatest interest. The determination of the domains must be driven by a theoretical model of the disease or condition, and how it will interact with the treatment.

Practical considerations should be taken into account. The mode of administration of the measure needs to be consistent with the overall design of the study. For example, it would be improper to have study participants self-administer a measure designed for use in a phone survey. Measures that have been used previously in similar studies should be given preference over infrequently used or new measures, provided they seem to capture the salient information on the effects being targeted. Widely used measures will facilitate comparisons of the results of the study with previous studies.

The investigator should also consider the distribution of expected scores in the study population. Measures which minimize the probability of floor or ceiling effects should be selected. For example, if the study population consists of frail elderly, measures designed for healthy populations should be avoided as much as possible.

Some measures require the use of complicated scoring algorithms. Some are also bulky or complicated. All other things equal, simpler and shorter is better.

The time frame of measures also varies. For example, the SF-36 asks about the previous 4 weeks. Other measures may ask about the previous 6 months. Some may ask about the present state. A measure should be selected with a time frame appropriate for the intervention and condition.

It is also worth considering how the results of the study will be analyzed. The method of analysis should be established prior to the beginning of the study. This allows the investigator to select appropriate statistical tests and thereby to conduct a power analysis and determine the necessary sample size.

CONCLUSION

The proper selection of the outcomes measure is key to a successful outcomes study. The best approach to picking a measure is to first acquire an understanding of the natural history of the condition and then develop a theory of how the intervention affects the condition. This allows for the discovery of domains where the intervention is expected to have an impact. Condition-specific measures are focused, precise measures that are able to delve deeply into the domains of greatest interest. Condition-specific measures should be teamed with appropriate generic measures so that the intervention can be evaluated, not just with regard to its narrow impact on the condition, but also for its impact on overall health across a multitude of domains. This enables the investigator to view results within the larger context of other competing populations and treatments.

Condition-specific measures play a central role in assessing the outcomes of care. Rather than engaging in a debate about their relative merits as compared with generic measures, condition-specific measures are best seen as complements to generic measures. Many condition-specific measures have their basis in clinical practice, and, as consequence, they are more acceptable to clinicians. Care must be exercised not to place undue confidence in the reliability of measures derived directly from practice.

REFERENCES

Acquadro, C., Joyce, C. R. B., Patrick, D. L., Ware, J. E., & Wu, A. W. (2004). *Linguistic validation manual for patient-reported outcomes (PRO) instruments.* Lyon, France: MAPI Research Trust.

Barry, M. J., Fowler, F., O'Leary, M. J., Bruskewitz, R. C., Holtgrewe, H. L., & Mebust, W. K. (1995). Measuring disease-specific health status in men with benign prostatic hyperplasia. *Medical Care, 33*(4 Supplement), AS145–AS155.

Bellamy, N., Buchanan, W. W., Goldsmith, C. H., Campbell, J., & Stitt, L. W. (1988). Validation study of WOMAC: A health status instrument for measuring clinically important patient relevant outcomes to antirheumatic drug therapy in patients with osteoarthritis of the hip or knee. *Journal of Rheumatology, 15*(12), 1833–1840.

Berlowitz, D. R., Ash, A. S., Hickey, E. C., Friedman, R. H., Kader, B., & Moskowitz, M. A. (1997). Outcomes of hypertension care: Simple measures are not that simple. *Medical Care, 35*(7), 742–746.

Bombardier, C., Melfi, C., Paul, J., Green, R., Hawker, G., Wright, J.,Coyte, P. (1995). Comparison of a generic and a disease specific measure of pain and physical function after knee replacement surgery. *Medical Care, 33*(4 Supplement), AS131–AS144.

Bowling, A. (2001). *Measuring disease: A review of disease-specific quality of life measurement scales* (2nd ed.). Buckingham, UK: Open University Press.

Brazier, J., & Fitzpatrick, R. (2002). Measures of health-related quality of life in an imperfect world: A comment on Dowie. *Health Economics, 11*(1), 17–19.

Damiano, A., Steinberg, E., Cassard, S., Bass, E., Diener-West, M., Legro, M., . . .Kolb, M. (1995). Comparison of generic versus disease specific measures of functional impairment in patients with cataract. *Medical Care, 33*(4 Supplement), AS120–AS130.

Dowie, J. (2002). Decision validity should determine whether a generic or condition specific HRQOL measure is used in health care decisions. *Health Economics, 11*(1), 1–8.

Elmore, J., Wells, C., Lee, C., Howard, D., & Feinstein, A. (1994). Variability in radiologists' interpretations of mammograms. *New England Journal of Medicine, 331*(22), 1493–1499.

Feinstein, A. R. (1987). *Clinimetrics.* New Haven, CT: Yale University Press.

Fishman, R. A. (1985). Normal-pressure hydrocephalus and arthritis. *New England Journal of Medicine, 312*(19), 1255–1256.

Fitzpatrick, R., Davey, C., Buxton, M., & Jones, D. (1998). Evaluating patient-based outcome measures for use in clinical trials. *Health Technology Assessment, 2*(14), 1–74.

Fletcher, R. H., & Fletcher, S. W. (2005). *Clinical epidemiology: The essentials* (4th ed.). Philadelphia: Lippincott Williams and Wilkins.

Guyatt, G. (2002). Commentary on Jack Dowie, "Decision validity should determine whether a generic or condition-specific HRQOL measure is used in health care decisions." *Health Economics, 11*(1), 13–16.

Guyatt, G. H., Feeny, D. H., & Patrick, D. L. (1991). Issues in quality-of-life measurement in clinical trials. *Controlled Clinical Trials, 12*(Supplement), 81S–91S.

Guyatt, G. H., Feeny, D. H., & Patrick, D. L. (1993). Measuring health-related quality of life. *Annals of Internal Medicine, 118*, 622–629.

Haynes, R. B., Sackett, D. L., Guyatt, G. H., & Tugwell, P. (2006). *Clinical epidemiology: How to do clinical practice research* (3rd ed.). Philadelphia: Lippincott Williams and Wilkins.

Idler, E. L., & Kasl, S. (1991). Health perceptions and survival: Do global evaluations of health status really predict mortality? *Journal of Gerontology, 46*(2), S55–S65.

Kane, R. L., Bershadsky, B., Rockwood, T., Saleh, K., & Islam, N. C. (2005). Visual Analog Scale pain reporting was standardized. *Journal of Clinical Epidemiology, 58*(6), 618–623.

Kazis, L. E., Anderson, J. J., & Meenan, R. F. (1989). Effect sizes for interpreting changes in health status. *Medical Care, 27*(3 Supplement), S178–S189.

Kessler, R., & Mroczek, D. (1995). Measuring the effects of medical interventions. *Medical Care, 33*(4 Supplement), AS109–AS119.

Kjerulff, K., & Langenberg, P. (1995). A comparison of alternative ways of measuring fatigue among patients having hysterectomy. *Medical Care, 33*(4 Supplement), AS156–AS163.

Koos, E. L. (1954). *The health of regionville.* New York: Columbia University Press.

Luepker, R. V., Apple, F. S., Christenson, R. H., Crow, R. S., Fortmann, S. P., Goff, D., . . .Tunstall-Pedoe, H. (2003). Case definitions for acute coronary heart disease in epidemiology and clinical research studies: A statement from the AHA Council on Epidemiology and Prevention; AHA Statistics Committee; World Heart Federation Council on Epidemiology and Prevention; the European Society of Cardiology Working Group on Epidemiology and Prevention; Centers for Disease Control and Prevention; and the National Heart, Lung, and Blood Institute. *Circulation, 108*(20), 2543–2549.

MAPI Research Trust. (2009). PROQOLID Patient Reported Outcome and Quality of Life Instruments Database. Available at: http://www.proqolid.org/. Accessed April 17, 2010.

McColl, E., Eccles, M. P., Rousseau, N. S., Steen, I. N., Parkin, D. W., & Grimshaw, J. M. (2003). From the generic to the condition-specific? Instrument order effects in quality of life assessment. *Medical Care, 41*(7), 777–790.

McDowell, I. (2006). *Measuring health: A guide to rating scales and questionnaires* (3rd ed.). New York: Oxford University Press.

Meredith, L. S., & Siu, A. L. (1995). Variation and quality of self-report health data: Asian and Pacific Islanders compared with other ethnic groups. *Medical Care, 33*(11), 1120–1131.

Patrick, D. L., & Deyo, R. A. (1989). Generic and disease-specific measures in assessing health status and quality of life. *Medical Care, 27*(3), S217–S232.

Pickering, T. G., Hall, J. E., Appel, L. J., Falkner, B. E., Graves, J., Hill, M. N., . . .Roccella, E. J. (2005). Recommendations for blood pressure measurement in human beings and experimental animals: Part 1: Blood pressure measurement in humans: A statement for professionals from the subcommittee of professional and public education of the American Heart Association Council on High Blood Pressure Research. *Hypertension, 45,* 142–161.

Roland, M. O., & Morris, R. W. (1983). A study of the natural history of back pain: Part 1: Development of a reliable and sensitive measure of disability in low back pain. *Spine, 8,* 141–144.

Sherbourne, C., & Meredith, L. (1992). Quality of self-report data: A comparison of older and younger chronically ill patients. *Journal of Gerontology, 47*(4), S204–S211.

Spiegel, J. S., Leakes, B., Spiegel, T. M., Paulus, H. E., Kane, R. L., Ward, N. B., & Ware, J. E. Jr. (1986). What are we measuring? An examination of self-reported functional status measures. *Arthritis and Rheumatism, 31*(6), 721–728.

Stroud, M. W., McKnight, P. E., & Jensen, M. P. (2004). Assessment of self-reported physical activity in patients with chronic pain: development of an abbreviated Roland-Morris disability scale. *Journal of Pain, 5*(5), 257–263.

Sudman, S., & Bradburn, N. (1974). *Response effects in surveys.* Chicago: Aldine Publishing.

Temkin, N. R., Dikmen, S., Machamer, J., & McLean, A. (1989). General versus disease-specific measures: Further work on the Sickness Impact Profile for head injury. *Medical Care, 27*(3), S44–S53.

Ware, J. E., Kosinski, M., & Keller, S. D. (1994). *SF-36 Physical and Mental Health Summary Scales: A user's manual.* Boston: The Health Institute.

Ware, J. E., Kosinski, M., & Keller, S. D. (1996). A 12-item Short-Form Health Survey: Construction of scales and preliminary tests of reliability and validity. *Medical Care, 34*(3), 220–233.

Ware, J. E., & Sherbourne, C. D. (1992). The MOS 36-Item Short-Form Health Survey (SF-36). *Medical Care, 30*(6), 473–483.

Ware, J. E., Snow, K., K, Kosinski, M., & Gandek, B. (1993). *SF-36 Health Survey: Manual and interpretation guide.* Boston: The Health Institute, New England Medical Center.

Zborowski, M. (1952). Cultural components in response to pain. *Journal of Social Issues, 8*, 16–30.

CHAPTER 8

Satisfaction with Care[1]

THE IMPORTANCE OF PATIENT SATISFACTION

Patient satisfaction is an important outcome of care. It may be viewed as a complement to more traditional clinical measures, but it is separate from quality of life. It can refer to satisfaction with the process of care or with the outcomes. It essentially reflects patients' reactions to their care experience (Pascoe, 1983). However, patients can be fickle and have short memories. The relative importance of care elements may change with time and subsequent experiences.

As medical care has come to be viewed as an economic commodity, patient satisfaction has taken on more salience. Initially, interest in patient satisfaction arose from sociological research, where it was seen as a clue to other aspects of care. For example, increased patient satisfaction was associated with improved compliance with appointment keeping, medication use, and following treatment recommendations (Williams, 1994). Satisfied patients were also less likely to sue for malpractice (Hickson et al., 1994).

But satisfaction has also been recognized as a valuable goal in itself. Many years ago, Donabedian (1966) noted that, "achieving and producing health and satisfaction, as defined for its individual members by a particular society or subculture, is the ultimate validation of the quality of care."

As market models were adopted for health care, satisfaction became a direct goal (Cleary & McNeil, 1988). Now that emphasis has been placed on a patient-centered approach to medicine with the patient recast in a

---

[1]Much of this chapter draws on an earlier version by Maureen Smith, Chris Schüssler-Fiorenza, and Todd Rockwood (2006).

159

more active role, the patient's perspective has become even more important (Mead & Bower, 2000). Active patient participation in the healthcare process is thought to promote better health outcomes (Greenfield, Kaplan, & Ware, 1985)

The rise in consumerism and the attempt to apply consumer models to health care reflect a market mentality in which patients (now retitled as "customers") shop for care and make insightful decisions based on good information about their health care (Hudak, McKeever, & Wright, 2003). At the other end, healthcare organizations may use patient satisfaction survey results as a marketing tool.

The rise of evidence-based medicine has placed new emphasis on evaluating the quality of medical care, including patient satisfaction. This information may be used directly, or patients' views and values can be used to weight different outcomes when defining quality care (Cleary & McNeil, 1988). Patient satisfaction surveys are currently implemented as a measure of healthcare quality, linked with national accreditation measures, and may be tied to financial reimbursements to providers.

THEORETIC MODELS OF SATISFACTION

Although there is no universally accepted theoretic model of patient satisfaction, most concepts are based on some variation of fulfilled or unfulfilled expectations. The expectancy–disconfirmation model is adapted from the customer service literature, in which the customer compares his or her expectations with the service performance. When service performance exceeds expectations, customers are satisfied; if it fails to meet expectations, the result is customer dissatisfaction. A modification of this model is called the cognitive–affect model of satisfaction, in which perception of service performance includes a cognitive evaluation, affective response, and a direct effect on satisfaction (Oliver, 1993). The affective response can be tempered or increased by attributions of causality and perceptions of equity, which may have special salience in the case of health care. Satisfaction can create feedback loops to the extent that a patient's satisfaction affects their subsequent behavior; it sends a message to the service provider, assuming the message is clear and correctly interpreted (Crow et al., 2002; Strasser, Aharony, & Greenberger, 1993). Patient characteristics, values, beliefs, and experiences affect both their expectations and their attributive style. Providers may also be able to shape patient expectations through information about treatment and outcomes.

Interpreting Satisfaction Ratings

Expectations and Psychosocial Determinants

Although the expectancy–disconfirmation model is frequently studied and critiqued, one review found that only 20% of patient satisfaction research articles included expectations in their study (Crow et al., 2002). Although some studies, particularly in the United States, have found positive association between expectations and satisfaction, the amount of variance of satisfaction explained by expectations remains low, at no more than 20% and often much less than that in some studies (Thompson & Sunol, 1995). There have been several theorized mechanisms for this. People may adjust their expectations if the discrepancy is modest, and express dissatisfaction only at the extremes (Thompson & Sunol, 1995). Satisfaction may reflect not just unexpected good performance; patients may also be satisfied if nothing unexpected happens. Thus, dissatisfaction may only be expressed at markedly unexpected negative performances (Williams et al., 1996). People may have a wide zone of tolerance and will be satisfied with any performance that falls inside. The less choice a consumer has, the wider their zone of tolerance (Edwards, Staniszweska, & Crichton, 2004).

Another critique of expectations is the argument that many patients come in with unformed expectations. This appears to occur more frequently in the United Kingdom than in the United States and is cited as a reason why expectations have not been found to correlate satisfaction in the United Kingdom, in contrast to the United States where a positive relationship has been found (Crow et al., 2002).

Satisfaction has several dimensions. One can be satisfied with the treatment provided or the outcomes achieved. The treatment provided may include technical quality and interpersonal skill. The latter is easier for most patients to assess and may influence any judgment about the former (Davies & Ware, 1988). However, even patients who do not have specific expectations with respect to medical testing, treatment, and outcome may still have expectations for the interpersonal interaction and information obtained during the visit. In addition, it is unclear how the healthcare experience and its results provide feedback to the patient and can inform his or her expectations and attributions in the future. Expectations in the context of medical care may be more complex because an important component of many medical care encounters is to provide patients with diagnostic information and expectations about treatments, complications, duration, and outcome. Thus, patients who start care with unformed expectations may then acquire expectations about their treatment and out-come, and patients with formed expectations about treatment that differ from the physician's preferred course of care may change their expectations in the face of a persuasive explanation from the physician. How these new expectations then correlate with satisfaction with treatment and outcomes has not been well studied. However, patients who obtain information about what to expect have increased satisfaction (Crow et al., 2002; Krupat, Fancey, & Cleary, 2000) and complaints of lack of information can result in the desire to switch physicians (Keating et al., 2002).

Expectations and satisfaction ratings are conditioned by social norms and people may become habituated to lowered expectations over time. People with poor care may be satisfied, because they have lowered expec-tations, not because they are receiving high quality care. If satisfaction surveys are used uncritically, high satisfaction rates can be cited to main-tain the status quo even if the quality of care is inadequate instead of serving to advance the patient/consumer perspective (Crow et al., 2002; Weithman, 1995). Thus, one may need to ask patients about their ideal expectations, especially in cases in which patients' desires differ from what is normatively available.

Attribution is also an important component of the conceptual model. When patients assign satisfaction ratings, they may consider the duty of the provider and whether the provider is culpable for the event (Williams, Coyle, & Healy, 1998). A client with a negative experience who perceives the service provider as not culpable for a bad experience or assumes that the service is outside the duty of the service provider may still be satisfied. Equity judgments can also modify satisfaction ratings of negative affective experiences if they are perceived as equitable and may be particularly salient in countries with a national health service (Thompson & Sunol, 1995). The attribution part of the model may explain why trust in provider and evidence of caring is highly associ-ated with satisfaction (Joffe, Manocchia, Weeks, & Cleary, 2003). If the patient trusts or believes that the provider has done his or her best and that negative performance is out of his or her control, the patient will still rate highly satisfied.

Not all patients accept an active consumer role. The consumer model assumes that patients consider their opinions legitimate and are willing to express their opinions (Williams, 1994). The higher satisfaction rates among older patients have been attributed to their assuming a more passive role with respect to medical authority, but this has never been directly tested (Crow et al., 2002; Sitzia & Wood, 1998). In addition, psychosocial pressures can work to transform patients' negative affective responses into positive ratings. Even a patient who accepts a more active role is still in a dependent position in the healthcare system. Patients' need for a positive working relationship with the healthcare system can exert psychological incentives for them to maintain a positive outlook about their care in part to maintain a positive outlook for their outcome (Edwards et al., 2004). This is in line with cognitive consistency theory in which patients need to justify their time, effort, and discomfort to themselves and thus report they are satisfied (Sitzia & Wood, 1997).

Dimensions of Satisfaction

Patient satisfaction appears to be simultaneously a unidimensional and a multidimensional construct. Patients' summary judgments about their overall experiences with care suggest that a global measure of satisfaction may be appropriate (Aharony & Strasser, 1993). However, there is substantial evidence that satisfaction is multidimensional (Abramowitz, Cote, & Berry, 1987; Meterko, Nelson, & Rubin, 1990). When satisfaction is broken down into different components, there is greater evidence of dissatisfaction with certain components (Sitzia & Wood, 1997). A review of the acute care setting listed interpersonal manner, technical quality of care, accessibility/convenience, finances, efficacy/outcomes of care, physical environment, and availability as the core dimensions of satisfaction (Ware, Snyder, Wright, & Davies, 1983).

The lack of a widely accepted conceptual framework for dimensions of satisfaction not only leads to considerable variation of the dimensions among studies but also leads to omission of certain dimensions (Hall & Dornan, 1988; Wensing, Grol, & Smits, 1994). Satisfaction may address a variety of elements of care. Table 8-1 lists a number of these potential areas. When using satisfaction as an outcome, it is important to be sure that the dimensions addressed are those likely to be affected by the intervention.

Table 8-1 **Dimensions of Satisfaction**

Access to care	Coordination of care	Participation in care
Interpersonal manner	Respect shown	Behavioral intention
Technical quality	Information	Listens to what is said
Access to case	Physical comfort	Level of trust
Continuity of care	Emotional support	Administrative burden
Finances/cost of services	Encouragement	Availability
Shared decision making		

Little information is available on the relative importance of the various dimensions to patients (Sitzia & Wood, 1998), although common themes across healthcare settings include interpersonal relations, communication, being treated with respect, and trust. These dimensions may be related to the overall conceptual model of satisfaction in terms of how patients attribute their experiences.

The Donabedian framework for quality assessment (structure, process, and outcome) provides a good basis for a conceptual model of satisfaction dimensions (Donabedian, 1988). This model incorporates components of health services access and cost into the structural aspect of satisfaction with care and health services quality into the process aspect of satisfaction with care. In different healthcare settings, the components of health are prioritized differently. For example, social environment is critical for nursing home satisfaction, whereas medical aspects may be more important for ambulatory care and inpatient care, or the physical environment may be relevant for nursing home and hospital care.

In this model, structural aspects of satisfaction include access, cost, and physical environment factors related more to the physical and social (access/cost) side of health care. Process aspects of satisfaction include technical quality that is mainly focused on physical (and sometimes mental) health, interpersonal relations/communications, and continuity/coordination of care reflective of the social side of medicine and important for psychosocial well-being and satisfaction. Outcomes aspects include satisfaction with physical and mental (and perhaps social) health (see Figure 8-1).

Priorities differ across different settings. For health plans, the structural aspects of quality (access, cost, and physical environment such as

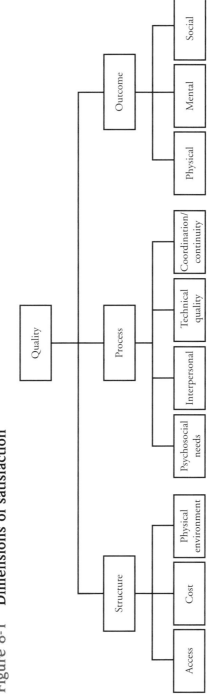

Figure 8-1   **Dimensions of satisfaction**

technology) are valued highly (Crow et al., 2002), whereas for inpatient care, the physical living environment and interpersonal interactions, particularly with nursing care, are more important (Crow et al., 2002; Rubin, 1990). The patient's condition may also affect their satisfaction. For example, patients who present with an acute physical complaint in an ambulatory setting may prioritize outcome, whereas patients who present with a chronic disease might prioritize the process dimensions of satisfaction.

Process of Care and Satisfaction

Satisfaction with the process of care can include several areas. Patients are probably least able to judge the technical quality of the care (unless they are given specific guidance about what to look for). Instead they focus on the way the care is provided. Did they have long waits to get an appointment or to be seen? Were people friendly? Did the doctor seem rushed? In the hospital, patients may comment on the food or whether nurses came quickly when summoned.

An interesting aspect of such satisfaction is the role of time. If you talk with a person just discharged from the hospital (or even still in it), they will likely tell you all about the food and the nursing. But as time passes, the salience of those aspects fades and they remember other elements of the experience that involve the care they received. Much of the judgment about such care over time may be clouded by the outcomes achieved.

Outcomes and Satisfaction

Although patient satisfaction is often considered as an outcome of health care, it is also affected by outcomes of care. One model of satisfaction argues that the major goal of patients who present with a health problem is not satisfaction but the resolution of their health problem (Sitzia & Wood, 1997). Despite this important insight, only a small minority of studies investigate the effect of outcomes on patient satisfaction (Hall & Dornan, 1988; Wensing et al., 1994). There is evidence, however, that outcomes affect satisfaction, although it is also possible for patients to be satisfied with their health care even when they experience poor outcomes.

Understanding these apparently contradictory results requires investigation of the feedback loops that influence satisfaction attitude formation. One study found that immediately after a visit to an acute care clinic, satisfaction was most related to lack of unmet expectations and receiving an explanation for a symptom's cause and an estimate of likely system duration, whereas at 2 weeks and 3 months, satisfaction was related to improvement of the underlying symptom (Jackson, Chamberlin, & Kroenke, 2001). In this study, satisfaction correlated with absolute symptom impairment as had been found previously (Kane, Maciejewski, & Finch, 1997). It appears that patient satisfaction with outcomes may be based more on their current status than on an appreciation of how much they have improved. One interpretation of these findings is that satisfaction at a later point in time "is really measuring satisfaction with the patient's health outcome rather than the individual physician" (Jackson et al., 2001). An alternative interpretation might be that for the types of health conditions studied, the patients (who were not asked about expectations with outcome) expected complete resolution of their symptoms and thus any residual symptom was a source of dissatisfaction. Another study that looked at sources of patients' unmet expectations found that half the patients they interviewed focused on length of symptom duration rather than on severity, and that these patients interpreted refractory symptoms as a sign that the physician was off track (Kravitz et al., 1996). In addition to physical outcomes, the way illness affects functional and emotional well-being is very important for patients, but can be overlooked by physicians (Kravitz et al., 1996). For certain disease states, the patients' relationship to the involved body part, the meanings attached to treatment outcome, as well as how significantly the impairment affects occupational and social function, may also greatly affect satisfaction (Hudak, McKeever, & Wright, 2004).

Methodology of Measuring Satisfaction

Measurement Methods

All of the standard social research methods are capable of measuring satisfaction: archival, ethnographic, focus groups, and survey research. The first two of these methods have received little attention in the study of satisfaction but can provide useful information. Data from existing sources (such as patient complaint records) can provide a means of identifying areas in which patients have expressed dissatisfaction with the performance of the organization or with healthcare professionals. Open-ended interviews with patients can provide a detailed understanding of the dynamics of the healthcare provision process from a patient's point of view and may be useful in exploring or generating hypotheses, particularly as an initial step in areas that have not been well researched. Focus groups have several advantages but share the generalizability problem also found with archival and ethnographic methods. Focus groups can provide qualitative as well as quantitative data; they permit detailed exploration of specific events and present an opportunity for spontaneous information to emerge. The most common method to assess satisfaction is by survey. A closed response format survey relies on the standardization of measurement whereby all respondents are presented with the same questions and are constrained to respond in a uniform manner. They allow a sample of the population to be studied and the findings to be generalized to an entire population.

The same issue can be approached in several different ways.

- One can ask how satisfied the patient is with this aspect of care.
- One can ask about how well this aspect is provided.
- One can ask how much the patient agrees with a value statement or rating about the aspect of care.

One scheme for measuring satisfaction discriminates between measures along diametrically opposed dimensions. Figure 8-2 illustrates these using four axes for satisfaction measurement (Hudak et al., 2004). To measure satisfaction in getting a doctor's appointment, several possible question versions are suggested. One approach that emphasizes *perception* asks the following:

> On a scale of 1 to 10, where 1 means very low and 10 means very high, how would you rate your ability to get a doctor's appointment when you want one?

An alternative approach stresses the behavioral or more observable aspects of getting an appointment.

> How many days did you wait to get an appointment with your doctor?

Either question could be appropriate for measuring satisfaction with getting an appointment with a physician. It will depend on the question.

Figure 8-2   Axes for satisfaction measurement

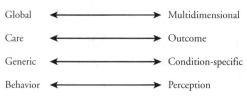

Methodological Issues

Selection bias can be a significant problem with satisfaction surveys. The response rates for mailed satisfaction surveys are often less than 50%, leading to questions about the representativeness of the survey results. Generally dissatisfied patients are likely to withdraw from care before treatment is completed and not return mailed surveys. Concerns about response bias mean one must interpret results with extreme caution. As a rule, it is better to target a subgroup of patients and pursue them diligently than to simply rely on large numbers of patients with small response rates.

An underappreciated problem with satisfaction measures is the inherent bias of patient responses. Acquiescence response bias refers to "the tendency to agree with statements of opinion regardless of content" (Ware, Davies-Avery, & Stewart, 1978). There is a tendency for favorably worded items and opinion questions to overestimate satisfaction and negatively worded items to underestimate satisfaction. Unfortunately, there is no specific method for estimating the extent to which acquiescence bias is operating. This threat can lead to high levels of apparent satisfaction and poor discrimination among comparison groups (skewed and clustered distributions). One outcome of satisfaction surveys is the high percentage (greater than 90%) of satisfied ratings for many aspects of health care. These results are inadequate for quality improvement and discriminating among comparison groups.

A number of approaches have been suggested for managing acquiescence response bias. What follows is a brief list of approaches

- Employ balanced measures; that is, positively and negatively worded items. This technique may cause problems if the respondents do not pay close attention to the wording or are easily confused.
- Use neutral wording in questions.
- Use response categories to evaluate various aspects of care. For evaluation rating scales, (such as poor, fair, good, very good, excellent) the number of response categories at the high end of the response continuum better discriminates between very good and excellent aspects of care. The problem is this no longer assesses satisfaction.
- Multi-item scales versus single-item measures provide better discrimination among patient group.
- Force the respondent to rank the various aspects of care from highest to lowest.

- Be cognizant that older patients and sicker patients are disposed to response biases.

Social desirability is most problematic when a personal interview is used to collect the data. There is some evidence that responses are affected by interviewer expectations. This, coupled with the privacy of the data collection setting, may be responsible for universally high ratings associated with interviews. A related potential bias is the *fear of retribution*. This is a potential bias whenever there is a positional difference between the patient completing the satisfaction measure and the person being evaluated. Potential for this problem underscores the importance of guaranteeing anonymity and confidentiality of responses. Each of these biases can be reduced by: (1) guaranteeing confidentiality and privacy of data collected, (2) using an external group for evaluation, and (3) using a neutral location or method for collecting the data, such as secured drop-boxes for place of service assessment and self-addressed stamped mailers.

Psychometric Testing

Reliability and Validity. The reliability and validity of measures of satisfaction are crucial, although in the past they were often not tested or reported. One review article found that only 6% of instruments met minimal reliability and validity testing criteria (Sitzia & Wood, 1998). The main types of reliability at issue are inter-item reliability or internal consistency reliability of multi-item scales (e.g., Cronbach's coefficient alpha), test–retest reliability, and interobserver reliability for those measures administered by telephone or in-person interview. Test–retest reliability is reported even less frequently than internal consistency reliability and it may be difficult to discern how it is affected by changing perceptions over time or poor recall.

Surveys also need to be tested against internal and external validation criteria. While measures are often tested for internal discriminant validity, which is the ability of patients to discriminate among different features of care, external discriminant validity or how patients' discriminations compare to independent ratings is rarely tested (Aharony & Strasser, 1993). Approaches to external validation include comparison of patient ratings of care to those of other sources, comparison of the ratings to other variables theoretically related to patient satisfaction, and experimental manipulation of features of care (Rubin, 1990). The external validation of patient satisfaction and ratings of technical quality is particularly important. At a minimum, satisfaction measures need face validity if they are to be used and accepted in the evaluations of health plans, hospitals, and clinicians (Ben-Sira, 1976; Davies & Ware, 1988; DiMatteo & Hays, 1980). Finally, satisfaction measures need to be validated in more than one population or setting of care. Cultural differences may affect perceptions of care. The same construct of satisfaction may have varying salience in different care settings. Many existing measures of satisfaction have not been validated in this way and ongoing research in this area is important.

The response format for individual items has an impact on reliability and validity. The five-point Likert-type *agree disagree* response scale requires more items per dimension to achieve validity and may be susceptible to acquiescent response bias. Ware and Hayes (1988) found that the *excellent poor* format produced responses that were less skewed, had greater variability, and performed better on validity tests compared to a six-point *very satisfied very dissatisfied* scale, although this finding was not replicated in a more recent study (Hendriks, Vrielink, Smets, van Es, & De Haes, 2001). Hendriks and colleagues did find that word responses next to the items resulted in fewer missing items (2001). Different subpopulations may respond better to certain response formats; for example, a study found that older adults preferred a 10-item visual analog form and this version had greater response variability (Castle & Engberg, 2004). The Consumer Assessment of Healthcare Providers and Systems (CAHPS; formerly called Consumer Assessment of Health Plan Study) program chose a 0–10 numeric scale after performing cognitive testing and psychometric field data analysis, because of its ease of use in telephone administration and greater distribution of responses compared to a five-point scale (Harris-Kojetin, Fowler, Brown, Schnaier, & Sweeny, 1999).

Bias. A number of biases, such as nonresponse bias, acquiescent response bias, and sociopsychological artifacts may affect survey measures. Especially in daily operations, satisfaction surveys are plagued by low response rates, often less than 50% (Aharony & Strasser, 1993; Barkley & Furse, 1996; Sitzia & Wood, 1998). Large organizations, like hospitals, frequently send out thousands of satisfaction surveys to all their discharged patients each month (obviously deceased patients cannot respond) and get back a small percentage. They may send out thousands and get back hundreds. They take pride in the large numbers of responses and do not think about the response rate. By contrast, the epidemiological literature considers a response rate that is less than 80% substandard. Nonresponse bias can greatly affect the validity of the results. Demographics, utilization patterns, and health status differ between respondents and nonrespondents (Fowler, Gallagher, Stringfellow, Zaslavsky, Thompson, & Cleary, 2002; Lasek, Barkley, Harper, & Rosenthal, 1997; Mazor, Clauser, Field, Yood, & Gurwitz, 2002; Zaslavsky, Zaborski, & Cleary, 2002). Because less satisfied patients may be less likely to respond, caution must be taken when interpreting the results of studies with satisfaction rates below 80% (Eisen & Grob, 1979; Ley, Bradshaw, Kincey, & Atherton, 1976; Mazor et al., 2002).

Acquiescent response bias is the tendency to agree with statements regardless of actual content. It can be reduced by varying positive and negative statements in a survey. However, there are risks in this strategy, especially with people with limited cognitive or literary skills—the reverse wording may lead to confusion and the respondents may not pick up on the subtle differences. Sociopsychologic artifacts refer to how responses may be affected by fear of retribution or social desirability. Social desirability is the tendency of respondents to offer answers that are consistent with values the respondent believes are held by the interviewer (Groves, 1989; Groves et al., 1988; Locander, Sudman, & Bradburn, 1976). This social influence, which pressures the respondent to provide an answer that is in line with normative expectations or self-enhancing presentation, is influenced both by the mode of survey administration as well as substantive content of questions; it is a greater risk in interviews. It can be reduced, but not eliminated, by guaranteeing confidentiality (Singer, Von Thurn, & Miller, 1995).

Utilization Patterns, Survey Timing, and Reference Group

Survey results may also be influenced by utilization patterns with high users of care and low or nonusers of care rating satisfaction differently. Thus, surveys that allow differentiation between the satisfaction survey results of users versus low or nonusers of care enable greater focus and, in addition, analysis of sicker subpopulations whose contact time and satisfaction with health care may differ. The timing of survey administration can also influence results because a patient's perceived satisfaction with care may change over time (Aharony & Strasser, 1993; Jackson et al., 2001). One cause of this change may be symptom improvement over time (Jackson et al., 2001).

The reference standpoint of a satisfaction instrument is also important. A general reference asks patients to rate health care given to people in general; whereas a personal reference asks them how satisfied they are with their own health care. The personal referent has been found to be more specific and useful as an evaluation measure. However, it must also be noted that people tend to rate satisfaction with their own care higher than they do when using a general referent (Pascoe, 1983; Ware et al., 1983). It is unclear whether the skewed response distributions of the personal referent measure may be in part influenced by psychosocial artifacts such as the tendency to give socially desirable responses, reluctance to criticize provider, or because of fear of retribution (Hays & Ware, 1986). Other possible explanations include rating the general referent more negatively because of biases against doctors and health care in general or, conversely, a positive bias toward rating one's own care higher because the tendency of people to think they are better off than others (Hall & Dornan, 1988).

Reporting Versus Rating

The CAHPS chose to have patients report their experiences with different attributes of health plans thought to be important to patient satisfaction rather than directly rating their satisfaction with these attributes. Thus, for example, instead of asking patients to rate their satisfaction with waiting time before seeing a doctor, the survey asks how long the patient had to wait. This avoids the problem that different patients may have different expectations of care and also avoids some of the subjectivity associated with rating. However, this study maintained the global satisfaction rating items. The advantage of this approach is that it provides more objective information about patients' experiences of the details of care and facilitates quality improvement projects. In addition, future customers of health plans can make their own value judgments about different aspects of care based on these reports. The disadvantage of this approach is that with only a summative rating of patient satisfaction, there is less information on the relative importance of various attributes of health plans to consumers.

Importance of Satisfaction Elements

It is possible to design a scoring system that captures the relative importance of each satisfaction element when creating weighted score. Table 8-2 shows an example of such an approach. Three levels of satisfaction and three of importance are used to illustrate the approach. Low satisfaction

Table 8-2   **Example of Weighting Satisfaction by Importance**

	Level of Satisfaction		
Importance	High (3)	Medium (1)	Low (−3)
High (3)	9	3	−9
Medium (2)	6	2	−6
Low (1)	3	1	−3

(or dissatisfaction) is given a negative weight. Thus, strong satisfaction with an important element of care would get a score of +9 and strong dissatisfaction with an important element would get a −9. Items of low importance would have a range of only +3 to −3.

Existing Satisfaction Measures

Health Plan

The major dimensions of patient satisfaction of health plans are access, cost, quality of physicians, and plan administration (see Table 8-3). In evaluating satisfaction of health plans, it is critical to also survey those no longer enrolled to get a more accurate assessment of satisfaction because the most dissatisfied members may have left the plan (Bender, Lance, & Guess, 2003).

Another issue that needs further study in evaluating the quality of and patient satisfaction with health plans is the relationship between provider satisfaction and patient satisfaction. Patient satisfaction has been found to be associated with provider satisfaction (Haas et al., 2000), although the mechanisms have not been fully elucidated. One study suggested that sources of provider dissatisfaction are associated with restriction of choice of hospitals, strong influences of the managed care plan on practice, and types of financial incentives (Landon et al., 2002). These are issues that patients care about but may not experience directly because it is not always possible to know the choices that are not offered. If the goal of patient satisfaction research is to assess health plan quality and provide a basis for informed choice for consumers, understanding the relationship between patient and provider satisfaction or assessing provider satisfaction directly, particularly with issues of access that the patient may not be fully aware of (such as problematic financial assessments, restrictions

Table 8-3 Measures of Health Plan Satisfaction

Name of instrument	Source(s)	Items/time	Dimension	Reliability	Validity evaluated	Notes
Consumer Assessment of Health Plans Study (CAHPS 2.0)	Hargraves, 2003	46 items/ 20 minutes	Getting care quickly	Plan Rel/ICC	Construct	Mail, telephone administration
			Doctors who communicate	$0.94/\alpha = 0.58$		Supplemental items
			Courteous/helpful office staff	$0.88/\alpha = 0.86$		Confirmatory factor analysis
			Getting needed care	$0.90/\alpha = 0.75$		
			Customer service	$0.95/\alpha = 0.62$		
			Overall ratings:	$0.94/\alpha = 0.51$		
			Personal doctor or nurse	$0.88/\text{na}$		
				$0.82/\text{na}$		
			Quality of health care	$0.93/\text{na}$		
			Specialist health plan	$0.96/\text{na}$		

(continues)

Table 8-3   *(continued)*

Name of instrument	Source(s)	Items/time	Dimension	Reliability	Validity evaluated	Notes
Consumer Satisfaction Survey (CSS)	Davies, 1991	47 items	Access Finances Technical quality Communication Choice and continuity Interpersonal care Services covered Information Paperwork Costs of care General satisfaction Overall care Time spent Outcomes Overall quality Overall plan Plan satisfaction	subscales $\alpha = 0.80 - 0.97$	Content claimed predictive	Self, telephone, face-to-face

na, not applicable.

on treatments, or referrals offered) may be a useful adjunct in assessment of quality.

Consumer Assessment of Healthcare Providers (CAHPS). In 1995, the Agency for Health Care Policy and Research (AHCPR) (now the Agency for Healthcare Research and Quality, or AHRQ) sponsored a major collaborative effort headed by the Research Triangle Institute, RAND, and Harvard Medical School to develop a set of standardized, psychometrically tested instruments to evaluate consumers' experiences of health plans. That program remains in effect and has now addressed several aspects of care delivery. Originally called the Consumer Assessment of Health Plans Study survey, its name has been changed to reflect its broader coverage (see https://www.cahps.ahrq.gov/default.asp). Table 8-4 lists the family of CAHPS measures. The CAHPS 2.0 (now CAHPS 4.0) has become the most widely used survey instrument to evaluate patients' experiences of health plans (Hargraves, Hays, & Cleary, 2003) and has served as a model for explorations of satisfaction with other aspects of care. It has undergone extensive psychometric testing and two revisions since it was first introduced. CAHPS is designed to provide information to consumers rather than purchasers of health plans (AHCPR, 1996). Items were developed through extensive cognitive testing and focus groups, which resulted in a higher concentration of items concerning access, interpersonal skills, and communication and fewer items on provider technical skills. Further projects to develop instruments evaluating hospital care, individual providers, ambulatory care experience, nursing home care experiences, and research into cultural comparability, and the use of CAHPS results for quality improvement is ongoing (AHRQ, 2003a)

Table 8-4 The Family of CAHPS Measures

• CAHPS health plan survey
• CAHPS surveys at the medical group and individual provider level
• ECHO® survey (the CAHPS survey of behavioral health services)
• CAHPS hospital survey
• CAHPS in-center hemodialysis survey
• CAHPS nursing home surveys
• CAHPS people with mobility impairments survey

Consumer Satisfaction Survey. The Consumer Satisfaction Survey (CSS) was originally developed in 1988 by the Group Health Association of America (GHAA; Davies & Ware, 1991) to allow employers and business coalitions to compare satisfaction across health plans and other employee health benefit options. It was developed with the advice and input of health plans and employers and also used a number of items from the Patient Satisfaction Questionnaire-III. It utilizes the *excellent* to *poor* response scale, which some research suggests has superior psychometric properties (Ware & Hays, 1988). A second version of the CSS was released in 1991 and was expanded to include more health plan-specific features, such as range of services covered, availability of information, paperwork, and costs. The CSS has been extensively fielded by both mail and telephone procedures; national norms for several items are now available.

CSS contributed substantially to the Annual Member Health Care Survey (AMHCS) developed by the National Committee on Quality Assurance (Kippen, Strasser, & Joshi, 1997; NCQA, 1995). After CAHPS 1.0 was developed, the NCQA working together with AHCPR and the CAHPS consortium merged the CAHPS survey and AMHCS which resulted in a new core set of items and developed a Health Plan Employer Data and Information Set (HEDIS) supplement to the revised CAHPS core. This new instrument was called the CAPHS 2.0H and has been used for NCQA accreditation and with HEDIS since 1999 (AHRQ, 2003a).

Hospital

Both the literature review by Rubin (1990) and the review by Crow and colleagues (2002) found that nursing, physicians, interpersonal relations, and communication were important to patient satisfaction in the hospital setting (see Table 8-5). Physical environment or ward atmosphere is also important. Several studies found that patient and staff ratings of quality of care were particularly associated with assessments of overall quality of nursing, overall quality of medical care, and ward atmosphere (Rubin, 1990).

Hospital CAHPS. Hospital CAHPS (H-CAHPS) covers eight domains that were chosen through an extensive literature review, use of consumer focus groups, domains that were previously covered by CAHPS, and domains that performed well in terms of reliability and validity on pilot tests. Domains that the H-CAHPS developers chose not to include are billing, emergency room/department, emotional support, family, food privacy, technical skills, and convenience. H-CAHPS may also be combined with surveys that

Table 8-5   **Measures of Hospital Satisfaction**

Name of instrument	Source(s)	Items/time	Dimension	Reliability	Validity evaluated	Notes
Patient Judgments Hospital Quality (PJHQ)	Meterko, 1990	106 items	Admissions Nursing and daily care Medical care Hospital environment Information discharge	$\alpha = 0.87 - 0.95$ for subscales	Content claimed; construct; convergent; discriminant; predictive	Mail or telephone administration
H-CAHPS (draft)	CAHPS II AHRQ	32 items	Concern for patient Doctor Communication Medication Nursing services Discharge Information Pain control Physical Environment Global ratings (hospital care, doctor care, nursing care)	$A = 0.51 - 0.89$ composites	Construct	Pilot studies early 2004; Mail, telephone implementation summer 2005

hospitals currently use for internal purposes, which has the advantage of allowing comparison between hospital results for the core items but allows individual hospitals to customize the survey to evaluate issues particular to that hospital. Internal consistency reliability, hospital level reliability, and construct validity were tested during the pilot study. The study also looked at case mix differences, and potential response bias (AHRQ, 2003b).

Patient Judgments on Hospital Quality. The Patient Judgments on Hospital Quality (PJHQ) does not focus exclusively on patient satisfaction but also looks at how patients judge key attributes of hospital quality (Nelson, Hays, Larson, & Batalden, 1989). The survey items were constructed from literature reviews, preexisting questionnaires, focus groups with patients, and interviews with hospital administrators, physicians, and nurses. The survey development process has been extensively described in an eight-article supplement to the journal *Medical Care* (Meterko et al., 1990). In addition to the standard form, a short form containing 69 items has also been developed (Hays, Larson, Nelson, & Batalden, 1991). The PJHQ system has been used extensively in nonpoor populations with adult patients as well as with the parents of pediatric patients (McGee, Goldfield, Riley, & Morton, 1997). There is less information on its use with inpatients who have psychiatric or organic brain syndrome diagnoses or in poor populations.

Ambulatory Care

Ambulatory care encompasses a variety of care including preventive care, acute symptom care, and chronic care (Table 8-6). Issues of interpersonal relationships with providers, access and waiting times, and continuity of care are important. Although the importance of outcomes of care may vary depending on type of problem, outcomes clearly influence the satisfaction of patients presenting with acute physical problems (Jackson et al., 2001; Marple, Kroenke, Lucey, Wilder, & Lucas, 1997). When asking about a primary provider, it is important to note that women may have additional difficulties in completing survey instruments that assume only one primary care doctor, because women often see a gynecologist regularly either as their only doctor or in conjunction with their internist. Thus, they may be confused on items asking them to rate their regular doctor. The Women's Primary Care Satisfaction Survey was designed to overcome this problem and to be more focused on attributes of primary care that affect women (Scholle, Weisman, Anderson, & Camacho, 2004).

Table 8-6   Measures of Ambulatory Satisfaction

Name of instrument	Source(s)	Items/time	Domains	Reliability	Validity evaluated	Notes
Patient Satisfaction Questionnaire-Form III (PSQ III)	Marshall, et al., 1993	50 items/ 9–12 minutes	Interpersonal manner Communication Technical competence Time spent with dr. Financial aspects Access to care General satisfaction	$\alpha = 0.82 - 0.89$	Construct	
Visit-Specific Satisfaction Questionnaire (VSQ)	Ware, 1988	7 items	General satisfaction Technical care Interpersonal care Waiting time	subscales $\alpha = 0.82 - 0.94$	Construct	
A-CAHPS	Consumer Assessment of Healthcare Providers and Systems, 2004b		Access Doctor communication Office staff courtesy, helpfulness, respect Shared decision making Coordination/ integration Health promotion, education Customer service			In development

Ambulatory CAHPS. Ambulatory CAHPS (A-CAHPS) is a set of surveys currently under development for the evaluation of patient experiences and satisfaction with ambulatory care. The goal of CAHPS is to develop instruments that can assess patient satisfaction at a number of levels in the healthcare system, including sites of care and clinicians. The CAHPS developers identified the following domains as important functional areas in ambulatory care: access, doctor communication, coordination of care, shared decision making, office staff courtesy, helpfulness and respect, cultural sensitivity, customer service, health promotion, and education. For each level of the healthcare system, the plan is to have a question-naire that will consist of core items that will enable comparisons of result across survey users. It also will have supplemental items to allow greater focus on a specific function of the healthcare system or specific attri-butes of respondents. In addition, the survey will collect information on patients' global evaluations and the characteristics of survey respondents. Although a number of planned items for the surveys have been developed and tested, the CAHPS development team is in the process of soliciting input from stakeholders with respect to further items for each function and for how the functions fit into the various levels of the healthcare system (Health and Human Services/Agency for Healthcare Research and Quality, 2004b). Given that the health plan and hospital versions of the CAHPS survey have set a standard for evaluation of patient satisfaction in these areas, it is likely that A-CAHPS will accomplish the same thing in the area of ambulatory care.

Visit-Specific Satisfaction Instrument. The Visit-Specific Satisfaction Instrument (VSQ) was designed to be a focused, short instrument to measure satisfaction with specific features of care at the time of a specific medical visit (Ware & Hays, 1988). It was developed using prior visit-spe-cific satisfaction surveys as a guide. Several response formats were tested with the VSQ and the *excellent poor* format was ultimately recommended (Ware & Hays, 1988). Both a 51-item version and a 7-item version were psychometrically tested. A 9-item version was developed for use in the Medical Outcomes Study and remains available (Davies & Ware, 1991).

Patient Satisfaction Questionnaire III. The original Patient Satisfaction Questionnaire (PSQ) was developed by Ware in the 1970s and it origi-nally contained 80 items that were selected from a large pool of items obtained through extensive literature reviews, focus groups, analyses of reasons for disenrollment, and analyses of open-ended questions. It is one of the most commonly used measures of patient satisfaction (Ware & Karmos, 1976; Ware, Snyder, & Wright, 1976; Ware et al., 1983; Ware & Young, 1976). The current version is a 50-item instrument that uses a 5-point Likert response scale (*strongly agree* to *strongly disagree*) that was developed for use in the Medical Outcomes Study (Marshall, Hays, Sherbourne, & Wells, 1993). A short form, the PSQ-18, also exists that takes 3–4 minutes to complete; its subscales substantially correlate with those of the PSQ-III (Marshall et al., 1993).

Long-Term Care

Patient satisfaction is a major goal of long-term nursing care, and the essential domains focus on elements required for well-being and quality of life (see Table 8-7). Perhaps because long-term care has not been traditionally under medical auspices, nursing homes do not fit as well under a medical model; instead, psychosocial and environmental aspects of care predominate. A literature review of 16 nursing home instruments found through content analysis that the essential domains for nursing home satisfaction surveys are activities, care and services, caregivers, environment, meals, and well-being (Robinson, Lucas, Castle, Lowe, & Crystal, 2004). They noted that only 25% of instruments had solicited the opinions of nursing home residents in their development. The authors also interviewed a sample of nursing home residents in three New Jersey nursing homes. They identified essential content areas and found that 25% of these areas were covered by the New Jersey residents but not by the survey instruments. Items not in published surveys but identified as important by these nursing home residents were availability of outdoor activities, consistency of staff, good personal/grooming care, being treated as an adult, close proximity to family and friends, and opportunities to discuss concerns and problems (Robinson et al., 2004). Nursing home and long-term care surveys have important differences from surveys of other types of care (e.g., hospital, ambulatory). The instruments tend to rely more on interviews that can be subject to more psychosocial artifacts. It is helpful to have an instrument that is suitable for those with cognitive impairments. Often, family members or caretakers may assist in filling out or answering the questionnaires. Family members and caretakers are also used at times as proxies, although caution needs to be taken that surveys do not mix the results of the two because one study found

Table 8-7   Measures of Long-Term Care Satisfaction

Name of instrument	Source(s)	Items/time	Dimension	Reliability	Validity evaluated	Notes
NH-CAHPS	AHRQ					In development
Nursing Home Resident Satisfaction Scale (NHRSS)	Zinn, 1993	11 items	Physician services Nursing services Environment Global satisfaction	$\alpha = 0.69$–74 for subscales	Not reported	In-person interview
American Health Care Association Satisfaction Assessment Questionnaires (SAQs)	Case, 1996	87–113 items	Domains vary depending on population studied	None	none	In-person or telephone
Home Care Satisfaction Measure (HCSM)	Geron, 1997	61 items	Homemaker	Subscales: $\alpha = 0.46$–0.87	Construct by factor analysis and Pearson correlations	In-person interview
			Home health aide	$\alpha = 0.26$–0.83		
			Case management	$\alpha = 0.54$–0.88		
			Meal	$\alpha = 0.58$–0.88		
			Grocery	$\alpha = 0.49$–0.79		

| Home Care and Terminal Care Satisfaction Scale (HCTC) | McCusker, 1984 | 58 items (home care); 34 items (terminal care) | General satisfaction
Availability of care
Continuity of care
Physician availability
Physician competence
Personal qualities of physician
Communication with physician
Involvement of patient and family in treatment decisions
Freedom from pain
Pain control | Home care subscales: $\alpha = 0.10$–0.75
Caretaker subscales: $\alpha = 0.50$–0.85
Term Care subscales: $\alpha = 0.59$–0.90 | Face validity claimed
Convergent for several subscales
Discriminant for several subscales | Patient and caretaker satisfaction
In-person interview with patient (home care)/ surviving relative(TC)
Self-administered; caretaker |

that regular visitors tended to rate nursing home care more highly than residents (Gasquet, Dehe, Gaudebout, & Falissard, 2003). Finally, the concerns and satisfaction of family members/caretakers themselves may be important in evaluating long-term and terminal care (Atherly, Kane, & Smith, 2004).

CAHPS Nursing Home Survey. The Centers for Medicare and Medicaid Services (CMS) and the Agency for Healthcare Research and Quality (AHRQ) are working together to develop an instrument that can provide information on experiences of both short-term and long-term nursing home residents. They have conducted a national field test of a draft instrument and have produced some elements for a national study using the Minimum Data Set. The CAHPS team (NH-CAHPS) is also exploring the possibility of surveying family members of nursing home residents and their experiences with nursing homes (Consumer Assessment of Healthcare Providers and Systems, 2004a).

Nursing Home Resident Satisfaction Scale. The Nursing Home Resident Satisfaction Scale (NHRSS) was designed to be used as an indicator of nursing home quality and to provide feedback to nursing home administrators (Zinn, Lavizzo-Mourey, & Taylor, 1993). The items were selected based on a literature review and then tested and refined using a pilot study. The advantages of the NHRSS are that the interview is short, easy to administer, and the results are not affected by mild levels of cognitive impairment. However, the instrument validity is not known. In addition, the small pilot sample limits the amount of information on the generalizability of the instrument to other populations and sensitivity of the instrument to discriminate between facilities.

American Health Care Association Satisfaction Assessment Questionnaires. The American Health Care Association (AHCA) developed a set of satisfaction assessment questionnaires (SAQs) to measure the satisfaction with care of nursing residents and their families. There are separate SAQs for cognitively intact residents, rehabilitation residents, medically complex residents, family members of the cognitively intact and cognitively impaired residents, and residents of assisted living facilities. Guided by the six core principles identified as appropriate for the long-term industry (Case, 1996), the AHCA used a development process that included in-person and phone interviews conducted by the University of Wisconsin and nationwide polling of customers by the Gallup association (American Health Care Association, 1999). The questionnaires cover many domains. For example, the SAQ for cognitively intact residents examines overall satisfaction, family and community involvement, independence and respect, programs, facility setting, meals and dining, health care, doctor's care, staff, safety and security, roommates and other residents, and moving in/out. The surveys use a five-point *excellent poor* rating scale. The SAQs are widely used; however, a major disadvantage is that no psychometric testing of the instruments has been undertaken and thus in the absence of reliability and validity data, it is difficult to know how to interpret the results.

Home Care Satisfaction Measure. The Home Care Satisfaction Measure (HCSM) is used to assess the satisfaction of older adults with five common home care services: homemaker, home health aide, home-delivered meals, grocery, and case management services (Geron, 1997). The survey was developed using focus groups that included ethnic minorities and preexisting satisfaction measures from other types of healthcare services, and underwent further testing and refinement. The incorporation of the perspectives of the service recipients, including those of ethnic minorities, is an advantage of the HCSM. By looking at satisfaction with specific services, this instrument can be used as a guide for quality improvement projects, which is another advantage. However, because the survey excluded older adults whose cognitive impairments precluded a structured interview and because all the sampled participants received case management services, its generalizability may be limited, particularly in the subset of the older adult population with greater memory and cognitive impairments. In addition some of the reliabilities of the subscales were low, requiring cautious interpretation of its results.

Home Care and Terminal Care Satisfaction Scale. The Home Care and Terminal Care (HCTC) satisfaction scale was developed to measure the satisfaction of chronically and terminally ill patients and their families with home care as well as their preferences for location of care (McCusker, 1984). Three instruments were developed: one to measure the satisfaction of the patients themselves, to measure the evaluations of the patients' caretakers, and a third postbereavement version designed to be administered to caretakers following the patients' death. The instruments adapted items from previous acute care satisfaction measures and added items suggested by project investigators and staff. The measures were tested and revised. However, some subscales did not perform well and their use was not recommended. In addition, the timing of the administration of interviews may matter, particularly with the postbereavement version.

LITERATURE REVIEWS

In addition to the reviews already discussed that examined patient satisfaction in a particular healthcare setting, a major literature review of the measurement of satisfaction in health care was performed by Crow and associates (2002) as part of the National Health Service's (NHS) Technology Assessment Program. The goal of the review was to examine and summarize results of methodological studies, studies on the determinants of satisfaction in health care in different settings, as well as to determine where the gaps are in existing knowledge in order to point to future research. For methodological issues, they looked at studies examining modes of surveying and response rates as well as survey design issues. For the determinants of satisfaction, they reviewed studies looking at patient-related determinants such as expectations, health status, socioeconomic and demographic characteristics, and health service-related determinants. They examine health service-related determinants by setting and including general/primary care, inpatient hospital satisfaction, and hospital outpatient care as well as studies examining the patient-practitioner relationship (Crow et al., 2002).

SUMMARY

The development of the CAHPS generated interest in and substantial effort toward rigorous assessment of patients' experiences with health care and their overall satisfaction. This work is important for looking at healthcare performance and quality, but there are still a number of areas in patient satisfaction research that need exploration. Given that patients today are inundated with health information from the media, Internet, drug company advertising, and other sources, more work needs to be done on how patients form expectations and how these are changed or formed through the healthcare encounter. Patients' preferences of care and their rank ordering of the attributes of health care that affect their satisfaction still remains to be explored. Current patient satisfaction research focuses almost exclusively on the processes of care to the exclusion of outcomes. Research into outcomes is particularly important because providers often only assess physical outcomes, but it may be that functional, psychological, and social outcomes play a larger role in patient satisfaction. One criticism of using outcomes as a measure of quality is that one can have a high-quality process and a bad outcome. It seems that assessment of patient satisfaction can bridge that gap to some extent, because patients can still be satisfied with overall health care, even in the face of poor outcomes if they perceive that the process was good and the outcome was beyond the provider's control. Given the increasing use of patient satisfaction as a proxy for quality, it is particularly important to understand the relationship between patient perceptions of quality processes and quality outcomes.

REFERENCES

Abramowitz, S., Cote, A. A., & Berry, E. (1987). Analyzing patient satisfaction: A multianalytic approach. *Quality Review Bulletin, 13*(4), 122–130.

Agency for Health Care Policy and Research. (1996). *Technical overview of Consumer Assessment of Health Plans (CAHPS)* (AHCPR Pub. No. 97-R013). Rockville, MD:, Author.

Agency for Healthcare Research and Quality. (2003a). CAHPS® and the National CAHPS® Benchmarking Database: Fact sheet. Available at: https://www.cahps.ahrq.gov/. Accessed March 1, 2010.

Agency for Healthcare Research and Quality. (2003b, February 2003). Update on Hospital CAHPS (HCAHPS). Available at: http://www.ahrq.gov/qual/cahps/hcahpsupdate.htm. Accessed January 24, 2005.

Aharony, L., & Strasser, S. (1993). Patient satisfaction: What we know about and what we still need to explore. *Medical Care Review, 50*(1), 49–79.

American Health Care Association (AHCA). (1999). SAQ of the cognitively intact resident. Available at: http://www.ahcancal.org/research_data/quality/Documents/2006SatisfactionSurvey.pdf. Accessed June 29, 2010.

Atherly, A., Kane, R. L., & Smith, M. A. (2004). Older adults' satisfaction with integrated capitated health and long-term care. *Gerontologist, 44*(3), 348–357.

Barkley, W. M., & Furse, D. H. (1996). Changing priorities for improvement: The impact of low response rates in patient satisfaction. *The Joint Commission Journal on Quality Improvement, 22*(6), 427–433.

Ben-Sira, Z. (1976). The function of the professional's affective behavior in client satisfaction: a revised approach to social interaction theory. *Journal of Health & Social Behavior, 17*(1), 3–11.

Bender, R. H., Lance, T. X., & Guess, L. L. (2003). Including disenrollees in CAHPS managed care health plan assessment reporting. *Health Care Finance Review, 25*(1), 67–79.

Case, T. (1996). A quality assessment and improvement system for long-term care. *Quality Management in Health Care, 4*(3), 15–21.

Castle, N. G., & Engberg, J. (2004). Response formats and satisfaction surveys for elders. *Gerontologist, 44*(3), 358–367.

Cleary, P. D., & McNeil, B. J. (1988). Patient satisfaction as an indicator of quality care. *Inquiry, 25*(1), 25–36.

Crow, R., Gage, H., Hampson, S., Hart, J., Kimber, A., Storey, L., Thomas, H. (2002). The measurement of satisfaction with healthcare: Implications for practice from a systematic review of the literature. *Health Technology Assessment, 6*(32), 1–244.

Davies, A. R., & Ware, J. E. Jr. (1988). Involving consumers in quality of care assessment. *Health Affairs, 7*(1), 33–48.

Davies, A. R., & Ware, J. E. Jr. (1991). *GHAA's consumer satisfaction survey and user's manual* (2nd ed.). Washington, DC: Group Health Association of America.

DiMatteo, M. R., & Hays, R. (1980). The significance of patients' perceptions of physician conduct: A study of patient satisfaction in a family practice center. *Journal of Community Health, 6*(1), 18–34.

Donabedian, A. (1966). Evaluating the quality of medical care. *Millbank Memorial Fund Quarterly, 40*(3), 166–206.

Donabedian, A. (1988). The quality of care. How can it be assessed? *Journal of the American Medical Association, 260*(12), 1743–1748.

Edwards, C., Staniszweska, S., & Crichton, N. (2004). Investigation of the ways in which patients' reports of their satisfaction with health-care are constructed. *Sociology of Health & Illness, 26*(2), 159–183.

Eisen, S. V., & Grob, M. C. (1979). Assessing consumer satisfaction from letters to the hospital. *Hospital & Community Psychiatry, 30*(5), 344–347.

Fowler, F. J., Jr., Gallagher, P. M., Stringfellow, V. L., Zaslavsky, A. M., Thompson, J. W., & Cleary, P. D. (2002). Using telephone interviews to reduce nonresponse bias to mail surveys of health plan members. *Medical Care, 40*(3), 190–200.

Gasquet, I., Dehe, S., Gaudebout, P., & Falissard, B. (2003). Regular visitors are not good substitutes for assessment of elderly patient satisfaction with nursing home care and services. *Journal of Gerontology: Biological Sciences and Medical Sciences, 58*(11), 1036–1041.

Geron, S. M. (1997). *The Home Care Satisfaction Measures (HCSM): Study design and initial results of item analyses.* Boston: Boston University School of Social Work.

Greenfield, S., Kaplan, S., & Ware, J. E., Jr. (1985). Expanding patient involvement in care. Effects on patient outcomes. *Annals of Internal Medicine, 102*(4), 520–528.

Groves, R. M. (1989). *Survey errors and survey costs.* New York: Wiley.

Groves, R. M., Biemer, P. P., Lyberg, L. E., Massey, J. T., Nicholls, W. L., & Waksberg, J. (Eds.). (1988). *Telephone survey methodology.* New York: Wiley.

Haas, J. S., Cook, E. F., Puopolo, A. L., Burstin, H. R., Cleary, P. D., & Brennan, T. A. (2000). Is the professional satisfaction of general internists associated with patient satisfaction? *Journal of General Internal Medicine, 15*(2), 122–128.

Hall, J. A., & Dornan, M. C. (1988). Meta-analysis of satisfaction with medical care: Description of research domain and analysis of overall satisfaction levels. *Social Science and Medicine, 27*(6), 637–644.

Hargraves, J. L., Hays, R. D., & Cleary, P. D. (2003). Psychometric properties of the Consumer Assessment of Health Plans Study (CAHPS) 2.0 adult core survey. *Health Services Research, 38*(6 Pt 1), 1509–1527.

Harris-Kojetin, L. D., Fowler, F. J., Jr., Brown, J. A., Schnaier, J. A., & Sweeny, S. F. (1999). The use of cognitive testing to develop and evaluate CAHPS 1.0 core survey items. Consumer Assessment of Health Plans Study. *Medical Care, 37*(3 Suppl), MS10–MS21.

Hays, R. D., Larson, C., Nelson, E. C., & Batalden, P. B. (1991). Hospital quality trends: A short-form patient-based measure. *Medical Care, 29*(7), 661–668.

Hays, R. D., & Ware, J. E., Jr. (1986). My medical care is better than yours: Social desirability and patient satisfaction ratings. *Medical Care, 24*(6), 519–524.

Hendriks, A. A., Vrielink, M. R., Smets, E. M., van Es, S. Q., & De Haes, J. C. (2001). Improving the assessment of (in)patients' satisfaction with hospital care. *Medical Care, 39*(3), 270–283.

Hickson, G. B., Clayton, E. W., Entman, S. S., Miller, C. S., Githens, P. B., Whetten-Goldstein, K., Sloan, F. A. (1994). Obstetricians' prior malpractice experience and patients' satisfaction with care. *Journal of the American Medical Association, 272*(20), 1583–1587.

Hudak, P. L., McKeever, P., & Wright, J. G. (2003). The metaphor of patients as customers: Implications for measuring satisfaction. *Journal of Clinical Epidemiology, 56*(2), 103–108.

Hudak, P. L., McKeever, P. D., & Wright, J. G. (2004). Understanding the meaning of satisfaction with treatment outcome. *Medical Care, 42*(8), 718–725.

Jackson, J. L., Chamberlin, J., & Kroenke, K. (2001). Predictors of patient satisfaction. *Social Science and Medicine, 52*(4), 609–620.

Joffe, S., Manocchia, M., Weeks, J. C., & Cleary, P. D. (2003). What do patients value in their hospital care? An empirical perspective on autonomy centred bioethics. *Journal of Medical Ethics, 29*(2), 103–108.

Kane, R. L., Maciejewski, M., & Finch, M. (1997). The relationship of patient satisfaction with care and clinical outcomes. *Medical Care*, *35*(7), 714–730.

Keating, N. L., Green, D. C., Kao, A. C., Gazmararian, J. A., Wu, V. Y., & Cleary, P. D. (2002). How are patients' specific ambulatory care experiences related to trust, satisfaction, and considering changing physicians? *Journal of General Internal Medicine*, *17*(1), 29–39.

Kippen, L. S., Strasser, S., & Joshi, M. (1997). Improving the quality of the NCQA (National Committee for Quality Assurance) Annual Member Health Care Survey Version 1.0. *American Journal of Managed Care*, *3*(5), 719–730.

Kravitz, R. L., Callahan, E. J., Paterniti, D., Antonius, D., Dunham, M., & Lewis, C. E. (1996). Prevalence and sources of patients' unmet expectations for care. *Annals of Internal Medicine*, *125*(9), 730–737.

Krupat, E., Fancey, M., & Cleary, P. D. (2000). Information and its impact on satisfaction among surgical patients. *Social Sciences Medicine*, *51*(12), 1817–1825.

Landon, B. E., Aseltine, R., Jr., Shaul, J. A., Miller, Y., Auerbach, B. A., & Cleary, P. D. (2002). Evolving dissatisfaction among primary care physicians. *American Journal of Managed Care*, *8*(10), 890–901.

Lasek, R. J., Barkley, W., Harper, D. L., & Rosenthal, G. E. (1997). An evaluation of the impact of nonresponse bias on patient satisfaction surveys. *Medical Care*, *35*(6), 646–652.

Ley, P., Bradshaw, P. W., Kincey, J. A., & Atherton, S. T. (1976). Increasing patients' satisfaction with communications. *British Journal of Social & Clinical Psychology*, *15*(4), 403–413.

Locander, W., Sudman, S., & Bradburn, N. (1976). An investigation of interview method, threat and response distortion. *Journal of the American Statistical Associations*, *71*(354), 269–275.

Marple, R. L., Kroenke, K., Lucey, C. R., Wilder, J., & Lucas, C. A. (1997). Concerns and expectations in patients presenting with physical complaints: Frequency, physician perceptions and actions, and 2-week outcome. *Archives of Internal Medicine,* *157*(13), 1482–1488.

Marshall, G. N., Hays, R. D., Sherbourne, C. D., & Wells, K. B. (1993). The structure of patient satisfaction with outpatient medical care. *Psychological Assessment, 5*(4), 477–483.

Mazor, K. M., Clauser, B. E., Field, T., Yood, R. A., & Gurwitz, J. H. (2002). A demonstration of the impact of response bias on the results of patient satisfaction surveys. *Health Services Research, 37*(5), 1403–1417.

McCusker, J. (1984). Development of scales to measure satisfaction and preferences regarding long-term and terminal care. *Medical Care, 22*(5), 476–493.

McGee, J., Goldfield, N., Riley, K., & Morton, J. (1997). *Collecting information from health care consumers: A resource manual of tested questionnaires and practical advice.* Gaithersburg, MD: Aspen Publishers, Inc.

Mead, N., & Bower, P. (2000). Patient-centredness: A conceptual framework and review of the empirical literature. *Social Sciences Medicine, 51*(7), 1087–1110.

Meterko, M., Nelson, E. C., & Rubin, H. R. (1990). Patient judgments of hospital quality: report of a pilot study. *Medical Care, 28*(9 Suppl), S1–S56.

National Committee for Quality Assurance. (1995). *Annual Member Health Care Survey Manual, Version 1.0.* Washington, DC: Author.

Nelson, E. C., Hays, R. D., Larson, C., & Batalden, P. B. (1989). The patient judgment system: Reliability and validity. *Quality Review Bulletin, 15*(6), 185–191.

Oliver, R. L. (1993). Cognitive, affective, and attribute bases of the satisfaction response. *Journal of Consumer Research, 20*(3), 418–430.

Pascoe, G. C. (1983). Patient satisfaction in primary health care: A literature review and analysis. *Evaluation & Program Planning, 6*(3–4), 185–210.

Robinson, J. P., Lucas, J. A., Castle, N. G., Lowe, T. J., & Crystal, S. (2004). Consumer satisfaction in nursing homes: Current practices and residence priorities. *Research on Aging, 26*(4), 454–481.

Rubin, H. R. (1990). Can patients evaluate the quality of hospital care? *Medical Care Review, 47*(3), 267–326.

Scholle, S. H., Weisman, C. S., Anderson, R. T., & Camacho, F. (2004). The development and validation of the primary care satisfaction survey for women. *Womens Health Issues, 14*(2), 35–50.

Singer, E., Von Thurn, D. R., & Miller, E. R. (1995). Confidentiality assurances and response: A qualitative review of the experimental literature. *Public Opinion Quarterly, 59*(1), 66–77.

Sitzia, J., & Wood, N. (1997). Patient satisfaction: A review of issues and concepts. *Social Science & Medicine, 45*(12), 1829–1843.

Sitzia, J., & Wood, N. (1998). Response rate in patient satisfaction research: An analysis of 210 published studies. *International Journal for Quality in Health Care, 10*(4), 311–317.

Smith, M. A., Shussler-Fiorenza, C., & Rockwood, T. (2005). Satisfaction with care. In R. L. Kane (Ed.), *Understanding healthcare outcomes research* (pp. 185–216). Sudbury, MA: Jones and Bartlett Publishers.

Strasser, S., Aharony, L., & Greenberger, D. (1993). The patient satisfaction process: Moving toward a comprehensive model. *Medical Care Review, 50*(2), 219–248.

Thompson, A. G., & Sunol, R. (1995). Expectations as determinants of patient satisfaction: Concepts, theory and evidence. *International Journal for Quality in Health Care, 7*(2), 127–141.

US Department of Health and Human Services, Agency for Health Care Policy and Research. (2004a, March 31). The CAHPS Nursing Home Survey. Available at: http://www.cahps-sun.org/Products/NHCAHPS/NHCAHPSIntro.asp. Accessed January 2005.

US Department of Health and Human Services, Agency for Health Care Policy and Research. (2004b). *An introduction to ambulatory CAHPS*. Rockville, MD: Author.

Ware, J. E. Jr., Davies-Avery, A., & Stewart, A. L. (1978). The measurement and meaning of patient satisfaction. *Health and Medical Care Review, 1,* 1–15.

Ware, J. E. Jr., & Hays, R. D. (1988). Methods for measuring patient satisfaction with specific medical encounters. *Medical Care, 26*(4), 393–402.

Ware, J. E. Jr., & Karmos, A. H. (1976). *Development and validation of scales to measure patient satisfaction with health care services: Volume II. Perceived health and patient role propensity* (Final rept. 30 Jun 72–31 Mar 76, Vol. 274). Carbondale, IL: Southern Illinois University.

Ware, J. E. Jr., Snyder, M. K., & Wright, W. R. (1976). *Development and validation of scales to measure patient satisfaction with health care services: Volume I. Part B. Results of scales constructed from the patient satisfaction questionnaire and other health care perceptions* (Final rept. 30 Jun 72–31 Mar 76, Vol. 447). Carbondale, IL: Southern Illinois University.

Ware, J. E. Jr., Snyder, M. K., Wright, W. R., & Davies, A. R. (1983). Defining and measuring patient satisfaction with medical care. *Evaluation & Program Planning, 6*(3–4), 247–263.

Ware, J. E. Jr., & Young, J. (1976). *Development and validation of scales to measure patient satisfaction with health care services: Volume III. Conceptualization and measurement of health as a value.* (Final rept. 30 Jun 72–31 Mar 76, Vol. 203). Carbondale, IL: Southern Illinois University.

Weithman, P. J. (1995). Contractualist liberalism and deliberative democracy. *Philosophy and Public Affairs, 24*(4), 314–343.

Wensing, M., Grol, R., & Smits, A. (1994). Quality judgements by patients on general practice care: A literature analysis. *Social Science & Medicine, 38*(1), 45–53.

Williams, B. (1994). Patient satisfaction: A valid concept? *Social Science & Medicine, 38*(4), 509–516.

Williams, B., Coyle, J., & Healy, D. (1998). The meaning of patient satisfaction: an explanation of high reported levels. *Social Science & Medicine, 47*(9), 1351–1359.

Williams, S., Pauly, M. V., Rosenbaum, P. R., Ross, R., Schwartz, J. S., Shpilsky, A., & Silber, J. H. (1996). Ranking hospitals by the quality of care for medical conditions: The role of complications. *Transactions of the American Clinical & Climatological Association, 107,* 263–273.

Zaslavsky, A. M., Zaborski, L. B., & Cleary, P. D. (2002). Factors affecting response rates to the Consumer Assessment of Health Plans Study survey. *Medical Care, 40*(6), 485–499.

Zinn, J. S., Lavizzo-Mourey, R., & Taylor, L. (1993). Measuring satisfaction with care in the nursing home setting: The nursing home resident satisfaction scale. *The Journal of Applied Gerontology, 12*(4), 452–465.

CHAPTER 9

Demographic, Psychologic, and Social Factors[1]

Almost every study design will include demographic factors. It is hard to imagine a proposal that does not include information on at least age and gender. It is virtually de rigueur, even when there is no clear reason to suspect that these factors will affect the outcomes of interest. One might almost say it is better to be safe than sorry.

At the other extreme, we know (or certainly strongly suspect) that demographic factors affect the outcomes of many interventions. Wealth, insurance coverage, and education, along with cultural values and beliefs, will influence the likelihood that people get treated and the extent to which they adhere to that treatment. It is often hard to separate racial disparity from cultural preference, but a growing literature suggests it is possible.

There is good evidence to show that social support, including marital status, can positively affect one's survival well-being.

On the flip side some sociodemographic factors may be outcomes in themselves, rather than independent variables. The ability to work, having meaningful social roles, and relationships may be outcomes on their own. In a perverse twist, one might argue that even your age, which reflects your survival, is an important outcome.

Thus, psychosocial variables can be outcomes (dependent variables), things that affect outcomes (independent variables), or things that one

---

[1]This chapter draws on material from an earlier work by Todd Rockwood and Melissa Constantine (2005).

controls for in the analysis (control variables). Figure 9-1 illustrates how depression might be used in each capacity. In the top part of the figure, depression is illustrated as the primary outcome of the research. The intent of the research is to focus on the impact that counseling and returning to work has on depression that emerges as a response to some type of traumatic loss. In the middle, depression is an independent variable; that is, returning to work after a traumatic loss could be influenced both by an individual receiving counseling as well as the severity of their depression, which is viewed here as not being the result per se of the loss. In the final instance, depression is used as a control variable; the purpose of the research is to evaluate how much influence counseling has on returning to work after a traumatic loss, controlling for the of severity of depression where the depression may result from the loss.

Psychosocial phenomena are not always straightforward (Blalock, 1974; Bohrnstedt & Borgatta, 1981; Campbell & Russo, 2001; Summers, 1970).

Figure 9-1   Depression as a dependent, independent, and control variable

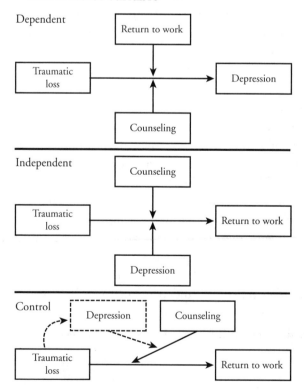

They can be objective and directly observable, subjective and not observable, or both. Thus, the use of these variables must be carefully thought out at all levels (conceptually, operationally, and analytically) (Campbell & Overman, 1988; Campbell & Russo, 2001). Simply measuring them because others do, or doing so because they might be relevant, can lead to problems.

Demographic, psychological, and social phenomena cover a wide range from directly observable characteristics or events, such as sex and social interaction, to abstract constructs, such as depression and anxiety. A brief example illustrates some of the complexity involved in the conceptualization, measurement, and analytic usage of demographic, psychological, and social variables. When one is asked about sex, a range of things could be considered relevant. It becomes important to think not just about what one means when one says "sex" but what its purpose is in research (dependent, independent, or control variable) and how one intends to measure it. Almost every study measures sex as male or female, but there are problems with such measurement. If the focus is on gender identity or role, it is not safe to assume that this is what has been measured if all one has determined is male or female. Alternatively, a significant difference among the sexes might reflect differences in how males versus females were treated, and thus the inference should be about treatment, not about sex. In an outcomes research study on fertility, reproductive physiology would be important. Alternatively, in a study focusing on depression, gender identity might be equally or more important.

In developing outcomes research, it is important to identify at the beginning of the research what role, if any, psychosocial variables play in the research. Their thoughtless inclusion can lead to spurious findings. If a psychosocial variable is not the outcome (dependent variable), then prior to including it in the study one needs to consider whether the variable is expected to have a relationship to the outcome or whether it is needed as a control variable. The latter role implies that it my either have an effect on the outcome or may affect the way another independent variable influences the outcome.

DEMOGRAPHIC FACTORS

Demography is the study of populations (Shryock, Siegel, & Stockwell, 1976; Weeks, 1981). The old joke goes that most people can be broken down by age and sex, but other variables should also be considered. The following discussion is not meant to be an exhaustive list of demographic variables, but instead highlights some of the major ones that are used in outcomes research.

Age

In outcomes research, and in fact almost all research, age is measured chronologically—the amount of time a person has been alive. How age is measured should depend primarily upon the nature of the research question. Most people think of age as the time that has elapsed since birth, but gerontologists view age in terms of the force of mortality or the likelihood of dying. This concept is more akin to the idea of real age (i.e., one's biological age taking into account factors that affect the likelihood of death). Thus, someone in good health may be "younger" than their chronological age and vice versa. However, current measures of real age have been primarily used for commercial purposes and have not yet demonstrated good validity, and thus should be used judiciously in outcomes research.

One can treat age as a continuous variable, which implies that its effect is more or less constant. Alternatively, one may expect that there is some inflection point, when the age effect is maximized. In the latter instance it would be better to treat age as categorical. The size of the categories should be commensurate with the effect one seeks. Typically, decades will suffice, but sometimes 5-year increments may be needed. In general, if you collect age as a continuous variable, you can create categories post hoc, but it is difficult to go the other way.

Residence

In outcomes research, two issues around residence can be of concern. Location can be used for many different purposes: as an indicator of access to health services, in general or particular types (e.g., a tertiary care facility), but also as a factor directly related to other issues associated with health (exposure). At the grossest level, it can be identified as rural or urban. Data with geographic distinctions often comes from secondary sources that are linked to primary data collection. The Area Resource File (www.arfsys.com) contains a wealth of information regarding healthcare issues at the county level from data available from the census bureau as well as health-related studies such as the Behavioral Risk Factor Surveillance Survey (www.cdc.gov/brfss). The key to using this data is ensuring that data collected from study participants allows one to link the primary data to these secondary resources, such as county of residence, zip code, actual street address (if permitted by the institutional review board [IRB]), or nearest intersection when an address cannot be obtained.

It has become increasingly popular to use geographic residence as an indirect measure of socioeconomic status (SES) by attributing the mean income value of the census track where a person lives to the individual. This works on average but raises a lot of problems in assuming that every resident shares the mean value.

The second, often ignored aspect of residence, is the characteristics of the dwelling in which one lives or the larger built environment that surrounds each resident (Diez Roux, 2003; Jackson, 2003; Northridge, Sclar, & Biswas, 2003; Rubin, 1998). The built environment can affect health, safety, and function (Lucy, 2003; Rubin, 1998). For example, in an outcomes study of recovery following hip surgery for individuals who return to home, having to climb stairs may make a big difference. As more attention is devoted to this area with a focus on public health and community (Perdue, Gostin, & Stone, 2003), the importance of the built environment is reflected in diverse research, from how hospitals are built to floor plans for homes (Douglas & Douglas, 2004).

Race

Although in health research, race and ethnicity are often mistakenly treated as synonymous, the historically assumed correlation between them is decreasing. The Census Bureau distinguishes them, and this classification is typically used. It is helpful to use consistent and familiar categories; however, the purpose of the variable in the analytic model in hand should ultimately determine the way the variable is measured (see Table 9-1 for the census classifications). The numerous definitions of race essentially converge around a common theme—a population that lives within a specified geographic area and shares the same gene pool. Given the mobility in contemporary society, the historical notion and importance of race is rapidly diminishing, although in a few instances— such as diabetes and obesity in the Pima community—race might be still be relevant (Bennett, 1999; Imperatore, Knowler, Nelson, & Hanson, 2001; Lillioja & Bogardus, 1988; Pratley, 1998; Ravussin, 1993). There is the danger of the ecologic fallacy, whereby characteristics or outcomes that are associated with a population are attributed to individuals within that population. Attention to race may focus on genetic factors, which are

Table 9-1   Census Bureau (National Institutes of Health)
Classifications of Race and Ethnicity

Ethnic Category	Racial Category
Hispanic or Latino	American Indian/Alaska Native
Non-Hispanic or Latino	Asian
	Native Hawaiian or Other Pacific Islander
	Black or African American
	White

attributes or characteristics of an individual, not a population. Although the genetic predisposition for a condition could be distributed throughout the population, it is critical to distinguish between genotypic attributes of an individual and the phenotypic attributes expressed in a population.

There are problems with trying to infer ethnicity from race (Snipp, 2003; Takeuchi & Gage, 2003). Ethnicity refers to a set of cultural factors that identify a person as belonging to a group. The historical correlation between race and ethnicity is declining, especially in industrialized nations. Thus, the temptation to infer ethnicity from race needs to be discouraged. African American is not a race; it is not necessarily even an ethnicity; it could even represent multiple subcultures within a single city. Even issues that might appear simple, such as the use of tobacco in Southeast Asians, demonstrate significant ethnic and cultural differences between Hmong, Vietnamese, Laotians, and Cambodians.

Marital Status

Marital status is generally loosely used to denote some sort of civil arrangement that reflects a legally binding relationship that is recognized by the state. Given the shifting pattern of arrangements between sexes, the term needs greater attention and the rules for inclusion should be carefully considered. In general, it classifies people's arrangement along a trichotomized axis: never, current, and past (divorced, widowed). In self-report (survey research), the variable is generally operationalized as: Are you currently: (1) married or living in a marriage-like relationship, (2) widowed, (3) divorced, or (4) single. Although options 2 and 3 are a subset of 4, those states can significantly impact the individual, and thus they are kept as separate categories. The simple nonjudged existence of a stable relationship has been shown to affect a variety of outcomes. In general, married people fare better than unmarried. Divorce and widowhood may represent life stresses.

Marriage may also have a deeper implication, reflecting the presence or absence of characteristics associated with relationship(s), intimacy, support (i.e., emotional, physical, fiduciary, etc.), and issues related to the stability and permanency in roles and behavior.

Marital status could be an outcome as well. For example, a study of caregiving or the death of a child might examine the toll it took on marital relationships.

Social Economic Status

Social economic status (SES) is most frequently used as an independent variable; it has been demonstrated to be related to a spectrum of health outcomes and diseases, from outcomes associated with cardiovascular disease (Kaplan & Keil, 1993) to dementia (Cobb, Wolf, Au, White, & D'Agostino, 1995). Measures of SES range from measures that utilize relatively few variables (such as residence, income, occupation, and education) to recently developed measures that focus on social capital (Oakes & Rossi, 2003) (see Table 9-2).

Table 9-2 Measures of Socioeconomic Status

Instrument	Description
Hollingshead Index of Social Position (Hollingshead, 1957; Hollingshead & Redlich, 1958)	SES measure originally based on three factors: residence (location), occupation, and education; given the complexity of coding residence, the two factor model in which residence is omitted is traditionally used.
Duncan Socioeconomic Index (Duncan, 1961)	SES measure based on three factors: occupation, income, and education; note that the coding of occupation is complex and revised frequently
Nam-Powers Socioeconomic Score (Nam & Powers, 1983)	SES measure based on three factors: education, occupation, and income (see www.ssc.wisc.edu/cde/cdewp/96-10.pdf for methodology)

Historically, measures of SES, such as the indexes developed by Hollingshead (1957; Hollingshead & Redlich, 1958), Duncan (1961), or Nam-Powers (Nam & E.W., 1986) have dominated the measurement of SES. Both Duncan's and Nam-Powers' indexes use three variables: income, education, and occupation. The instruments vary in terms of the weight assigned to each of the three different variables. Both draw on the US Census Bureau's coding system for occupation; and, as a result, if the methodology is used, it is essential to use the most recent coding for occupation. In comparison, the Hollingshead index uses two variables: income and a relatively simple coding of occupation (seven levels). What is often ignored in the usage of these indexes is the original intent behind the development of the measures; they were developed as measures of social stratification and social class. These measures reflect a notion of class that dominated social thought from the late 1800s to the mid-1900s. Recent studies have demonstrated the importance of moving away from such classical notions by noting the importance of economic variables in the study of health and SES (Daly, Duncan, McDonough, & Williams, 2002). Alternatively, new concepts, such as social capital, have emerged, which may prove to be more useful in the study of outcomes than the traditional concept of SES.

PSYCHOLOGIC FACTORS

Mind–Body Connection

Psychological factors are complicated. The mind–body concept can be related to traditional Western medical research, but it is especially strong in complementary and alternative medicine.

Measures regarding the mind–body connection can be useful in outcomes research in particular areas, such as behavioral medicine (e.g., irritable bowel syndrome, fibromyalgia, etc.). One especially relevant area is the placebo effect, which can apply to all sorts of practice, including surgery (Moseley et al., 2002).

A number of constructs can be subsumed under the general heading of mind–body connection. Table 9-3 summarizes these; they are discussed as follows.

Table 9-3 Mind–Body Measures

Domain	Instrument	Description
Well-being	General Well-Being Schedule (Fazio, 1977)	Developed for the National Center for Health Statistics, this is intended to measure well-being in the general population.
	Index of Well-Being (Campbell et al., 1976)	Composed of eight semantic differential items and one life satisfaction item
Locus of Control		
General	Spheres of Control Battery (Paulhus, 1983)	Three dimensional measures focusing on: 1. Personal efficacy (control over one's own life) 2. Interpersonal control (expectancies of outcomes in social situations) 3. Sociopolitical control (perception of ability to influence society)
	Internality, Powerful Others, and Chance Scales (Levenson, 1981)	Three scales focusing on different aspects of life: 1. Internality (perception of control over one's own life) 2. Powerful others (belief that others control events in one's life) 3. Chance (belief that chance determines events and outcomes in life)
Health Locus of Control	Multidimensional Health Locus of Control Scale (Wallston & Wallston, 1981)	Three dimensional instrument for health-specific locus of control based upon Levenson's (Levenson, 1981) conceptual framework: 1. Internal (individual is in control of their own health) 2. Chance (health/illness are because of chance) 3. Powerful others (health/illness are in control of external agents)

(continues)

Table 9-3 *(continued)*

Domain	Instrument	Description
	Mental Health Locus of Control Scale (Hill & Bale, 1980)	Bipolar instrument focused on beliefs about control relative to therapeutic changes. Pole 1: internal (patient is responsible for changes) Pole 2: therapist (therapist is responsible for changes)
Pain		
General	Visual Analog Scales (VAS) and Numeric Rating Scales (NRS) (McDowell & Newell, 1996) Standardization of Self-Reported Pain (Kane et al., 2002)	VAS includes a range of methods from 10 on horizontal or vertical lines. NRS usually range from 0 to 10. Poles in both versions are usually labeled *no pain* (0) and *pain* as bad as it could be, worst pain imaginable, or unbearable (10).
	McGill Pain Questionnaire (Turk & Melzack, 1992; Turk et al., 1985)	Weighted scale designed to profile three aspects of pain: 1. Sensory–discriminative 2. Motivational–affective 3. Cognitive–evaluative
	Medical Outcomes Study Pain Measures (Stewart & Ware, 1992)	Basic multi-item measure intended to measure the impact of pain on daily living; not intended to provide a detailed measure of pain
	Pain and Distress Scale (Zung, 1983)	Measure intended to assess mood and behavior changes associated with acute pain
Specific		
Cancer	Brief Pain Inventory (Cleeland, 1991)	Measures two aspects of pain: 1. Sensory 2. Functional limitations arising from pain

Back	Oswestry Low Back Pain Disability Questionnaire (Fairbank et al., 1980)	Instrument focuses on the impact of pain and contains a rating of pain intensity and assessment of the impact of pain in nine areas: personal care, lifting, walking, sitting, standing, sleeping, sex life, social life, and traveling.
	Back Pain Classification Scale (Leavitt & Garron, 1979a, 1979b)	Screening tool developed for clinical use to discriminate between back pain arising from psychological versus physiological factors
Fatigue/ Insomnia	Fatigue, Energy, Consciousness, Energized and Sleepiness (Shapiro et al., 2002)	Adjective checklist developed to assess function in five areas: fatigue, energy, consciousness, energized, and sleepiness.
Stress		
Perceived	Perceived Stress Questionnaire (Cohen et al., 1983)	Short 10-item survey focused on perception of stress and ability to deal with stress
	Perceived Stress Questionnaire (Levenstein et al., 1993)	Longer instrument assessing perceived stress; contains seven subscales: harassment, overload, irritability, lack of joy, fatigue, worries, and tension
Experiences	Social Readjustment Rating Scale (Holmes & Rahe, 1967)	Event checklist that contains a weighted value of the amount of stress for each event
	Life Stressors and Social Resources Inventory (LISRES; Impara & Plake, 1998)	The LISRES measures two aspects: life stressors (nine subscales) and social resources (seven subscales). Assessment occurs for eight domains: physical health status, housing and neighborhood, finances, work, relationship with spouse or partner, relationships with children, relationships with extended family, and relationships with friends and social groups.

(continues)

Table 9-3   *(continued)*

Domain	Instrument	Description
	Life Stressor Checklist–Revised (Wolfe & Kimerling, 1997)	Screen of life events that meet the definition of a trauma according to *DSM-IV*; assess occurrence, symptomatology, and functioning for 30 events
Other	Illness Behavior Questionnaire (Pilowsky & Spence, 1983)	Assessment of adjustment/responses to illness that are not functional, including hypochondriacal, denial, and changes in effect.
	Readiness to Change–Alcohol (Rollnick et al., 1992) –Drugs (Hodgins, 2001) –Smoking (McConnaughy et al., 1983)	Instruments have been developed to assess a wide range of health-related issues based on the model of readiness by Prochaska and colleagues (Prochaska et al., 1992; Prochaska & Norcross, 2001)

Well-Being

Well-being can range widely, from economic well-being to emotional well-being. Measures of well-being overlap substantially with the construct of health-related quality of life (HRQL) is discussed in Chapter 6. Measures of well-being, while health influenced, do not specifically measure a direct relationship between health status and well-being. The measures are general in nature and thus should be used only when general well-being is relevant; otherwise measures of HRQL should be used. Two commonly used measures of well-being are the General Well-Being Schedule (Fazio, 1977) and the Index of Well-Being (Campbell, Converse, & Rodgers, 1976).

Locus of Control

Locus of control in health research is an outgrowth of psychological work on mastery and efficacy (Rotter, 1966). Many scales have been developed to represent different conceptualizations of the concept of control. Although most share internal and external aspects ("my life is under my control," "my life is controlled by the environment around me"), others recognize the role of chance (see Levenson, 1981) and environmental influence (the ability of individuals to change their social environment; see Paulhus, 1983).

Instruments created in this area, which emerged 30 years ago, have been used extensively for health research. Such instruments can be sued as dependent variables (programs to empower patients), independent variables (to explain the success of intervention), and as controls (to evaluate the outcomes of an intervention controlling for the subjects' beliefs about who or what is responsible for their health). The two most commonly utilized instruments are the Multidimensional Health Locus of Control scale (MHLCS; Wallston & Wallston, 1981) and the Mental Health Locus of Control (MHLC; Hill & Bale, 1980). The MHLC is drawn primarily from conceptualizations of locus of control (Levenson, 1981).

Pain

Pain is a frequently used measure, but remains poorly understood. Few individuals have not experienced pain, but the pain experience is not necessarily shared. Pain is a complex construct that reflects combined physiological, psychological, and social forces.

The most commonly used measures of pain are simple visual analog scale (VAS), usually 10cm long or numeric rating scale (NRS; e.g., 0–10) with the ends anchored with no pain and worst pain imaginable (McDowell & Newell, 1996). Although these scales are useful in assessing pain for treatment and even demonstrate utility in research, they have drawbacks. Given the personal differences in the pain experience, the ability to compare pain scores among individuals or across populations is limited. Methods have been proposed by which responses to VAS or NRS could be standardized to facilitate such comparisons, using relatively few items (Kane, Bershadsky, Lin, Rockwood, & Wood, 2002).

Pain measurement may be simple or researchers may opt to describe the nature of the pain in great detail, including many attributes of the pain. The decision is based on the nature of the outcome sought. Because clinicians are usually interested in large effects, simple measures may suffice. Frequency and intensity may be the most relevant elements. Many diverse instruments have been developed to assess pain. The Brief Pain Inventory (Daut, Cleeland, & Flanery, 1983) includes information on the location(s) of pain, its severity, and its quality. The McGill Pain

Questionnaire focuses on the sensory nature of the pain (Turk & Melzack, 1992; Turk, Rudy, & Salovey, 1985). Several instruments address pain and function, such as the MOS Pain Measure (Stewart & Ware, 1992). Some general measures have been adapted for specific purposes. For example, in orthopedics research, the Low Back Pain Disability Questionnaire (Fairbank, Couper, Davies, & O'Brien, 1980) focuses on the relationship between pain and function. Alternatively, research in fibromyalgia would probably be better served by combining several measures, such as the Brief Pain Inventory, which focuses on severity and quality of the pain, and the McGill Pain Questionnaire, which would provide information regarding the sensory aspect of the pain experience.

Stress

The concept of stress is often unrecognized in outcomes research, perhaps because of the diversity in conceptualization and content. Types of stress can range from emotional, physiological, social, and even economic. Stress is subjective; it can be either perceive or experienced. If stress is a focus of the research, it is often important to include measures of both perception of stress and stressful experiences, as well as measures of resources that can be used to deal with stress (such as the Life Stressors and Social Resources Inventory; Impara & Plake, 1998). One widely used, but potentially flawed measure ranked a series of life events on perceptions of individuals' ability to deal with stressful events—the Social Readjustment Rating Scale (Holmes & Rahe, 1967). The Perceived Stress Questionnaire (Cohen, Kamarck, & Mermelstein, 1983) instrument would be more consistent with their conceptual definition of stress.

Other

Instruments such as the Illness Behavior Questionnaire (Pilowsky & Spence, 1983) focus on nonfunctional adjustment or responses to illnesses such as those just identified.

A frequently salient concept is readiness to change. Primarily based on the work of Prochaska, "stages of change" research classifies people in terms of their readiness to adopt a new behavior, such as stopping smoking or starting to exercise (Hodgins, 2001; McConnaughy, Prochaska, & Velicer, 1983; Prochaska, DiClemente, & Norcross, 1992; Prochaska & Norcross, 2001; Rollnick, Heather, Gold, & Hall, 1992).

Affect

Among psychological factors, affect has received the most attention in outcomes research. Again, this construct can be used as both a dependent and an independent variable. Construct validity becomes very important with regard to affect states like depression, where physiological manifestations, such as sleep, diet, alertness, and awareness, are often associated with the state. It is not always clear when the physiological symptom is attributable to the affect or even possibly its cause. Moreover, they may be in contradiction with one another; sleeping a lot as well as sleep disruptions, or increased and decreased appetite, are both considered signs of depression. Most affect concepts involved in health outcomes research are characterized as "negative emotions," but there can be positive feelings as well. Affect can be both a state and a diagnosis. Most of the time health outcomes researchers are concerned about the state and do not require a certified diagnosis. For example, a researcher who wanted to include "depression" as an independent variable could conceptualize depression in terms of a diagnostic state, but would more likely use tools that captured the person's status at a point in time. One such tool is the Center for Epidemiologic Studies Depression Scale (CES-D) or geriatric depression scale. Conversely, if the measure is supposed to indicate a clinical diagnosis of depression, then screening tools for depression are not the appropriate measurement strategy.

As with any measure, the measures of affect should be reliable and valid. They should also be capable of detecting meaningful change (Lieberson, 1985). The difficulty lies in determining what is meaningful change. Is it clinical, lifestyle, or functional? In a study of a depression intervention like serum serotonin reuptake inhibitors (SSRIs) in patients who manifest signs of depression but do not necessarily have a formal diagnosis of depression, one would likely focus on either the reduction in symptoms or the consequences of those symptoms in terms of overall functioning or utilization of reacted services. Table 9-4 presents a brief list of some of the measurement instruments discussed.

Depression and anxiety are the most common affect domains addressed in outcomes research. Anxiety is most often used as an independent variable. For example, both anxiety and depression can influence recovery from surgery and other medical procedures.

Table 9-4   **Psychological Measures**

Domain	Instrument	Description
Depression		
Screening	Self-Rating Depression Scale (Zung, 1965)	Assesses affective, somatic, psychomotor, and psychological aspects of depression in general population
	Center for Epidemiologic Studies Depression Scale (CES-D; Radloff, 1977)	Instrument emphasizes measurement of affective components of depression: mood, guilt, worthlessness, helplessness, as well as psychomotor, appetite, and sleep
	Geriatric Depression Scale (Yesavage et al., 1982)	Instrument specifically for administration in geriatric populations in the clinical setting
Other	Carroll Rating Scale (Carroll et al., 1981)	Based on the work of Hamilton (1960), this instrument was designed to assess severity of depression for 17 symptoms associated with depression.
	Depressive Experiences Questionnaire (Blatt et al., 1976)	Measures two aspects of depression: anaclitic (emotional dependence on others) and introjective (stringent standards for self, guilt, self-esteem, etc.)
Anxiety		
	Self-Rating Anxiety Scale (Zung, 1971)	A 20-item instrument that focuses on psychological as well as physiological factors associated with stress.
	Hamilton Anxiety Scale (HAMA; Bruss et al., 1994; Hamilton, 1959)	Developed to quantify the severity of anxiety symptomatology, often used in psychotropic drug evaluation; generally used for clinical administration
	State Trait Anxiety Measure (Spielberger, 1983)	The self-report inventory consists of 20 items to assess state anxiety and another 20 items to assess trait anxiety; these two parts differ in the item wording and in the response format (intensity versus frequency)

	Endler Multidimensional Anxiety Scales (EMAS; Endler et al., 1991)	The instrument has three modules: the EMAS-S that assesses state anxiety, the EMAS-T that assesses trait anxiety, and the EMAS-P that assesses perception of threat (what is causing the anxiety).
Other Measures		
	Affect Balance Scale (Bradburn, 1969)	Short instrument assessing reaction to events as well as state over the past 2 weeks; includes measures of positive and negative affect
	Memorial University of Newfoundland Scale of Happiness (MUNSH; Kozma & Stones, 1980)	Developed to assess general mental health in the elderly, includes four subscales: positive effect, negative effect, general positive experience, and general negative experience
	PGC Moral Scale (Lawton, 1975)	Developed to assess well-being in the elderly; instrument has 22 items and contains measures in three areas: dissatisfaction-loneliness, agitation, and attitudes toward one's own aging
	Mini-Mental State Exam (Folstein et al., 1975)	Instrument contains 11 items and assesses a range of issues, including orientation to time and place, recall, addition, ability to follow instruction, as well as motor skills
	Short Portable Mental Status Questionnaire (Pfeiffer, 1975)	Instrument adapted from the Mental Status Questionnaire (Kahn et al., 1984) for administration in the community setting as brief screen for cognitive function; mental status questionnaire has been demonstrated to be effective in institutional settings, but not in community settings; Short Portable Mental Status Questionnaire adapted from the Mental Status Questionnaire for administration in the community.

Depression

Depression is the most prevalent mental health problem in the United States (Shaver & Brennan, 1991). Clinically, depression is usually defined as a complex of symptoms generally characterized by dysphoria and loss of interest and pleasure in "things." It is related to loneliness and social isolation.

The manifestations of depression can range from suicidal ideation to sadness or feeling "blue." The *Diagnostic and Statistical Manual of Mental Disorders - Fourth Edition* (American Psychiatric Association, 1994) has a stringent diagnosis of major depressive episodes, but most outcomes research relies on symptoms that are less than diagnostic, such as the Self-Rating Depression Scale (Zung, 1965) or the Center for Epidemiologic Studies Depression Scale (CESD; Radloff, 1977).

Specialized instruments, such as the Geriatric Depression Scale (Yesavage et al., 1982), have been developed to target the depressive effect in particular populations; a number of tools have emerged to assess depression in particular populations (e.g. cancer, such as the Functional Assessment of Chronic Illness Inventory; Cella et al., 1993).

Alternatively, some instruments have focused on environmental factors that contribute to depression. Generally these instruments have been either a direct adaptation of a clinical tool, such as the adaptation of the Hamilton Rating Scale (Hamilton, 1960) for nonclinical administration, Carroll Rating Scale (Carroll, Feinberg, Smouse, Rawson, & Greden, 1981), or based more on psychosocial theory, such as the Depressive Experiences Questionnaire (Blatt, D'Afflitti, & Quinlan, 1976). The choice of an instrument should reflect what the investigator wants to assess. Regardless of which approach to measurement is used, it is important that the content of the instrument reflects the concept being targeted.

Anxiety

The distinction between depression and anxiety is becoming somewhat blurred (Hamilton, 1983), especially as anxiety is increasingly viewed as an affective state or trait of an individual. Even more than depression, anxiety has a range of conceptual and operational definitions in outcomes research, from situational and well defined (e.g., "white-coat anxiety") to a vague state experienced in anticipation of some ill-defined pending doom, to one that is based in social phenomena characterized by perceived danger and powerlessness. As a result, a wide range of descriptors is commonly utilized in measuring aspects of anxiety: "How often do you feel apprehensive?" "How often do you find that you can't stop worrying?" Thus, despite being a widely used term, anxiety is rarely clearly defined. However, such a clear definition is necessary prior to selecting how to measure the construct.

The vagueness of the construct leads to diverse approaches to measuring it. Most of the early measures focused on adjective checklists, such as the Anxiety Adjective Checklist (Zuckerman & Lubin, 1965). Later measures included a more diverse set of measures, including physiological conditions and social isolation (Zung's Self-Rating Anxiety Scale; Zung, 1971), (Hamilton Anxiety Scale; Bruss, Gruenberg, Goldstein, & Barber, 1994; Hamilton, 1959).

Later work has attempted to differentiate state from trait anxiety. The State-Trait Anxiety Inventory (STAI; Spielberger, 1983) was initially conceptualized as a research instrument to study anxiety in adults. It is a self-report assessment device that includes separate measures of state and trait anxiety. State anxiety is characterized as a transitory response in which the individual experiences anxiety, apprehension, or tension. It can manifest both emotionally as well as physiologically, but is regarded as being short term. By contrast, trait anxiety is identified as a persistent and stable anxiety response to the environmental factors. The Endler Multidimensional Anxiety Scales (EMAS; Endler, Edwards, & Vitelli, 1991) assess state and trait anxiety as well, but also include a measure regarding the perception of what is causing anxiety.

Given the overlap that often occurs when dealing with psychologic phenomena such as depression and anxiety, an alternative is to utilize more general instruments to assess psychologic states. A number of instruments, such as the Affect Balance Scale (Bradburn, 1969) and the Multiple Affect Adjective Checklist (Zuckerman & Lubin, 1965), provide multidimensional assessments. Although they lack some of the specificity of depression or anxiety scales, they represent an integrative approach to the assessment of affect. Such an approach has advantages in that it recognizes the similarity between constructs and attempts to look at effect generally, without attempting to make direct attributions.

An affect measure that approaches but is distinct from depression and anxiety is morale. The PGC Morale Scale (Lawton, 1975) utilizes measures of depression, anxiety, usefulness, and loneliness, as well as other issues to develop three scores: agitation, attitude toward one's own aging, and lonely dissatisfaction.

Positive emotions are much less often studied in health research, but concepts like happiness are certainly legitimate. Instruments such as the Rosenburg Self-Esteem Scale (Rosenburg, 1965), the Memorial University of Newfoundland Scale of Happiness (Kozma & Stones, 1980), or the Affectometer 2 (Kammann & Flett, 1983) can be used to assess happiness and related positive emotions.

Cognitive Function

Measures of cognitive function are not intended to assess intelligence; rather they address a range of areas, including judgment, memory, and the ability to perform interpretative and related tasks. Cognition may be an outcome in its own right, it may be an independent variable, or it may be a criterion for inclusion in a study. For example, a study used a battery of function measures to assess the impact of dialysis on the cognitive abilities of patients undergoing treatment. This research demonstrated a significant change in cognitive ability, not just during the dialysis process, but also in the time between treatments (Murray et al., 2006).

Establishing a person's cognitive status may involve only basic measures of orientation, such as knowing who they are, where they are, or what day it is, but usually cognition involves some level of more formal testing. A number of tests have evolved as screens for cognitive function. The Minimental State Exam (MMSE; Folstein, Folstein, & McHugh, 1975) assesses recall, addition, and the ability to follow instruction, as well as motor skills and some executive functions. The shorter Mental Status Questionnaire (Kahn, Goldfarb, Pollack, & Peck, 1984) and its close cousin, the Short Portable Mental Status Questionnaire (Pfeiffer, 1975) can be used for simple screening and crude identification of those with cognitive impairments.

Social Function

Social functioning usually refers to one's ability to fulfill various roles expected of a person. It may involve both giving and receiving help. In general, we think of a person's role in relation to employment or some other major activity (like going to school). But people have other roles as well. They participate in organizations and groups. They have friends. They interact. Some of these activities may be salient to certain types of health care. For example, a person's goal may be to get well enough to sing in a choir or attend her daughter's wedding.

An important outcome for many medical problems is how the individual fulfills social roles. To some extent, the effect of illness on social role depends on what that role had been previously. For example, a physical limitation will have a bigger effect on a laborer's ability to return to work than an executive's ability, but the effect on filling the role of husband or father may be the same.

Social Support

There are many conceptual definitions of social support, social function, and related measures. Social support may address objective data on the type and amount of assistance rendered to a person's perceptions of whether they are supported. The extent to which they give social support or assistance reflects social role and functioning. Assessing social support in outcomes research can range from very simple items, such as "Is there anyone who can help you change your bandages at home?" to more complex measures that attempt to identify who provides what type of support and how satisfied the individual is with that support. Three different measures of social support are presented in Table 9-5. The social support questionnaire asks the respondents if they have someone they can rely on for support; it uses 27 different items and also asks the person to rate their satisfaction with the support provided by that person (Sarason, Levine, Basham, & Sarason, 1983). The Medical Outcomes Study Social Support Survey measures functional social support and resources (Sarason et al., 1983). The measurement of social support and resources is broken into four subscales that assess: tangible, affectionate, positive social interaction, and emotional or informational support. The Duke-UNC (University of North Carolina) Functional Social Support Survey is intended primarily as a measure of satisfaction with support in eight social and emotional areas (Broadhead, Gehlbach, de Gruy, & Kaplan, 1988). Finally, the Duke Social Support and Scale combines an assessment of both the amount of support received from as well as stress caused by family and nonfamily sources (Parkerson et al., 1989).

Social Function/Adjustment

Measures of social support focus on the dynamic relationship between the individual and the environment, whereas measures of social function and adjustment focus on assessing the individual's status and function. Instruments assessing social function tend to be long due to the complexity of the phenomenon. The Social Functioning Schedule

Table 9-5   Social Measures

Domain	Instrument	Description
Social Support	The Social Support Questionnaire (Sarason et al., 1983)	Instrument asks the respondents to indicate if they (1) have someone they can turn to for support for 27 items and (2) asks them how satisfied they are with that support.
	Medical Outcomes Study Social Support Survey (Sherbourne & Stewart, 1991)	Instrument is focused on the measurement of functional social support and resources; has four subscales: tangible support, affectionate, positive social interaction, and emotional or informational support
	Duke-UNC Functional Social Support Survey (Broadhead et al., 1988)	Intended as a measure of satisfaction with functional and emotional social support; assess satisfaction of eight areas
	Duke Social Support and Stress Scale (Parkerson et al., 1989)	Instrument provides a rating for support received from and the amount of stress caused by family and nonfamily sources
Social Functioning/ Adjustment	Social Functioning Schedule (Remington & Tyrer, 1979)	Instrument assesses function in 12 areas: employment, household chores, contribution to household, money, self-care, material relationships, care of children, patient–child relationships, patient–parent relationships, household relationships, hobbies, and spare time activities; is conducted as a semi-structured interview and is a large instrument
	Social Adjustment Schedule (Weissman & Bothwell, 1976)	Intended to assess the quality of social relationships and role performance in a number of areas: work (outside and inside the home), spare time, family, and financial; for each of the areas, five aspects assessed

	Social Maladjustment Scale (Clare & Cairns, 1978)	Scale assesses three issues (material condition, social management, and satisfaction) for six different areas (housing, occupation, economic situation, leisure/social activities, family and domestic relationships, and marriage)
	Social Dysfunction Scale (Linn, Sculthorpe, Evje, Slater, & Goodman, 1969)	Instrument designed to assess function in three areas: self-esteem, interpersonal, and performance; primarily focuses on negative aspects
Complex Organizations		
Commitment	Organizational Commitment Questionnaire (Mowday, Steers, & Porter, 1979)	A 15-item instrument to assess global organizational commitment; has also been modified to assess professional commitment or commitment to job as well (Gunz & Gunz, 1994; Millward & Hopkins, 1998)
	Affective, Normative, and Continuance Commitment (Meyer & Allen, 1997)	Instrument is designed to assess three aspects of commitment to an organization: effect (sense of belonging, attachment), normative (loyalty, job tenure), and continuance; continuance scale has two subscales to assess: (1) level of sacrifice the individual is willing to make to remain in the organization and (2) alternative work possibilities
Work Control	Work Control (Dwyer & Ganster, 1991)	Designed to assess a worker's perception of control over work environment, including control over performance, timing, and procedures associated with work tasks

(continues)

Table 9-5 *(continued)*

Domain	Instrument	Description
	Job Routinization and Formalization (Bacharach, Bamberger, & Conley, 1990)	Instrument is designed to assess aspects of conflict between employee preference and organizational needs; instrument has measures in four areas: routinization, pervasiveness of rules, record keeping, and formalization
	Role Overload (Bacharach et al., 1990)	Intended to measure inconsistencies between activities and tasks demanded and the time and resources available for completing the task
	Job Overload (Caplan et al., 1980)	An 11-item instrument designed to measure quantitative aspects of pace and amount of work
	Job Interdependence (Pearce & Gregersen, 1991)	Two dimensions assessed in this measure: interdependence and independence; interdependence measures focus on reciprocal relationships and independence measures address autonomy
	Inventory of Stressful Events (Motowidlo, Packard, & Manning, 1986)	Instrument developed to assess stressful events for nurses; measures composed of 45 items that focus on the stress associated with events associated with the provision of nursing care
	Frustration with Work (Peters, O'Connor, & Rudolf, 1980)	Short three-item instrument assessing frustration with job/work
	Job Stress Scale (Parker & Decotiis, 1983)	Instrument assesses job stress for two dimensions: time and anxiety; measures of time stress include measures related to work as well as impact of work on nonwork life; anxiety measures focus solely on anxiety arising from job

(Remington & Tyrer, 1979) assesses function in 12 areas including, work, home/family, and hobbies. Within each area, a number of aspects are addressed, including behavioral (frequency of event), as well as psychological (stress associated with activity). It is a good instrument to assess social function, but involves a long, semistructured interview.

Measures of social adjustment tend to either take a positive (adjustment) or negative (maladjustment) approach. The Social Adjustment Schedule (Weissman & Bothwell, 1976) focuses on a range of social relationships, including community, work, and home for each area in which the five aspects are assessed. The Social Maladjustment Scale (Clare & Cairns, 1978) focuses on six areas ranging from occupation to housing and marriage. For each area, the material conditions, the individual's ability to manage it, and overall satisfaction are assessed.

SUMMARY

Psychosocial and demographic variables can play different roles in outcomes research. While they are typically used to control for patient characteristics, they can also be outcomes in their own right. As with most measures, choosing the right measure involves understanding what aspects of the phenomenon you want to assess. Social and psychological variables may be especially sensitive to this problem because they represent often vague social constructs.

A number of excellent resources are available to researchers when looking for measures in this area. Some of focus primarily on health (McDowell & Newell, 1996); others are more general in nature (Robinson, Shaver, & Wrightsman, 1991).

REFERENCES

American Psychiatric Association. (1994). *Diagnostic and statistical manual of mental disorders (DMS-IV)*. Washington, DC: Author.

Bacharach, S. B., Bamberger, P., & Conley, S. C. (1990). Work processes, role conflict, and role overload: The case of nurses and engineers in the public sector. *Work and Occupations, 17,* 199–228.

Bennett, P. H. (1999). Type 2 diabetes among the Pima Indians of Arizona: An epidemic attributable to environmental change? *Nutrition Reviews, 57*(5 Pt 2), S51–S54.

Blalock, H. M. (1974). *Measurement in the social sciences: Theories and strategies.* Chicago: Aldine Publishing Company

Blatt, S. J., D'Afflitti, J. P., & Quinlan, D. M. (1976). *Depressive experiences questionnaire.* New Haven, CT: Yale University Press.

Bohrnstedt, G. W., & Borgatta, E. F. (1981). *Social measurement: Current issues.* Beverly Hills, CA: Sage Publications Inc.

Bradburn, N. M. (1969). *The stucture of psychological well-being.* Chicago: Aldine.

Broadhead, W. E., Gehlbach, S. H., de Gruy, F. V., & Kaplan, B. H. (1988). The Duke-UNC Functional Social Support Questionnaire. Measurement of social support in family medicine patients. *Medical Care, 26*(7), 709–723.

Bruss, G. S., Gruenberg, A. M., Goldstein, R. D., & Barber, J. P. (1994). Hamilton Anxiety Rating Scale Interview guide: Joint interview and test-retest methods for interrater reliability. *Psychiatry Research, 53*(2), 191–202.

Campbell, A., Converse, P. E., & Rodgers, W. L. (1976). *The quality of American life: Perceptions, evaluations, and satisfactions.* New York: Russell Sage Foundation.

Campbell, D. T., & Overman, E. S. (1988). *Methodology and epistemology for social science: Selected papers.* Chicago: University of Chicago Press.

Campbell, D. T., & Russo, M. J. (2001). *Social measurement.* Thousand Oaks, CA: Sage Publications.

Caplan, R. D., Cobb, S., French, J. R. P., Van Harrison, R., & Pinneau, S. R. (1980). *Job demands and worker health.* Ann Arbor, MI: University of Michigan, Institute for Social Research.

Carroll, B. J., Feinberg, M., Smouse, P. E., Rawson, S. G., & Greden, J. F. (1981). The Carroll rating scale for depression.

I. Development, reliability and validation. *British Journal of Psychiatry, 138,* 194–200.

Cella, D. F., Tulsky, D. S., Gray, G., Sarafian, B., Linn, E., Bonomi, A., . . .Brannon, J. (1993). The Functional Assessment of Cancer Therapy scale: Development and validation of the general measure. *Journal of Clinical Oncology, 11*(3), 570–579.

Clare, A. W., & Cairns, V. E. (1978). Design, development and use of a standardized interview to assess social maladjustment and dysfunction in community studies. *Psychological Medicine, 8*(4), 589–604.

Cleeland, C. S. (1991). Pain assessement in cancer. In D. Osoba (Ed.), *Effect of cancer on quality of life* (pp. 293–305). Boca Raton, FL: CRC Press.

Cobb, J. L., Wolf, P. A., Au, R., White, R., & D'Agostino, R. B. (1995). The effect of education on the incidence of dementia and Alzheimer's disease in the Framingham Study. *Neurology, 45*(9), 1707–1712.

Cohen, S., Kamarck, T., & Mermelstein, R. (1983). A global measure of perceived stress. *Journal of Health and Social Behavior, 24,* 385–396.

Daly, M. C., Duncan, G. J., McDonough, P., & Williams, D. R. (2002). Optimal indicators of socioeconomic status for health research. *American Journal of Public Health, 92*(7), 1151–1157.

Daut, R. L., Cleeland, C. S., & Flanery, R. C. (1983). Development of the Wisconsin Brief Pain Questionnaire to assess pain in cancer and other diseases. *Pain, 17,* 197–210.

Diez Roux, A. V. (2003). Residential environments and cardiovascular risk. *Journal of Urban Health, 80,* 569–589.

Douglas, C. H., & Douglas, M. R. (2004). Patient-friendly hospital environments: Exploring the patients' perspective. *Health Expectations, 7*(1), 61–73.

Duncan, O. D. (1961). A socioeconomic index for all occupations. In A. J. Reiss, O. D. Duncan, P. K. Hatt & C. C. North (Eds.), *Occupations and social status.* Glencoe, IL: The Free Press.

Dwyer, D. J., & Ganster, D. C. (1991). The effects of job demands and control on employee attendeance and satisfaction. *Journal of Organizational Behavior, 12,* 595–608.

Endler, N. S., Edwards, J. M., & Vitelli, R. (1991). *Endler Multidimensional Anxiety Scales (EMAS): Manual.* Los Angeles: Western Psychological Services.

Fairbank, J. C., Couper, J., Davies, J. B., & O'Brien, J. P. (1980). The Oswestry low back pain disability questionnaire. *Physiotherapy, 66*(8), 271–273.

Fazio, A. F. (1977). A concurrent validational study of the NCHS general well-being schedule. *Vital and Health Statistics. Series 2, Data Evaluation and Methods Research, 73,* 1–53.

Folstein, M. F., Folstein, S. E., & McHugh, P. R. (1975). "Mini-mental state." A practical method for grading the cognitive state of patients for the clinician. *Journal of Psychiatric Research, 12*(3), 189–198.

Gunz, H. P., & Gunz, S. P. (1994). Professional/organizational committment and job satisfaction for employed lawyers. *Human Relations, 47,* 801–828.

Hamilton, M. (1959). The assessment of anxiety scales by rating. *British Journal of Psychology, 32,* 50.

Hamilton, M. (1983). The clinical distinction between anxiety and depression. *British Journal of Clinical Pharmacology, 15*(Suppl 2), 165S–169S.

Hamilton, M. A. (1960). A rating scale for depression. *Journal of Neurology, Neurosurgery, and Psychiatry, 23,* 56–62.

Hill, D. J., & Bale, R. M. (1980). Development of the mental health locus of control and mental health locus of origin scales. *Journal of Personality Asssement, 44,* 148–156.

Hodgins, D. C. (2001). Stage of change assessments in alcohol problems: Agreement across self and clinician reports. *Substance Abuse, 22,* 87–96.

Hollingshead, A. B. (1957). *Two factor index of social position*. New Haven, CT: Hollingshead.

Hollingshead, A. B., & Redlich, F. C. (1958). *Social class and mental illness*. New York: John Wiley.

Holmes, T. H., & Rahe, R. H. (1967). The social readjustment rating scale. *Journal of Psychosomatic Research, 11*(2), 213–218.

Impara, J. C., & Plake, B. S. (Eds.). (1998). *The thirteenth mental measurements yearbook*. Lincoln, NE: Buros Institute of Mental Measurements.

Imperatore, G., Knowler, W. C., Nelson, R. G., & Hanson, R. L. (2001). Genetics of diabetic nephropathy in the Pima Indians. *Current Diabetes Reports, 1*(3), 275–281.

Jackson, R. J. (2003). The impact of the built environment on health: An emerging field. *American Journal of Public Health, 93*(9), 1382–1384.

Kahn, R. L., Goldfarb A. I., Pollack M., & Peck, A. (1984). Mental status questionnaire. In D. J. Mangen & W. A. Peterson (Eds.), *Research instruments in social gerontology: Health, program evaluation, and demography* (Vol. 3). Minneapolis: University of Minnesota Press.

Kammann, R., & Flett, R. (1983). Affectometer 2: A scale to measure current level of general happiness. *Australian Journal of Psychology, 35*, 259–265.

Kane, R. L., Bershadsky, B., Lin, W. C., Rockwood, T., & Wood, K. (2002). Efforts to standardize the reporting of pain. *Journal of Clinical Epidemiology, 55*(2), 105–110.

Kaplan, G. A., & Keil, J. E. (1993). Socioeconomic factors and cardiovascular disease: A review of the literature. *Circulation, 88*(4 Pt 1), 1973–1998.

Kozma, A., & Stones, M. J. (1980). The measurement of happiness: Development of the Memorial University of Newfoundland Scale of Happiness (MUNSH). *Journal of Gerontology, 35*, 906–912.

Lawton, M. P. (1975). The Philadelphia Geriatric Center moral scale: A revision. *Journal of Gerontology, 30*, 85–89.

Leavitt, F., & Garron, D. C. (1979a). The detection of psychological disturbance in patients with low back pain. *Journal of Psychosomatic Research, 23*(2), 149–154.

Leavitt, F., & Garron, D. C. (1979b). Validity of a Back Pain Classification Scale among patients with low back pain not associated with demonstrable organic disease. *Journal of Psychosomatic Research, 23*(5), 301–306.

Levenson, H. (1981). Differentiating among internality, powerful others, and chance. In H. M. Lefcourt (Ed.), *Research with the locus of control construct* (Vol. 1, pp. 15–63). New York: Academic Press.

Levenstein, S., Prantera, C., Varvo, V., Scribano, M. L., Berto, E., Luzi, C., Andreoli, A. (1993). Development of the perceived stress questionnaire: A new tool for psychosomatic research. *Journal of Psychosomatic Research, 37*(1), 19–32.

Lieberson, S. (1985). *Making it count: The improvement of social research and theory.* Berkeley, CA: University of California Press.

Lillioja, S., & Bogardus, C. (1988). Insulin resistance in Pima Indians. A combined effect of genetic predisposition and obesity-related skeletal muscle cell hypertrophy. *Acta Medica Scandinavica - Supplementum, 723*, 103–119.

Linn, M. W., Sculthorpe, W. B., Evje, M., Slater, P. H., & Goodman, S. P. (1969). A social dysfunction rating scale. *Journal of Psychiatric Research, 6*(4), 299–306.

Lucy, W. H. (2003). Mortality risk associated with leaving home: Recognizing the relevance of the built environment. *American Journal of Public Health, 93*(9), 1564–1569.

McConnaughy, E. N., Prochaska, J. O., & Velicer, W. F. (1983). Stages of change in psychotherapy: Measurement and sample profiles. *Psychotherapy: Theory, Research and Practice, 20*, 368–375.

McDowell, I., & Newell, C. (1996). *Measuring health: A guide to rating scales and questionnaires* (2nd ed.). New York: Oxford University Press.

Meyer, J. P., & Allen, N. J. (1997). *Commitment in the workplace.* Thousand Oaks, CA: Sage Publicatinos.

Millward, L. J., & Hopkins, L. J. (1998). Psychological contracts and job committment. *Journal of Applied Social Psychology, 28,* 1530–1556.

Moseley, J. B., O'Malley, K., Petersen, N. J., Menke, T. J., Brody, B. A., Kuykendall, D. H., . . .Wray, N. P. (2002). A controlled trial of arthroscopic surgery for osteoarthritis of the knee. *New England Journal of Medicine, 347*(2), 81–88.

Motowidlo, S. J., Packard, J. S., & Manning, M. R. (1986). Occupational stress: Its causes and consequences for job performance. *Journal of Applied Psychology, 71,* 618–629.

Mowday, R. T., Steers, R. M., & Porter, L. W. (1979). The measurement of organizational commitment. *Journal of Vocational Behavior, 14,* 224–247.

Murray, A. M., Tupper, D. E., Knopman, D. S., Gilbertson, D. T., Pederson, S. L., Li, S., . . .Kane, R. L. (2006). Cognitive impairment in hemodialysis patients is common. *Neurology, 67*(2), 216–223.

Nam, C. B., & Powers, M. G. (1983). *The socioeconomic approach to status measurement (with a guide to occupational and socioeconomic status scores).* Houston, TX: Cap and Gown Press.

Northridge, M. E., Sclar, E. D., & Biswas, P. (2003). Sorting out the connections between the built environment and health: A conceptual framework for navigating pathways and planning healthy cities. *Journal of Urban Health, 80,* 556–568.

Oakes, J. M., & Rossi, P. H. (2003). The measurement of SES in health research: Current practice and steps toward a new approach. *Social Science & Medicine, 56*(4), 769–784.

Parker, D. F., & Decotiis, T. A. (1983). Organizational determinants of job stress. *Organizational Behavior and Human Performance, 32*, 160–177.

Parkerson, G. R. Jr., Michener, J. L., Wu, L. R., Finch, J. N., Muhlbaier, L. H., Magruder-Habib, K., . . .Jokerst, E. (1989). Associations among family support, family stress, and personal functional health status. *Journal of Clinical Epidemiology, 42*(3), 217–229.

Paulhus, D. (1983). Sphere-specific measures of perceived control. *Journal of Personality and Social Psychology, 44*, 1253–1265.

Pearce, J. L., & Gregersen, H. B. (1991). Task interdependence and extra-role behavior: A test of the mediating effects of felt responsibility. *Journal of Applied Psychology, 76*, 838–844.

Perdue, W. C., Gostin, L. O., & Stone, L. A. (2003). Public health and the built environment: Historical, empirical, and theoretical foundations for an expanded role. *Journal of Law, Medicine & Ethics, 31*(4), 557–566.

Peters, L. H., O'Connor, E. J., & Rudolf, C. J. (1980). The behavioral and affective consequences of performance-relevant situational variables. *Organizational Behavior and Human Performance, 25*, 79–96.

Pfeiffer, E. (1975). A short portable mental status questionnaire for the assessment of organic brain deficit in elderly patients. *Journal of the American Geriatrics Society, 23*(10), 433–441.

Pilowsky, I., & Spence, N. D. (1983). *Manual for the Illness Behavior Questionnaire (IBQ)* (2nd ed.). Adelaide, Australia: University of Adelaide.

Pratley, R. E. (1998). Gene-environment interactions in the pathogenesis of type 2 diabetes mellitus: Lessons learned from the Pima Indians. *Proceedings of the Nutrition Society, 57*(2), 175–181.

Prochaska, J. O., DiClemente, C. C., & Norcross, J. C. (1992). In search of how people change. Applications to addictive behaviors. *American Psychologist, 47*(9), 1102–1114.

Prochaska, J. O., & Norcross, J. C. (2001). Stages of change. *Psychotherapy: Theory, research, practice, training, 38*(4), 443–448.

Radloff, L. S. (1977). The CES-D scale: A self-report depression scale for research in the general population. *Applied Psychological Measurement, 1*(385–701).

Ravussin, E. (1993). Energy metabolism in obesity. Studies in the Pima Indians. *Diabetes Care, 16*(1), 232–238.

Remington, M., & Tyrer, P. J. (1979). The social functioning schedule: A brief semi-structured interview. *Social Psychiatry, 14*(3), 151–157.

Robinson, J. P., Shaver, P. R., & Wrightsman, L. S. (1991). *Measures of personality and social psychological attitudes.* London: Academic Press.

Rockwood, T., & Constantine, M. (2005). Demographic, psychological and social factors. In R. L. Kane (Ed.), *Understanding healthcare outcomes research.* Sudbury, MA: Jones and Bartlett Publishers.

Rollnick, S., Heather, N., Gold, R., & Hall, W. (1992). Development of a short "readiness to change" questionnaire for use in brief, opportunistic interventions among excessive drinkers. *British Journal of Addiction, 87*(5), 743–754.

Rosenburg, M. (1965). *Soceity and the adolescent self-image.* Princeton, NJ: Princeton University Press.

Rotter, J. B. (1966). Generalized expectancies for internal versus external control of reinforcement. *Psychological Monographs: General & Applied, 80*(1), 1–28.

Rubin, H. R. (1998). Status report—An investigation to determine whether the built environment affects patients' medical outcomes. *Journal of Healthcare Design, 10*, 11–13.

Sarason, I. G., Levine, H. M., Basham, R. B., & Sarason, B. R. (1983). Assessing social support: The Social Support Questionnaire. *Journal of Personality & Social Psychology, 44*(1), 127–139.

Shapiro, C. M., Flanigan, M., Fleming, J. A., Morehouse, R., Moscovitch, A., Plamondon, J., . . .Devins, G. M. (2002). Development of an adjective checklist to measure five FACES of fatigue and sleepiness. Data from a national survey of insomniacs. *Journal of Psychosomatic Research, 52*(6), 467–473.

Shaver, P. R., & Brennan, K. A. (1991). Measures of depression and loneliness. In J. P. Robinson, P. R. Shaver, & L. S. Wrightsman (Eds.), *Measures of personality and social psychological attitudes*. London: Academic Press.

Sherbourne, C. D., & Stewart, A. L. (1991). The MOS social support survey. *Social Science & Medicine, 32*(6), 705–714.

Shryock, H. S., Siegel, J. S., & Stockwell, E. G. (Eds.). (1976). *The methods and materials of demography* (Condensed). New York: Academic Press.

Snipp, C. M. (2003). Racial measurement in the American census: Past practices and implications for the future. *Annual Review of Sociology, 29*, 563–588.

Spielberger, C. D. (1983). *Manual for the state-trait anxiety inventory (STAI)*. Palo Alto, CA: Consulting Psychologists Press.

Stewart, A. L., & Ware, J. E. (1992). *Measuring functioning and well-being: The medical outcomes study approach*. Durham, NC: Duke University Press.

Summers, G. F. (1970). *Attitude measurement*. Chicago: Rand McNally.

Takeuchi, D. T., & Gage, S.-J. L. (2003). What to do with race? Changing notions of race in the social sciences. *Culture, Medicine and Psychiatry, 27*(4), 435–445.

Turk, D. C., & Melzack, R. (1992). *Handbook of pain assessment*. New York: Guilford Press.

Turk, D. C., Rudy, T. E., & Salovey, P. (1985). The McGill Pain Questionnaire reconsidered: Confirming the factor structure and examining appropriate uses. *Pain, 21*(4), 385–397.

Wallston, K. A., & Wallston, B. S. (1981). Health locus of control scales. In H. M. Lefcourt (Ed.), *Research with the locus of control construct* (Vol. 1, pp. 189–243). New York: Academic Press.

Weeks, J. R. (1981). *Population: An introduction to concepts and issues* (2d ed.). Belmont, CA: Wadsworth Publishing Company.

Weissman, M. M., & Bothwell, S. (1976). Assessment of social adjustment by patient self-report. *Archives of General Psychiatry, 33*(9), 1111–1115.

Wolfe, J., & Kimerling, R. (1997). Gender issues in the assessment of post-traumatic stress disorder. In J. P. Wilson & T. M. Keane (Eds.), *Assessing psychological trauma and PTSD* (pp. xiv, 577). New York: Guilford Press.

Yesavage, J. A., Brink, T. L., Rose, T. L., Lum, O., Huang, V., Adey, M., & Leirer, V. O. (1982). Development and validation of a geriatric depression screening scale: A preliminary report. *Journal of Psychiatric Research, 17*(1), 37–49.

Zuckerman, M., & Lubin, B. (1965). *Manual for the multiple affect adjective check list.* San Diego, CA: Educational and Industrial Testing Service.

Zung, W. W. (1965). A self-rating depression scale. *Archives of General Psychiatry, 12*, 63–70.

Zung, W. W. (1971). A rating instrument for anxiety disorders. *Psychosomatics, 12*(6), 371–379.

Zung, W. W. (1983). A self-rating pain and distress scale. *Psychosomatics, 24*(10), 887–890.

10

Treatment and Interventions[1]

IMPORTANCE OF UNDERSTANDING TREATMENT

The goal of outcomes research is to identify the effects of treatment (or some type of intervention). It is thus especially ironic that so little attention is paid to how to measure that treatment. We can think of treatment in either an absolute or relative sense. For example, an absolute question would be: Does "X" work (i.e., does it produce a desired result, perhaps without incurring great harms)? A related question would be: Does "X" produce a better result than "Y"? The latter comparison is typically referred to as comparative effectiveness.

WHAT IS A TREATMENT?

One way to think of outcomes research is to view it as an extension of epidemiology. In classical epidemiology, the questions posed generally address the potential causes of a specific disease. In outcomes research, we typically start with disease and test whether interventions can change the clinical course.

A treatment is essentially an intervention designed to improve a person's health state. It can come in many forms. It could be an effort at

---

[1]This chapter draws on earlier work by Jeremy Holtzman (2005).

cure or prevention. It could involve a procedure performed, a substance ingested, or a behavioral change. It could be a change in the way health care is organized or even paid for.[2]

Increasingly, more attention is being paid to the importance of systems thinking in improving healthcare delivery. What is done by an individual must be viewed in the larger context of the delivery system. Such a view makes defining treatment even harder. Simple models that isolate treatment must give way to more complex models that view treatment in the context of the practice environment. Thus, the effectiveness of the care rendered by a specific clinician may be influenced by the site of practice. For example, the care of physicians working in a clinic or a hospital may be influenced by the overall care in the facility. More sophisticated analytic models that take into account this nesting must be applied.

Any potentially modifiable factor that may impact health might be considered a treatment within outcomes research. This could be as simple as using a single medication as in the question "Does the use of aspirin reduce mortality following heart attacks?" or it could be as complex as an entire health delivery system, such as "Is the mortality after heart attacks greater for patients receiving health care on a fee-for-service basis or from an HMO?" Excluded from this definition are only those things that cannot even in theory be changed. Hence, insurance status, which could be very difficult to change for any given individual, could be a treatment, whereas age, which cannot be changed, would not be.

Although outcomes research may deal with a wide range of "treatments," from the very simple to the extraordinarily complex, all of health care ultimately may be distilled down to more basic elements. For example, when the effect of insurance status (fee-for-service versus health maintenance organization) on mortality for individuals with myocardial infarctions is examined, the treatment is in effect composed of thousands of other treatments that add up to the whole observed treatment. In both groups, individuals receive medications, procedures, nursing care, and counseling. Any differences seen in the outcome of the patients (after appropriately accounting for other patient factors) ultimately results from differences in the delivery of medications, procedures, nursing care, and all of those other elements of care that make up health care; but the main variable of interest is whether insurance coverage made a difference. Presumably

[2]For a description of an elaborate test of the effects of health insurance, see Newhouse (1993).

that difference would be mitigated by its effects on the delivery of care elements. That potential effect of those factors, or at least differences in their presence, should be examined in the analysis.

Components of Treatment

The "controlled" component of randomized controlled trials refers to an effort to standardize the intervention. Sometimes this standardization is expressed explicitly, such as a predefined number of doses of a specific drug at prescribed times, or performance of a procedure in a given way, or use of a standardized treatment protocol. In some cases, some flexibility is permitted, such as adjusting the dose to the size of the patient (e.g. mg/m^2) or even allowing dosage to tolerance (i.e., giving the drug until some threshold of intolerance is reached).

Frequently in an outcomes study, the treatment is specified generically but many details are omitted. For example, what does it mean to say a patient received a hip replacement? What surgical technique was used? What type of prosthesis was implanted? What kind of postoperative care did he or she receive? Was there physical therapy? What type of anesthetic was used? Provider characteristics may include amount of training, specialty, board certification, or years since graduation. Recently, substantial attention has been paid to the volume of procedures performed, under a tacit assumption that higher volumes reflect more skill or at least a better system of care.

Personal characteristics of the provider may also affect both the quality and type of treatment provided. For example, the gender of physicians has been associated with the provision of Pap smears and mammography to their female patients (Lurie et al., 1993). Patients who were treated by female physicians were more likely to receive diagnostic procedures than were patients treated by male physicians, although this difference ameliorated with the age of the physician. Likewise female surgeons are more likely to recommend prophylactic mastectomy (Arrington, Jarosek, Virnig, Habermann, & Tuttle, 2009).

It quickly becomes evident that the variable labeled "treatment" can be handled at many levels with quite different amounts of specificity. For practical purposes, most studies do not consider every element of the care provided, but rather focus on some areas of interest. Obviously, no single study can assess all of these components, but some may be especially salient to answering given question about outcomes.

However, they run the risk of overlooking a salient component. For example, postoperative physical therapy may dramatically change the short-term course of recovery from a hip replacement. It is therefore important that those designing outcomes studies have some feel for the components of care involved and appreciate the risks of omitting some details. Researchers need to have enough clinical insight (or be able to get relevant assistance with such insight) to be sure they do not miss an important dimension.

Different specialties emphasize different aspects of a study. For example, in a review of the treatment of a hip fracture, we observed that the studies conducted by orthopedists gave a great deal of attention to the nature of the surgical procedure and the prosthesis implanted but gave short shrift to the characteristics of the patients. Indeed, once they compared them in an introductory table they rarely used these variables in the analysis. By contrast, epidemiologists lavished great attention on the role of patient factors but glossed over variations in treatment (Butler et al., 2009). Neither approach was adequate on its own to provide a clear answer to the question about what accounts for differences in outcomes among hip fracture patients.

The growing popularity of what are termed "complementary and alternative medicine (CAM)" treatments, such as acupuncture, massage, or meditation, has raised an interesting debate about whether the allopathically familiar empirical approach to assessing effectiveness should apply. Some proponents of these alternative modalities argue the evaluation design should reflect the more spiritual nature of the treatment and use looser end-points and more inclusive research designs that allow for more subjectivity. Increasingly, however, these nontraditional approaches are being subjected to the same tests of outcomes as more familiar treatments. In some cases, the results are surprising. For example, there is surprisingly mixed evidence about the effects of intercessional prayer (i.e., prayer on your behalf by a third party without your direct knowledge) (Matthews, Conti, & Sireci, 2001; Palmer, Katerndahl, & Morgan-Kidd, 2004).

Ironically, despite the centrality of treatment, there are few widely used taxonomies to describe it. The most well developed taxonomy comes from pharmacology. Table 10-1 offers a generic approach to assessing treatment, based largely on the approach used for medications, and applies to three generic classes of treatment: medications, procedures (typically

Table 10-1   Elements Relevant for Each Type of Treatment

Treatment Element	Treatment Type		
	Medications	**Procedures**	**Counseling**
Type	X	X	X
Dosage	X		X
Route	X		
Frequency	X	X	X
Duration	X	X	X
Onset/Timing	X	X	X
Technical Aspects/ Provider Characteristics		X	X

surgery but increasingly noninvasive treatments), and counseling. Some elements apply to only certain classes of treatment.

When we think about drug therapy, we talk in terms of type of drug, dosage, frequency, and duration. It is fairly clear what is meant by dose for drugs, and perhaps even for counseling. Dosage may be represented by treatment intensity. Table 10-2 depicts various study questions that compare treatments according to intensity, timing, and duration. Comparisons of one treatment versus another is called comparative effectiveness; it can be either direct (Treatment A vs Treatment B), or indirect (each treatment vs its own control). The latter is less satisfactory for several reasons, including the potential lack of comparability of the samples. Comparisons based on the duration of treatment could examine how duration of antibiotic use affects recovery from urinary tract infections (i.e., medications; Elhanan, Tabenkin, Yahalom, & Raz, 1994); how the duration of electrical stimulation affects relief of back pain (i.e., procedure) (Hamza et al., 1999); or how a longer smoking cessation program affects the likelihood of quitting (i.e., counseling; Gilbert et al., 1992). Dose is less clear for procedures like surgery. It could include the type of surgery, for example, the nature of the incision or the use of specific prostheses. It could include the extent and nature of the resection and perhaps surgical time (what surgeons call time from skin to skin), but the latter may raise questions of endogeneity if complications lengthened the procedure. Issues like duration and frequency can apply more readily to counseling than to surgery. Duration in

Table 10-2   Bases for Comparing Treatments

1. Comparison of different treatment regimens
   a. Treatment A versus no treatment (placebo)
   b. Treatment B versus no treatment versus Treatment A versus no treatment
   c. Treatment A versus Treatment B
   d. Treatment A + B versus Treatment B alone

2. Comparison of the intensity of treatment
3. Comparison of the duration of treatment
4. Comparison of the timing of treatment

5. Comparison of the setting of the treatment
   a. Financial setting (e.g., HMO vs FFS)
   b. Physical setting (e.g., Hospital A vs Hospital B)
   c. Social/organizational setting (e.g., teaching hospitals vs community hospitals; hospice vs home care)
   d. Geographic setting (e.g., rural vs urban clinics)

6. Comparison of the characteristics of the provider
   a. Training
   b. Experience (volume)
   c. Personal characteristics

this context refers less to how long a session lasted (which is more akin to OR time) than to how long the full episode of care lasted.

A salient factor may be when in the course of the illness the treatment was begun; this may correlate with the severity of the illness, but it may also reflect points of clinical susceptibility to the treatment. For example, in the case of cancer, treating an early stage may be quite different from an advanced stage. Attempts are made to narrowly define the treatment. It would not be unusual for the treatment examined in such a trial to consist of one specific drug given at one specific dosage on one specific schedule. Many outcomes studies involve much more complex and less disciplined treatments. For example, managing a given disease may involve multiple components. Providing better insurance coverage is simply a start in a complex chain of events that will be influenced by available care.

In an experiment the investigator creates an intervention, but many health services research studies analyze the effects of different ways to delivering care that occur "naturally." These studies are more akin to evaluations.

Diagnosis Versus Treatment

Medical care of an individual is premised on a general process of care that involves first making a diagnosis in order to determine the patient's problem and then delivering a treatment to address the problem identified. The outcome of care can be the result of both of these steps. In this sense, both the diagnosis and the treatment of a medical condition may be components of the treatment. In many instances, the validity of the diagnosis is simply assumed. One presumes that the correct diagnosis has been made. Indeed, most medical care assumes that a treatment is effective for only specific diagnoses. For example, in the hypothetical study of differences in outcomes seen between patients in health maintenance organizations and fee-for-service medicine, the use of preventive diagnostic testing (e.g., mammography) might be expected to play a role in differences in outcomes seen, given that one hypothesized advantage of health maintenance organizations is their more diligent use of preventive diagnostic testing. Thus, more aggressive screening would presumably yield more positive finding, which should lead to more effective care. However, the better outcomes could result from identification of cases that would of themselves never lead to serious outcomes.

It might be argued that diagnosis has an effect only when it changes treatment; at a fundamental level, this is true. However, diagnosis and treatment are frequently so inextricably linked that attempting to focus solely on the treatment leads to less understanding rather than more. Thus, it is important to understand both the diagnostic and treatment components of the treatment in the outcome study. Because the treatment components of the treatment in the outcomes study are usually more important, they will be discussed first and the diagnostic components after.

Treatment Components

There are three basic components of treatment in allopathic (i.e., Western) medicine: medications, procedures, and counseling/education.[3] Within each of these components, a number of characteristics further define the

---

[3]Other medical belief systems, such as spiritual healing or chiropractic may have other types of components. These may be reasonable elements for an outcome study but the specifics of such are beyond the scope of this text. The general principles of understanding those interventions on a basic level outlined in this section would still apply to those other types of care. The basic level may, however, be different.

component. There are common patterns within the characteristics. All include the type and most include some measure of amount and timing. The components and their characteristics are described later. These individual pieces then fit together as the treatment studied.

Medications

Medications include everything that a patient physically takes into his or her system that has some causal, nontrivial relationship to health status. The type of medication could be a specific prescription or nonprescription drug, but could also include nutritional supplements, herbal remedies, or even nutritional intake itself. Other substances that an individual takes into his or her system could be a type of medication. For example, the type of anesthesia used during surgery could be considered medication. An early outcomes study compared the outcomes of patients who were given different anesthetics during surgery (Moses & Mosteller, 1968).

Another important aspect of medications is the dosage. Different amounts of a medication may be expected to have different effects. Likewise, the duration of treatment is important; many antibiotics are discontinued prematurely. Medications may also be characterized by the route of delivery (e.g., by mouth or intravenously) and the frequency of the medication. The point in the course of the illness when treatment begins can also be important.

Procedures

Procedures include anything physically done to the patient. Procedures share some characteristics with medications and have characteristics that are unique. Further, some characteristics may apply to certain procedures but not to others. For example, it makes more sense to think about the frequency of physical therapy than it does for open heart surgery. Technical aspects of the procedure (e.g., specific technique, devices used, how well it was done) can be very important. Usually, diseases are more responsive to treatment when caught earlier. The nature of a treatment can range anywhere from a noninvasive massage from a physical therapist to very invasive open heart surgery. For many procedures, the timing of the procedure may have an important effect on outcome. For example, the outcomes of total hip arthroplasty are better if it is done before patients become too disabled (Holtzman, Saleh, & Kane, 2002).

Many procedures are done only one time, but some involve multiple treatments, and for these, the frequency of the procedure is an important characteristic.

Unlike medications, many of the technical aspects involved in procedures may affect outcomes. The same procedure may be done with different techniques, with different degrees of skill, and with different devices. Technical skill is hard to assess. It typically relies on someone presumed to be skilled directly observing the performance of the procedure and rating it. Frequently, skill is approximated by using characteristics of the providers (for example, comparing novice operators to those with extensive experience). Because the information is readily available for administrative records, a frequent proxy for skill is volume. Using approximation requires some careful thought. For example, years of training or practice may not always correlate with specific experience performing a given procedure. Volume may reflect many different aspects of care. Surgeon volume needs to be distinguished from hospital volume. The latter more likely reflects care after surgery, whereas surgeon volume is believed to reflect acquired skill. But not every busy surgeon is skillful.

Counseling/Education

Counseling and educating patients involves exchanging information between the patient and the clinician for a therapeutic purpose, either being directly beneficial or by leading to a change in health environment or behaviors.

The nature of counseling or education can vary widely. What does it mean when a doctor said he talked to a patient about smoking? Is this simply an admonition or an in-depth discussion? This can range anywhere from an educational poster on health to intensive psychotherapy. It may also include instruction on other therapies such as how to take medications. The total dose of the counseling/education may be important. Was the discussion the full extent of the action or was there an organized follow-up and support effort? The medium is often the message. Handing someone a pamphlet, or showing them a video may produce very different results from having a physician (or a trained counselor) sit and talk with them. In some circumstances there is reason to believe that doctors carry more clout than other practitioners, but that effect may vary with the physician's skill and interest.

Understanding the Components of Treatment

Randomized controlled trials make special efforts to standardize the intervention in order to assure the impact being assessed can be reliability related to a given treatment. In daily practice, there is much more variation in the treatment provided and hence it is more difficult to identify precisely what elements of care given in what way are the determinants of the outcomes of interest. The more complex the treatment, the more difficult it is to assign the precise causal relationship.

One effort to standardize treatment has been the development of clinical guidelines. These guidelines vary widely in their precision. Some are, in effect, algorithms; others offer only general suggestions. Critics warn about the feasibility, and even the dangers, of forcing excessively strict adherence without adapting them to the individual patient's circumstances (Boyd et al., 2005).

For example, Odderson and McKenna (1993) examined whether the outcomes of patients were better after the introduction of guidelines for stroke care. After implementing the pathway, they noted a decrease in the rate of urinary tract infections (UTIs) of nearly two thirds. Can one conclude from that decrease that clinical pathways for stroke care are effective, at least in avoiding the complications of UTIs? For patients with strokes, the component of care that was most directly related to preventing the development of UTIs was early diagnosis of difficulty voiding through the use of an ultrasound of the bladder. The clinical pathway included an ultrasound of the bladder, which had not been routine care prior to the use of the pathway. Hence, the pathway appeared to be effective. Can one conclude that patients are now getting bladder ultrasounds because of the pathway? If so, would a more focused approach that simply emphasized bladder ultrasounds be as effective?

In order to implement the clinical pathway for stroke, it was first necessary to write the pathway. This task might require that representatives of all of the clinical staff get together and compose the pathway and reach consensus on the proper care of patients admitted with stroke. So, what is the treatment? Is it bringing nurses and doctors together to derive a plan of best care or is it actually using the piece of paper, the pathway, in clinical care? Indeed, in another study, the improvement in care associated with implementing a guideline actually began before the guideline was initiated (Holtzman, Bjerke, & Kane, 1998). The implications of this distinction are far reaching. If it was the process of developing the pathway that was important, how critical is actually using the pathway? On the other hand, can one expect to simply develop pathways that are never implemented? Further, one may not expect the same results if one adopts a pathway developed elsewhere and implements it. To draw a reasonable conclusion, one must become aware of the components of treatment and, having done so, isolate the specific treatment of interest.

Although much is said about evidence-based practice, in truth, most guidelines rely in whole or in part on opinion. Indeed, one way to make guidelines more empirical would be to reverse the process. Instead of using established research findings as the basis for a guideline, test the effects of using guidelines by comparing the outcomes of care delivered using the guidelines and not.

Getting guidelines implemented may not be easy. Major systems changes typically require strong administrative support and attention to how to improve the overall performance structure, including communication (especially at interfaces and hand-offs). Sometimes relatively simple interventions, like getting staff to systematically use checklists can produce big dividends (Pronovost et al., 2006).

Does the Type of Physician Matter?

American medicine has become very specialized, but it is not clear for what which kinds of specialists are needed. Jollis and colleagues (1996) found that patients who were admitted to the hospital with acute myocardial infarction by a cardiologist were less likely to die in the coming year than those who were admitted by other types of physicians. However, the patients admitted by cardiologists may differ in terms of severity of disease, comorbidities, and demographic factors that may independently influence the probability of death. In this study, the differences were still present when those factors were accounted for through statistical means. Can one conclude that care for patients admitted by cardiologists is better?

Here again, it is helpful to examine the components that make up the intervention. Care of the patient with a myocardial infarction involves multiple treatment components, but all of these components are not universally available and where available may not be of similar quality everywhere. For example, cardiac procedures such as cardiac catheterization and coronary artery bypass grafting are not available at all hospitals. Further, care in a coronary care unit might be expected to vary from a hospital that routinely cares for multiple patients with myocardial infarction at a time versus one that rarely cares for a patient with a myocardial infarction. To what extent do the improved results reflect greater access to or quality of these components of treatment in institutions where cardiologists practice versus the institutions where other physicians practice? In some instances, the presence of a cardiologist is inherently linked to the preferred service. For example, cardiac procedures are more likely to be available in institutions where cardiologists admit patients. Only by understanding the components of care and taking them into account in the execution and analysis of the study, can one conclude whether the treatment "admission by a cardiologist" leads to better outcomes.

Isolating the Treatment of Interest

The most straightforward way to isolate the effect of the treatment of interest is to use a comparison group that differs from the group that gets the treatment only by not getting the treatment. Because most treatments involve several components, designing a study that examines each component may prove very difficult. Most of the time we resort to what has been labeled "black box" evaluations, in which we test the effect of the overall treatment as though it were a large black box we could not see into. Interpreting and presenting the results of such a study requires great care. One does not want to exceed the actual findings and limitations, but there is great pressure to say something of value, which will catch people's attention. Results cast entirely in limitations will not attract a wide audience.

For treatments that occur over time, it may prove feasible to examine the effect at different points in time. As in the clinical pathway example, one might examine the change in outcome between the time before the pathway project was undertaken and the time when the pathway had been developed but not yet not implemented. A second analysis could focus on changes after pathway development but before and after it was implemented. Such an approach could isolate the effect of developing the pathway from the use of the pathway. (This technique for examining treatment would be much stronger if one can also include a group that is not exposed to the development or implementation of the pathway to account for any changes occurring over time.)

At least part of the success of many treatments may be attributed to what is termed the "placebo effect." Basically, the belief that one is getting treatment may in and of itself produce a positive effect. This is why drug trials always use placebos for control patients. A variation on this theme is the so-called attention control. Especially in counseling situations, clients may respond positively to the attention they receive, even if the specific counseling technique is ineffective. To guard against this risk, study designers routinely build in some sort of attention control, whereby the control group participates in an equally intense experience that is not expected to affect the outcomes of interest.

It is relatively easy to imagine a placebo control for a drug study (although the placebo may have fewer side effects and hence not be totally interchangeable). It is much harder to conceive an acceptable placebo for surgical interventions, even though surgery likely exerts a very potent placebo effect. It is hard to believe that someone who goes through a surgical procedure that is presented as a way to improve their condition would not be influenced by the experience. Not surprisingly, there have been very few sham surgery studies, wherein the control group received a deliberately ineffective procedure. One early example was the internal mammary ligation trial in which the control patients had their sternums split and reclosed without ligating the internal mammary arteries, a procedure believed then to increase collateral circulation to the coronary vessels. To everyone's chagrin, the control patients did slightly better than the experimental subjects on cardiac performance measures of the time (Cobb, Thomas, Dillard, Merendino, & Bruce, 1959). A more recent example was the double blinded study of knee arthroscopy, which again showed no benefit from the surgery (and generated a great deal of controversy) (Moseley et al., 2002). Needless to say, such studies are few and far between.

No recipe for a study design will work to isolate the treatment effect for every outcomes study. The important process is to examine the components of the treatment and with that knowledge design the study to isolate the effect.

Statistically Isolating the Effect of Treatment

For observational studies, the challenge of isolating the effects of treatment depends on both study design (are the right variables captured, is the sample adequate) and analysis. As noted earlier in this book, isolating the effects of treatment requires controlling for the effects of other potential influences. Chapter 3 addresses the various approaches that have been used to achieve this goal. Here we note, in particular, the need to think about potential interactions between the treatment of interest and other variables. Some treatments are likely to work better with some patients. The whole concept of individualized treatment has been spurred by the appreciation of the potential role of genetics in determining the effectiveness of various treatments, but many simpler factors can also be in play.

Age, gender, and race may influence the response to treatment in some circumstances because of biological differences. Prior experience with a disease will likely affect the response to the current treatment.

Variation in Treatment

Investigating the effect of treatment requires that there be variation in the treatment within the study. In other words, it is necessary to have a comparison group. Without some sort of comparison, one cannot assess the treatment effect. Three dimensions of comparison can be identified:

1. **Treatment versus no treatment.** Do elderly individuals who receive medication for isolated systolic hypertension have a lower incidence of cardiovascular disease than those receiving no treatment? (SHEP Cooperative Research Group, 1991)

2. **Treatment A versus Treatment B.** Is one antihypertensive medication more effective at preventing heart attack than another? (ALLHAT Collaborative Research Group, 2002)

3. **Treatment A + B versus Treatment B alone.** Do beta-blockers provide additional benefit for patients with congestive heart failure already on angiotensin converting enzyme inhibitors? (CIBIS-II Investigators and Committees, 1999)

Table 10-3 gives examples of each model of comparison for different types of treatment.

Treatments may also vary by intensity, timing, or duration. Table 10-4 shows examples of such variation for different types of interventions.

One challenge for a new treatment is the belief that it represents a substantial step forward. If that is the case, there will be a push to implement it for everyone rather than restrict its use to afford comparisons. This was the case with AIDS drugs. Since people were dying, the effectiveness of a new treatment was felt to not need a control. Survival was proof enough. Unfortunately, establishing efficacy without a strong

Table 10-3 Studies of Various Treatment Regimens

Treatment	Basis of Comparison		
	Treatment A vs No Treatment	Treatment A vs Treatment B (best current practice)	Treatment A + B vs Treatment A alone
Medication	SHEP trial; investigated whether it is better to treat isolated systolic hypertension in the elderly than to leave it untreated (Anonymous, 1991b)	ALLHAT trial compared the outcomes of different medications for hypertension with no placebo group (Anonymous, 2002)	CIBIS-II examined whether beta-blockers were beneficial in addition to ACE inhibitors for congestive heart failure (Anonymous, 1999)
Procedure	Macular Photocoagulation Study; investigated the use of photocoagulation vs no treatment for eyes with choroidal revascularization (Anonymous, 1991a)	The National Cancer Institute conducted a study examining whether outcomes were different for mastectomy or breast conservation surgery for breast cancer (Poggi et al., 2003)	Allen et al. examined whether a transmyocardial revascularization procedure provided additional benefit to patients undergoing coronary artery bypass grafting (Allen et al., 2000)
Counseling/ Education of patient	Hypertension Prevention Trial; addressed the effects of counseling changes in	Teri and Lewinsohn examined whether individual or group treatment was more effective	Lovibond, Birrell, and Langeluddecke examined whether more personalized counseling on

(continues)

Table 10-3   *(continued)*

Basis of Comparison			
Treatment	**Treatment A vs No Treatment**	**Treatment A vs Treatment B (best current practice)**	**Treatment A + B vs Treatment A alone**
	health behaviors on controlling mild hypertension (Anonymous, 1990)	for depression (Teri & Lewinsohn, 1986)	exercise provided benefit in addition to general counseling (Lovibond, Birrell, & Langeluddecke, 1986)
Combinations	The Lung Health Study; examined whether medications and counseling were more effective for smoking cessation than no intervention (Hughes, Lindgren, Connett, & Nides, 2004)	The Veterans Affairs cooperative urologic study group; examined surgical orchiectomy versus medications for prostate cancer (Anonymous, 1967)	Hurt et al. examined whether adding bupropion to counseling was more effective than counseling alone for smoking cessation (Hurt et al., 1997)

research design proved difficult, and ultimately the program retreated back to clinical trials.

Conversely, it may be hard to recruit patients to take a less effective treatment or especially to forgo care. In many instances, the best you can do is to adapt some form of quasi-experiment design in which the comparison is drawn from extant data. A number of designs are feasible (see Chapter 2). Basic strategies (each with its own limitations) include historical contrasts (basically before and after, but hopefully with more data

Table 10-4 Studies of Comparing Treatment Intensity, Timing, or Duration

Treatment	Basis of Comparison		
	Intensity	**Timing**	**Duration**
Medication	Kearon et al. examined more intensive versus less intensive warfarin therapy to prevent recurrent deep venous thrombosis (Kearon et al., 2003)	Cook, Zachariah, Cree, and Harrison examined the effectiveness of twice daily dosing of amoxicillin and clavulanate compared to three times a day for childhood respiratory tract infections (Cook, Zachariah, Cree, & Harrison, 1996)	Elhanan et al. examined 1 day versus 5 days of antibiotics of urinary tract infections in women (Elhanan et al., 1994)
Procedure	Helmhout, Harts, Staal, Candel, and de Bie examined whether high-intensity or low-intensity training was more effective for low back pain (Helmhout, Harts, Staal, Candel, & de Bie, 2004)	Rainville, Jouve, Hartigan, Martinez, and Hipona examined the effectiveness of twice a week versus three times a week physical therapy for back pain (Rainville, Jouve, Hartigan, Martinez, & Hipona, 2002)	Hamza et al. examined the effect of different durations of electrical stimulation to relieve low back pain (Hamza et al., 1999)

(continues)

Table 10-4 *(continued)*

Basis of Comparison			
Treatment	**Intensity**	**Timing**	**Duration**
Counseling/ Education of patient/ provider	Alterman, Gariti, and Mulvaney examined varying intensity of counseling for smoking cessation (Alterman, Gariti, & Mulvaney, 2001)	Joseph, Willenbring, Nelson, and Nugent examined the optimal timing of smoking cessation counseling in individuals undergoing alcohol dependence treatment (Joseph, Willenbring, Nelson, & Nugent, 2002)	Gilbert et al. examined the effect of the duration of a smoking cessation program on quitting (Gilbert et al., 1992)
Combinations	The UKPDS (UK Prospective Diabetes Study) examined whether a more intensive regimen of blood glucose control for diabetics reduced diabetic complications (Anonymous, 1998)		

points both pre- and postevent), comparison groups (comparable groups getting different treatments with analysis of change between them (what is sometimes called differences of differences), and franchises (wherein one part of a unit pursues the new treatment and others maintain the old approach).

Each approach has drawbacks. The more prospective the study, usually, the stronger the design. Historical designs typically must rely on extant records that may not capture the most relevant detail and certainly will not capture it consistently or in equal detail. One may end up using some unsatisfactory lowest common denominator approach to standardize data across observation points.

Combinations of different classes of treatments can also be compared. For example, Hurt and colleagues examined whether adding the medication bupropion to counseling for smoking cessation was more effective than counseling alone (Hurt et al., 1997).

Because the critical issue is comparing what was done, investigators should take steps to control for how well the treatment was administered. For example, if the study compares one surgical procedure versus another, investigators should take steps to ensure that the two procedures were performed by equally competent surgeons. A poorly executed coronary artery bypass graft (CABG) may have worse outcomes than a competently executed angioplasty regardless of the merits of the two procedures. The effect of variations in surgical skill can be disentangled from the effects of the treatments by manipulating the experimental design or by accounting for these variations statistically. Solutions based on experimental design include randomizing surgeons to surgical procedures so that there is no systematic correlation between surgeon characteristics and type of procedure. Statistical solutions involve estimating a multiple regression that includes dummy variables to indicate which physician performed the surgery or using other results from these surgeons as a proxy for their skills. In this way, any special skills that a given surgeon brings to the experiment can be statistically disentangled from the effect of the surgery itself. Dummy variables that represent interactions between the surgeon and the surgical procedure he or she performed may also be necessary if some surgeons tend to be skilled in one surgical procedure but not the other.

A more controversial element of treatment is the role of patient adherence. On the one hand, it seems intuitive that a drug not taken is unlikely to work. Hence, the rate of actually taking the drug should be considered. However, the reasons for not taking the drug may be related to the drug itself (e.g., taste, side effects). Thus, adherence is part of the picture. In formal drug trials, adherence is not allowed as an intervening variable. Indeed, there are formal rules about using intention to treat (ITT), whereby every subject assigned to a study condition must be retained in the analysis, even if they did not complete the course of treatment.

Nonetheless, examining adherence may prove useful in understanding why a particular drug regimen was not successful.

Quality Improvement

A special case of treatment may be found in connection with quality improvement (QI). QI projects may be very focused on a given element in the delivery process or they may address large system-wide changes. There is some controversy about how they should be judged. One school of thought holds that they should be viewed as any other interventions designed to improve care (Kane & Mosser, 2007). The other approach holds that QI is heavily contextual and can only be judged by understanding the full range of factors that affect the outcomes (Berwick, 2008).

SUMMARY

Health outcomes research is designed to identify the effects of treatment, but treatment is often poorly measured. It can have many facets. No single study can capture them all, but as much effort should be expended measuring what constitutes the treatment of interest as goes into assessing outcomes. There is no consensus about what constitutes treatment, but most measures should capture information about the type and the dosage (and perhaps also include the duration).

Drawing meaningful conclusions about the effect of treatment requires attending to three things about the treatment and its assessment in the study:

1. Understand the components of the treatment and how they go together—what elements are of interest and what elements need to be addressed in some other way.

2. Include variation in treatment in the study—some sort of comparison group or comparison within the treatment group (e.g., varying doses of medication).

3. Understand that the effect of the treatment observed is the difference in outcomes between the treatment group and the comparison group after the effects of other factors have been eliminated (or controlled for).

REFERENCES

Allen, K. B., Dowling, R. D., DelRossi, A. J., Realyvasques, F., Lefrak, E. A., Pfeffer, T. A., et al. (2000). Transmyocardial laser revascularization combined with coronary artery bypass grafting: A multicenter, blinded, prospective, randomized, controlled trial. *J Thorac Cardiovasc Surg, 119*(3), 540–549.

ALLHAT Collaborative Research Group. (2002). Major outcomes in high-risk hypertensive patients randomized to angiotensin-converting enzyme inhibitor or calcium channel blocker vs diuretic: The Antihypertensive and Lipid-Lowering Treatment to Prevent Heart Attack Trial (ALLHAT). *Journal of the American Medical Association, 288*(23), 2981–2997.

Alterman, A. I., Gariti, P., & Mulvaney, F. (2001). Short- and long-term smoking cessation for three levels of intensity of behavioral treatment. *Psychol Addict Behav, 15*(3), 261–264.

Anonymous. (1967). Treatment and survival of patients with cancer of the prostate. The Veterans Administration Co-operative Urological Research Group. *Surg Gynecol Obstet, 124*(5), 1011–1017.

Anonymous. (1990). The Hypertension Prevention Trial: Three-year effects of dietary changes on blood pressure. Hypertension Prevention Trial Research Group. *Arch Intern Med, 150*(1), 153–162.

Anonymous. (1991a). Laser photocoagulation of subfoveal neovascular lesions in age-related macular degeneration. Results of a randomized clinical trial. Macular Photocoagulation Study Group. *Arch Ophthalmol, 109*(9), 1220–1231.

Anonymous. (1998). Intensive blood-glucose control with sulphonylureas or insulin compared with conventional treatment and risk of complications in patients with type 2 diabetes (UKPDS 33). UK Prospective Diabetes Study (UKPDS) Group. *Lancet, 352*(9131), 837–853.

Arrington, A. K., Jarosek, S. L., Virnig, B. A., Habermann, E. B., & Tuttle, T. M. (2009). Patient and surgeon characteristics associated with increased use of contralateral prophylactic mastectomy in patients with breast cancer. *Annals of Surgical Oncology, 16*(10), 2697–2704.

Berwick, D. M. (2008). The science of improvement. *Journal of the American Medical Association, 299*(10), 1182–1184.

Boyd, C. M., Darer, J., Boult, C., Fried, L. P., Boult, L., & Wu, A. W. (2005). Clinical practice guidelines and quality of care for older patients with multiple comorbid diseases: Implications for pay for performance. *Journal of the American Medical Association, 294*(6), 716–724.

Butler, M., Forte, M., Kane, R. L., Joglekar, S., Duval, S. J., Swiontkowski, M., . . .Wilt, T. (2009). *Treatment of common hip fractures.* Rockville, MD: Agency for Healthcare Research and Quality. Available at: www.ahrq.gov/clinic/hipfractp.htm. Accessed May 3, 2010.

CIBIS-II Investigators and Committees. (1999). The Cardiac Insufficiency Bisoprolol Study II (CIBIS-II): A randomised trial. *Lancet, 353*(9146), 9–13.

Cobb, L. A., Thomas, G. I., Dillard, D. H., Merendino, K. A., & Bruce, R. A. (1959). An evaluation of internal-mammary-artery ligation by a double-blind technic. *New England Journal of Medicine, 260*(22), 1115–1118.

Cook, R. C., Zachariah, J., Cree, F., & Harrison, H. E. (1996). Efficacy of twice-daily amoxycillin/clavulanate ('Augmentin-Duo' 400/57) in mild to moderate lower respiratory tract infection in children. *British Journal of Clinical Practice, 50*(3), 125–128.

Elhanan, G., Tabenkin, H., Yahalom, R., & Raz, R. (1994). Single-dose fosfomycin trometamol versus 5-day cephalexin regimen for treatment of uncomplicated lower urinary tract infections in women. *Antimicrobial Agents and Chemotherapy, 38*(11), 2612–2614.

Gilbert, J. R., Wilson, D. M., Singer, J., Lindsay, E. A., Willms, D. G., Best, J. A., & Taylor, D. W. (1992). A family physician smoking cessation program: An evaluation of the role of follow-up visits. *American Journal of Preventive Medicine, 8*(2), 91–95.

Hamza, M. A., Ghoname, E. A., White, P. F., Craig, W. F., Ahmed, H. E., Gajraj, N. M., . . .Noe, C. E. (1999). Effect of the duration of electrical stimulation on the analgesic response in patients with low back pain. *Anesthesiology, 91*(6), 1622–1627.

Helmhout, P. H., Harts, C. C., Staal, J. B., Candel, M. J., & de Bie, R. A. (2004). Comparison of a high-intensity and a low-intensity lumbar extensor training program as minimal intervention treatment in low back pain: A randomized trial. *European Spine Journal, 13*(6), 537–547.

Holtzman, J. (2005). Capturing the effects of treatment In R. L. Kane (Ed.). *Understanding health care outcomes research* (2nd ed.). Sudbury, MA: Jones and Bartlett Publishers.

Holtzman, J., Bjerke, T., & Kane, R. (1998). The effects of clinical pathways for renal transplant on patient outcomes and length of stay. *Medical Care, 36*(6), 826–834.

Holtzman, J., Saleh, K., & Kane, R. (2002). Effect of baseline functional status and pain on outcomes of total hip arthroplasty. *The Journal of Bone and Joint Surgery, 84-A*(11), 1942–1948.

Hughes, J., Lindgren, P., Connett, J., & Nides, M. (2004). Smoking reduction in the Lung Health Study. *Nicotine & Tobacco Research, 6*(2), 275–280.

Hurt, R. D., Sachs, D. P., Glover, E. D., Offord, K. P., Johnston, J. A., Dale, L. C., . . .Sullivan, P. M. (1997). A comparison of sustained-release bupropion and placebo for smoking cessation. *New England Journal of Medicine, 337*(17), 1195–1202.

Jollis, J. G., DeLong, E. R., Peterson, E. D., Muhlbaier, L. H., Fortin, D. F., Califf, R. M., . . .Mark, D. B. (1996). Outcome of acute myocardial infarction according to the specialty of the admitting physician. *New England Journal of Medicine, 335*(25), 1880–1887.

Joseph, A. M., Willenbring, M. L., Nelson, D., & Nugent, S. M. (2002). Timing of alcohol and smoking cessation study. *Alcoholism and Clinical Experimental Research, 26*(12), 1945–1946.

Kane, R. L., & Mosser, G. (2007). The challenge of explaining why quality improvement has not done better. *International Journal for Quality in Health Care, 19*(1), 8–10.

Kearon, C., Ginsberg, J. S., Kovacs, M. J., Anderson, D. R., Wells, P., Julian, J. A., . . .Gent, M. (2003). Comparison of low-intensity warfarin therapy with conventional-intensity warfarin therapy for long-term prevention of recurrent venous thrombo-embolism. *New England Journal of Medicine, 349*(7), 631–639.

Lovibond, S. H., Birrell, P. C., & Langeluddecke, P. (1986). Changing coronary heart disease risk-factor status: the effects of three behavioral programs. *Journal of Behavioral Medicine, 9*(5), 415–437.

Lurie, N., Slater, J., McGovern, P., Ekstrum, J., Quam, L., & Margolis, K. (1993). Preventive care for women. Does the sex of the physician matter? *New England Journal of Medicine, 329*, 478–482.

Matthews, W. J., Conti, J. M., & Sireci, S. G. (2001). The effects of intercessory prayer, positive visualization, and expectancy on the well-being of kidney dialysis patients. *Alternative Therapies in Health & Medicine, 7*(5), 42–52.

Moseley, J. B., O'Malley, K., Petersen, N. J., Menke, T. J., Brody, B. A., Kuykendall, D. H., . . .Wray, N. P. (2002). A controlled trial of arthroscopic surgery for osteoarthritis of the knee. *New England Journal of Medicine, 347*(2), 81–88.

Moses, L. E., & Mosteller, F. (1968). Institutional differences in post-operative death rates. Commentary on some of the findings of the National Halothane Study. *Journal of the American Medical Association, 203*(7), 492–494.

Newhouse, J. P. (1993). *Free for all? Lessons from the RAND health insurance experiment.* Cambridge, MA: Harvard University Press.

Odderson, I. R., & McKenna, B. S. (1993). A model for manage-ment of patients with stroke during the acute phase. Outcome and economic implications. *Stroke, 24*(12), 1823–1827.

Palmer, R. F., Katerndahl, D., & Morgan-Kidd, J. (2004). A randomized trial of the effects of remote intercessory prayer: Interactions with personal beliefs on problem-specific outcomes and functional status. *Journal of Alternative & Complementary Medicine*, *10*(3), 438–448.

Poggi, M. M., Danforth, D. N., Sciuto, L. C., Smith, S. L., Steinberg, S. M., Liewehr, D. J., . . .Altemus, R. M. (2003). Eighteen-year results in the treatment of early breast carcinoma with mastectomy versus breast conservation therapy: The National Cancer Institute Randomized Trial. *Cancer*, *98*(4), 697–702.

Pronovost, P., Needham, D., Berenholtz, S., Sinopoli, D., Chu, H., Cosgrove, S., . . .Goeschel, C. (2006). An intervention to decrease catheter-related bloodstream infections in the ICU. *New England Journal of Medicine*, *355*(26), 2725–2732.

Rainville, J., Jouve, C. A., Hartigan, C., Martinez, E., & Hipona, M. (2002). Comparison of short- and long-term outcomes for aggressive spine rehabilitation delivered two versus three times per week. *The Spine Journal*, *2*(6), 402–407.

SHEP Cooperative Research Group. (1991). Prevention of stroke by antihypertensive drug treatment in older persons with isolated systolic hypertension. Final results of the Systolic Hypertension in the Elderly Program (SHEP). SHEP Cooperative Research Group. *Journal of the American Medical Association*, *265*(24), 3255–3264.

Teri, L., & Lewinsohn, P. M. (1986). Individual and group treatment of unipolar depression: Comparison of treatment outcomes and identification of predictors of successful treatment outcomes. *Behavior Therapy*, *17*(3), 217–228.

Risk Adjustment

There is an aphorism that every doctor believes he treats the toughest patients. When the results of a quality performance analysis are reported, those who fared poorly are quick to suggest that the difference was due to case mix. Especially in instances where there is no random assignment to treatment conditions, concerns over differences in risk will inevitably arise.

Ideally, every test of an intervention would compare it to a control condition on the same patients at the same time; this is called the counterfactual case. It is obviously possible only in theory. Instead, we must rely on statistical adjustment to account for the differences in the composition of the two groups.

This problem is not new. Florence Nightingale noted variation in the "106 principal hospitals of England" in the 19th century (Iezzoni, 1996). Just over 100 years later, US analysts working with Medicare data suggested that there were substantial variations in mortality across American hospitals (Jencks et al., 1988). This work was soon criticized for ignoring the role of comorbid diseases (Greenfield, Aronow, Elashoff, & Watanabe, 1988).

Any discussion of health outcomes must be prepared to contend with risk adjustment. The real question is risk of what to adjust for over how long a period. Alas, there is no simple answer; it depends on one's purpose (Iezzoni, 2003).

"The purpose. . .establishes the logical criterion for judging the validity and consistency of alternative measures. Without a clearly defined purpose, measurement becomes arbitrary" (Hornbrook, 1985).

Answering questions about outcomes requires specifying the outcomes of interest and a method to operationally define them. The second step involves devising ways to ascertain what caused the outcome. Iezzoni (2003) refers to this latter step as the "algebra of effectiveness." Patient outcomes are the result of a complex process, not the least of which involves the medical services provided, quality of care, random events, and patients' clinical attributes. The latter includes the severity of illness, coexisting diseases, and risk factors. Risk adjustment takes into account relevant patient attributes for making valid inferences about effectiveness and quality of care.

The term *risk adjustment* is inconsistently defined. It is used synonymously with terms like *severity, risk, case mix, sickness, intensity, complexity, comorbidity*, and *health status*. Risk adjustment implies the prediction of health outcomes based on the assessment of risk characteristics. The following broad set of characteristics can reflect risk:

- Age
- Sex
- Race and ethnicity
- Acute clinical stability
- Principal diagnosis ("case mix")
- Extent and severity of principal diagnosis
- Extent and severity of comorbidities (coexisting diseases)
- Physical functional status
- Psychological, cognitive, and psychosocial functioning
- Cultural, ethnic, and socioeconomic attributes and behaviors
- Health status and quality of life
- Patient attitudes and preferences for outcomes

SEVERITY AND COMORBIDITY

Severity and comorbidity are two closely related but distinct concepts. *Severity* refers to classifying the patient's primary problem in terms of prognosis. "'Severity' typifies the concept of 'risk'—the higher the severity, the higher patients' risk (or likelihood) of poor outcomes, variously defined" (Iezzoni, 2003). By contrast, *comorbidity* refers to coexisting conditions, aside from the patient's primary problem, that predict health outcomes. These are diseases and conditions unrelated etiologically to the principal diagnosis.

Severity can be approached in several ways. Gonella and colleagues developed a staging concept for a variety of diseases based on the long-standing approach to staging cancer. The first stage was a local or mild occurrence and the last stage was death (Gonnella, Hornbrook, & Louis, 1984).

A widely used generic severity measure is the APACHE II, which relies largely on physiologic data to predict the risk of death in ICU patients (Knaus, Draper, & Wagner, 1985) It sums values from the following three components:

- **A**cute **P**hysiology Score: 12 variables reflecting physiologic functioning, worse value over first 24 hours, and each variable assigned a weight
- **A**ge
- **C**hronic **H**ealth **E**valuation

Another generic risk measure designed for a specific-patient group is the probability of repeated hospital admissions (P_{ra}). It was developed to identify elderly patients who might benefit from a comprehensive geriatric evaluation. It predicts repeated admission to the hospital within 4 years and use of health-related services. It uses information derived from patient reports on self-rated health, disability, illnesses, and prior utilization (Boult et al., 1993; Boult, Pacala, & Boult, 1995; Pacala, Boult, & Boult, 1995).

A widely used diagnosis-specific severity measure is the Diagnosis-Related Grouping (DRG), which Medicare uses as the basis for hospital payment. It relies on studies that have related diagnoses and other readily available administrative data to length of stay in hospital patients. It groups patients with similar clinical attributes and output utilization patterns. It assigns the major group from primary diagnosis. Subgroups are created by examining comorbidities. Procedures and patient age are then used to refine groups. This approach was designed primarily for reimbursement purposes. It has limited use for risk adjustment.

DIAGNOSIS-SPECIFIC SEVERITY

One frequently used measure of diagnosis-specific severity is the American Heart Association (AHA) Stroke Outcome Classification (Kelly-Hayes et al., 1998). This measure is built around six clinical domains: motor, sensory, vision, language, cognition, and affect. Each of the domains is documented in terms of frequency and severity of the deficits. Patients are classified according to number of domains impaired, the severity, and functional classification.

The Canadian Neurological Scale (CNS) is an alternative measure that focuses on assessments of mentation and motor function (Cote et al., 1989; Cote, Hachinski, Shurvell, Norris, & Wolfson, 1986). The CNS has been shown to predict patient outcomes and identifies the presence of symptoms specific to acute stroke (e.g., consciousness, paralysis, and speech difficulty). Scoring is simply the sum of the individual scores within each assessment area (see Table 11-1).

Another example of a more complicated approach to a diagnosis-specific severity measure can be seen in the Low Back Classification system that incorporates the type of back pain (radicular pain versus regional low back pain), previous history of low back problems (no history of back problems versus previous history of back problems versus history of previous back surgeries), and length of time with back pain (less than 6 weeks versus 6 weeks or more).

Grade I – no history of back problems and regional low back pain on the date of visit.

Grade II – no previous history of back problems and radicular low back pain on the date of visit.

Grade III – previous history of back problems, regional or radicular low back pain on the date of visit, and current back pain for less than 6 weeks.

Grade IV – previous history of back problems, regional or radicular low back pain on the date of visit, and current back pain for more than 6 weeks.

Grade V – one or more back surgeries.

Generic Comorbidity Measures

Comorbidities can be expressed simply by listing each diagnosis a patient has and creating a dummy code (i.e., absent, present) for each, but that requires a lot of variables. Sometimes the researcher may simply limit the loss to those he or she feels are of greatest salience. A typical list might include asthma, congestive heart failure, angina, myocardial infarction, diabetes mellitus, hypertension, cancer, knee pain, osteoarthritis, visual impairment, and hearing impairment, although the latter two may not affect some outcomes.

Table 11-1   Canadian Neurological Scale

Mentation		Score
Level of consciousness	Alert	3.0
	Drowsy	1.0
Orientation	Oriented	1.5
	Disoriented/NA	0.0
Speech	Normal	1.0
	Expressive Deficit	0.5
	Receptive Deficit	0.0
Motor Functions: If There is **No** *Comprehension Deficit*		

Motor Functions	Weakness	Score
Face	None	0.5
	Present	0.0
Arm: Proximal	None	1.5
	Mild	1.0
	Significant	0.5
	Total	0.0
Arm: Distal	None	1.5
	Mild	1.0
	Significant	0.5
	Total	0.0
Leg: Proximal	None	1.5
	Mild	1.0
	Significant	0.5
	Total	0.0
Leg: Distal	None	1.5
	Mild	1.0
	Significant	0.5
	Total	0.0
Motor Functions: If There is a Comprehension Deficit		

Motor Functions	Weakness	Score
Face	Symmetrical	0.5
	Asymmetrical	0.0
Arms	Equal	1.5
	Unequal	0.0
Legs	Equal	1.5
	Unequal	0.0

NA, not applicable.

Sometimes he or she may simply count the number of comorbidities, in effect weighting each one equally. Probably the most commonly used measure of comorbidity was developed by Mary Charlson, who created a weighted comorbidity score. She originally estimated the risk of each of a number of conditions on hospital mortality and used those coefficients as the basis for the weights (Charlson, Pompei, Ales, & MacKenzie, 1987).

The Charlson score assigns weights, based on relative risk, to 23 possible conditions (the number of conditions varies slightly because of modifications in the index) and creates a final index based on summing the individual weights. The overall score reflects the increased likelihood of 1-year mortality (see Table 11-2).

Charlson and others later used the same approach to develop a weighted comorbidity score for ambulatory care (Charlson et al., 2008; D'Hoore, Sicotte, & Tilquin, 1993; Deyo, Cherkin, & Ciol, 1992; Romano, Roos, Luft, Jollis, & Doliszny, 1994).

The next progression was to move from chart review to administrative data sources. Table 11-3 compares three adaptations of the Charlson scale for use with administrative databases. As can be readily seen, each approach is a little different.

The list of comorbidities used to construct the Charlson Comorbidity Index has been expanded to include 30 diagnosis subgroups (Elixhauser, Steiner, Harris, & Coffey, 1998). The Elixhauser Comorbidity Index has seen wide use in health services and epidemiological research. Compared with the Charlson, it has broader application across a range of conditions

Table 11-2 Charlson Comorbidity Index Weights

Weights	Conditions
1	Myocardial infarct, congestive heart failure, peripheral vascular disease, cerebrovascular disease, dementia, chronic pulmonary disease, connective tissue disease, ulcer disease, mild liver disease, diabetes
2	Hemiplegia, moderate or severe renal disease, diabetes with end organ damage, any tumor, leukemia, lymphoma
3	Moderate or severe liver disease
6	Metastatic solid tumor, acquired immunodeficiency syndrome

Table 11-3   Comparison of Three Modifications of the Charlson Comorbidity Index Using ICD-9-CM Administrative Data

Weight	Diagnostic Category	Deyo	Romano	D'Hoore
1	Myocardial infarct	410.xx, 412*	410.xx, 412*	410, 411
	Congestive heart failure	428.x	402.01, 402.11, 402.91, 425.x, 428.x, 429.3	398, 402, 428
	Peripheral vascular disease	443.9,* 441–441.9,* 785.4,* V43.4,* 38.48	440.x,* 441.x,* 442.x,* 443.1–443.9,* 447.1,* 785.4,* 38.13–38.14,* 38.16,* 38.18,* 38.33–38.34,* 38.36,* 38.38,* 38.43–38.44,* 38.46,* 38.48,* 39.22–39.26,* 39.29*	440–447
	Dementia	290.x	290.x,* 331–331.2*	290, 291, 294
	Cerebrovascular disease	430–438	362.34, 430–436, 437–437.1, 437.9, 438, 781.4, 784.3, 997.0, 38.12, 38.42	430–433, 435
	Chronic pulmonary disease	490–496,* 500–505,* 506.4*	415.0,* 416.8–416.9,* 491.x–494,* 496	491–493
	Connective tissue disease	na	na	710, 714, 725

(continued)

Table 11-3 *(continued)*

Weight	Diagnostic Category	Deyo	Romano	D'Hoore
	Rheumatologic disease	710.0,* 710.1,* 710.4,* 714–714.2,* 714.81,* 725*	na	na
	Ulcer disease	531–534.9, 531.4–531.7, 532.4–532.7, 533.4–533.7, 534.4–534.7	531.xx–534.xx	531–534
	Mild liver disease	571.2,* 571.5, 571.6,* 571.4–571.49*	571.2,* 571.5–571.6, 571.8–571.9*	571, 573
	Diabetes	250–250.3, 250.7	250.0x–250.3x*	na
2	Hemiplegia	344.1,* 342–342.9*	342.x, 344.x	342, 434, 436, 437
	Moderate and severe renal disease	582–582.9,* 583–583.7,* 585,* 586,* 588–588.9*	582–586,* 42.0,* 45.1,* 56.x,* 39.27,* 39.42,* 39.9–39.95,* 54.98*	403, 404, 580–586

	Condition			
	Diabetes with complications	250–250.3, 250.7,* 250.4–250.6*	250–250.3, 250.7,* 250.4–250.6*	250
	Any tumor including leukemia and lymphoma	140–172.9, 174–195.8, 200–208.9	140–171.x,* 174.x–195.x,* 200.xx–208.x,* 273.0,* 273.3,* 10.46,* 60.5,* 62.4–62.41*	140–195
	Leukemia	na	na	204–208
3	Lymphoma	na	na	200, 202, 203
	Moderate or severe liver disease	572.2–572.8,* 456.0–456.2x*	572.2–572.4,* 456.0–456.2x,* 39.1,* 42.91*	070, 570, 572
6	Metastatic solid tumor	196–199.1	196–199.1	196–199
	AIDS	042.0–44.9	na	na

*Included if listed during index or prior hospitalizations.

AIDS, acquired immunodeficiency syndrome; na, not applicable.

and outcomes. With changes in the coding of administrative data from ICD-9 to ICD-10, both the Charlson and Elixhauser appear to have prognostic validity (Li, Evans, Faris, Dean, & Quan, 2008).

The problem of comorbidities becomes more complex when we realize that each comorbidity can also have a severity. Comorbidities might then be classified according to severity. Earlier work tried to capture the severity of the morbidities, but these approaches have failed to catch on in general use, perhaps because they were too complex (Greenfield, Apolone, McNeil, & Cleary, 1993; Kaplan & Feinstein, 1974; Linn, Linn, & Gurel, 1968).

It is important to distinguish comorbidities from complications. Comorbidities are present at the onset of the episode in question, whereas complications arise during the episode. Unfortunately, most administrative databases do not distinguish between these two types of additional diagnoses, and hence one risks adjusting away important differences in care. Medicare has recognized the salience of this distinction and now requires separate identification of a prescribed list of hospital acquired conditions. They will no longer allow an increase in case mix severity for these conditions, which were presumably the result of inadequate care. In the case of diabetes, many diagnoses included in risk adjustment are potential complications of the condition (e.g., end-stage nephropathy, retinopathy, and neuropathy). This is especially the case for some of the diagnoses found on the Charlson Comorbidity Index. In the case of diabetes, the investigator might choose to treat these triopathy of complications as a severity index of diabetes.

Why Should We Measure Comorbidity (or the Severity of Illness)?

Control for Selection Bias

In essence, case mix adjustment represents one step toward addressing selection bias (see Chapters 2 and 3). Adjusting for the presence of various diseases is one way to level the playing field. As the diagram below (Figure 11-1) suggests, severity and comorbidity might influence both the choice of treatment and its outcome. This problem is also referred to as confounding in epidemiological studies. Another way of looking at this is that treatments are differentially distributed across groups according to the severity of illness. Two conditions are necessary for confounding: (1) severity of illness

Figure 11-1   **Control for selection bias**

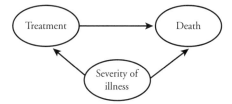

is associated with the outcome and (2) severity of illness is associated with the treatment, but it is not a consequence of the treatment (i.e., it is not an intermediate variable or a complication of the treatment).

Improve Prediction of Outcomes

Even in a randomized controlled trial, where selection bias is not assumed to be an issue, controlling for, or addressing case mix can be worthwhile (Figure 11-2). Accounting for severity of illness might reveal the effects of other independent risk factors controlling for severity of illness. Age and gender are typically included. These factors are related to the health outcome but do not influence which patients receive the treatment. Overall, the inclusion of these factors improves the precision of the risk adjustment strategy. In this scenario, the severity of illness is not a confounder for the treatment–outcome relationship. It is deemed to play a direct role.

Form a Basis for Subgroup Analysis

It may be useful to separately examine the effects of treatment-specific subgroups defined by severity. Clinicians think in terms of one treatment working better than another treatment for particular patients. The severity of illness may influence which patients respond favorably to treatment (Figure 11-3). Subgroup analysis permits investigating the effects of treatments for particular

Figure 11-2   **Improve prediction of outcomes**

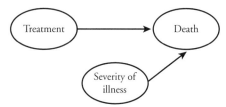

Figure 11-3 **Form a basis for subgroup analysis**

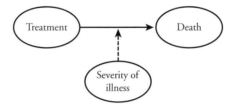

patients. We describe this type of analysis as looking for an interaction effect. One can include an interaction term in the analysis or analyze each subgroup separately. (The latter is, in effect, a complete interaction.)

Data Sources

Data on which to base risk adjustments can come from several sources. The two most common are medical records and administrative data. Each has advantages and limitations. Medical records offer a rich source of information in some detail, but they are not necessarily consistently completed. Moreover, they require substantial work to abstract the information. By contrast, administrative data, typically some variant of billing records, use systematic coding and are easier to use (once you get access to them). The standard coding systems include *International Classification of Disease*, Ninth Revision, Clinical Modification (*ICD-9-CM*), Current Procedural Terminology (CPT), and DRG. It is important to bear in mind that billing records are designed to maximize revenue. Hence, the choice of diagnoses may reflect those that are reimbursed highest. Moreover, there may be wide variation in the number and precision of diagnoses allowed in the administrative databases.

Some investigators have developed ways to use medications prescribed as a proxy for diseases a patient has. This can be a difficult cross walk because some medications can be used to treat a variety of diseases.

The National Drug Code (NDC) has been used for two purposes. The first is to identify individuals, or surveillance, with a high probability of having specific diseases, for example, by using insulin use as an indicator of diabetes mellitus. The difficulty in using drugs as proxies for diagnoses occurs when the same drug can be used to treat multiple conditions. The other use has been to coarsely grade the severity of a known condition;

for example, oral hypoglycemic versus oral hypoglycemic plus insulin to reflect the severity level of the diabetes. The latter example is flawed, but in the absence of clinical data it provides a rudimentary metric.

CONSIDERATIONS IN SELECTING A RISK-ADJUSTMENT STRATEGY

In many studies, risk adjustment is handled intuitively, largely by taking available measures off the shelf. But good risk adjustment needs careful thought. While developing a risk-adjustment method is difficult, a few basic principles may be helpful.

1. *Purpose of Risk Adjustment.* As noted at the outset of this chapter, the role of risk adjustment will vary with the purpose of the analysis and the question being asked. Is the risk-adjustment strategy appropriate to the outcome studied? Is the risk-adjustment strategy being inappropriately applied?

2. *Relative importance of diagnosis to risk adjustment.* Generic approaches are simple but lack the clinical credibility demanded by clinicians. It has been observed that the importance of diagnosis varies according to the outcome. For generic end-points, such as physical function, baseline functioning is prognostically more important than the patient's diagnostic status. But such an approach to risk adjustment may lack medical meaning for clinicians. If there is a lack of agreement in terms of the approach to risk adjustment, clinicians are likely to be critical of the effects of adjusting for risk differences. While risk adjustment might be viewed as a statistical process, a failure to consider the clinical validity of approaches is likely to result in defensiveness regarding the results reported. We recommend over-attention to risk adjustment, just to be able to respond to critics of the study (usually those who did not fare well) who challenge the results because of a failure to adjust for some esoteric variable, "we looked at that and it made no difference."

3. *Data-related considerations.* The data required are an early, important consideration in making risk adjustments (i.e., data acquisition, source of data, and its accessibility). Data sources include:

   Primary data – collected expressly for the purpose of making risk adjustments. Primary data could include chart data or patient completed survey data. Very detailed data can be collected, but the investigator needs to:

- Operationally define the study variables, whether from a medical record or from a patient survey;
- Deal with the completeness of the data, its accuracy and its lack of structure (if chart);
- Adequately address questions of reliability of the information gathered (self-reported measures might be unreliable, but the abstraction of chart data might equally pose lack of interrater agreement); and
- Deal with biases inherent in using that source of data, for example the medical record may not reflect a complete picture of the patient.

Secondary data – data collected for purposes such as risk adjustment. Administrative data is the best known example of these types of data. Examples include data from the Uniform Billing Form (UB-92), the HCFA 1500. The investigator needs to pay close attention to:

- Completeness of data
- Differences in coding practices
- Consider that since these data are used for billing purposes, they might be viewed with suspicion
- Less likely to be carefully collected in managed care/capitated plans, where they are not used for payment

Risk adjustment strategies must be given the same considerations as those of other measures. Reliable medical record and administrative data contribute to the potential usefulness of the risk-adjustment strategy. Sources of reliability include the following:

- Clarity of the definition pertaining to the data elements,
- Operational definition of the data elements,
- Extent of review, eligibility, completeness, and organization of charts (i.e., use of shadow records),
- Training of medical records reviewers, and
- Environment for reviewing medical records (e.g. on their lap and inadequate lighting).

4. *Role of competing risks.* To what extent does the risk adjustment strategy consider competing risks? Many strategies, such as DRGs, group cases with similarities in terms of cost but ignore other procedures that might be inappropriate or contribute to overall cost.

STATISTICAL PERFORMANCE: HOW DO YOU EVALUATE THE PERFORMANCE OF A RISK MODEL?

The value of a risk factor lies in its ability to predict an outcome of interest. The choice of statistical model depends on the type of outcome being tested. Predicting continuous risk factors typically relies on a simple general linear model.

$$Y_i = a + \Sigma_j b_j X_{ij}$$

where, the predicted outcome is a function of an intercept and coefficients associated with the independent variables (i.e., the risk factors).

The coefficient of determination is the standard measure for model performance when the outcome is a continuous variable.

<u>Inclusion or exclusion of outliers.</u> The overall performance of the model can vary according to whether outliers were included or excluded in the model. The coefficient of determination is generally higher when cases are analyzed. The coefficient of determination provides little information about the ability of the model to discriminate among cases with high and low values. One approach suggested by Iezzoni (2003) is to examine actual and predicted means at the extreme deciles (i.e., the upper and lower 10%). Larger ratios generally suggest better discrimination.

Many outcomes important to clinicians are dichotomous; for example, mortality within 30 days of a surgery, incidence of posttreatment complication, and hospital admission. The performance of models predicting dichotomous outcomes is slightly different from the techniques used for the continuous model. One approach uses the same technique used to assess the validity of a test. Figure 11-4 shows how the predicted outcome can be compared to the actual outcome.

The major problem using this sort of sensitivity and specificity approach to evaluate the performance of dichotomous models is that, like measures discussed earlier (e.g., CES-D, SPMSQ), a cut-point has

Figure 11-4 **Comparing a dichotomous outcome with a dichotomous prediction.**

	Outcome	
Risk score prediction	Dead	Alive
Dead	*True positives* a	*False positives* b
Alive	*False negatives* c	*True negatives* d

to be selected. Choosing a cut off point is rarely clear cut. It typically involves trade-offs between properties, such as how inclusive and exclusive you desire, and the availability of resources. Many risk adjustment methods use different cut points.

Logistic regression is the most widely used approach for modeling health outcomes data that are dichotomous. These models are evaluated by comparing the observed outcomes with predictions of the model using a logit of risk. The logit function is expressed by the following formula:

$$P_i = \frac{1}{1 + e^{-(\alpha + \beta_1 x_{i1} + \ldots + \beta_k x_{ik})}}$$

where the probability of the outcome, as predicted by the model, is a function of the linear combination of risk adjusters.

- The goodness of the model is evaluated for how well the model fits the data and whether the model distinguishes between those that have a higher and lower probability of the outcome. This defines the calibration and discrimination of the model respectively. Model calibration – the average of the predicted values match the average of the actual outcomes.
- Model discrimination – the extent to which higher probabilities of the outcome are predicted among those with the outcome.

Having a well calibrated model is desirable, but discrimination is more important. Consider the case of two different risk adjustment methods— one is well calibrated, the other predicts perfectly. In general medical practice, the prevalence of major depression is thought to be approximately 15%. If your risk adjustment method assigns a 15% probability of major depression to everyone seen in the practice, it is perfectly calibrated but cannot discriminate between patients with major depression and those without major depression. If the risk adjustment method assigns a predicted risk of 50% to patients who are depressed and 40% to those who are not depressed, one can say that your risk adjustment method predicts perfectly. However, the latter is poorly calibrated since it overestimates the degree of risk in the population. In general, calibration can be fixed, but for discrimination there is little hope.

In most statistical programs, discrimination is quantified using the c-statistic. The c-statistic is equivalent to the area under the receiver operating characteristic (ROC) curve. As rule of thumb, c-statistic values of 0.70 or greater for a logistic model are required for adequate discrimination. Model calibration typically uses the Hosmer and Lemeshow Goodness-of-Fit Test (Hosmer & Lemeshow, 1980). This test arranges the data into deciles of risk and calculates whether there is a significant difference in the proportion of observed and expected across the deciles using the chi square test. A negative finding, or a p value >0.05, reflects a good fit or well calibrated model.

SUMMARY

Risk adjustment is important in leveling the playing field to maximize the fairness of comparisons. It should be done thoughtfully with the ultimate goal clearly in mind. Most of the attention is fixed on adjusting for severity and comorbidity. These are different but potentially related concepts. It is important to distinguish comorbidity, which refers to diagnoses the patient brings to the intervention from complications that arise during or after the intervention. The latter are outcomes and should not be adjusted away.

REFERENCES

Boult, C., Dowd, B., McCaffrey, D., Boult, L., Hernandez, R., & Krulewitch, H. (1993). Screening elders for risk of hospital admission. *Journal of the American Geriatrics Society, 41*, 811–817.

Boult, C., Pacala, J. T., & Boult, L. (1995). Targeting elders for geriatric evaluation and management: Reliability, predictive validity and practicality of a questionnaire. *Aging: Clinical and Experimental Research, 7*(3), 159–164.

Charlson, M. E., Charlson, R. E., Peterson, J. C., Marinopoulos, S. S., Briggs, W. M., & Hollenberg, J. P. (2008). The Charlson comorbidity index is adapted to predict costs of chronic disease in primary care patients. *Journal of Clinical Epidemiology*, *61*(12), 1234–1240.

Charlson, M. E., Pompei, P., Ales, K. L., & MacKenzie, C. R. (1987). A new method of classifying prognostic comorbidity in longitudinal studies: Development and validation. *Journal of Chronic Diseases*, *40*, 373–383.

Cote, R., Battista, R. N., Wolfson, C., Boucher, J., Adam, J., & Hachinski, V. (1989). The Canadian Neurological Scale: Validation and reliability assessment. *Neurology*, *39*(5), 638–643.

Cote, R., Hachinski, V. C., Shurvell, B. L., Norris, J. W., & Wolfson, C. (1986). The Canadian Neurological Scale: A preliminary study in acute stroke. *Stroke*, *17*(4), 731–737.

D'Hoore, W., Sicotte, C., & Tilquin, C. (1993). Risk adjustment in outcome assessment: the Charlson comorbidity index. *Methods of Information in Medicine*, *32*(5), 382–387.

Deyo, R. A., Cherkin, D. C., & Ciol, M. A. (1992). Adapting a clinical comorbidity index for use with ICD-9-CM administrative databases. *Journal of Clinical Epidemiology*, *45*(6), 613–619.

Elixhauser, A., Steiner, C., Harris, D. R., & Coffey, R. M. (1998). Comorbidity measures for use with administrative data. *Med Care*, *36*(1), 8–27.

Gonnella, J. S., Hornbrook, M. C., & Louis, D. Z. (1984). Staging of disease: A case-mix measurement. *Journal of the American Medical Association*, *251*(5), 637–644.

Greenfield, S., Apolone, G., McNeil, B. J., & Cleary, P. D. (1993). The importance of co-existent disease in the occurrence of postoperative complications and one-year recovery in patients undergoing total hip replacement. Comorbidity and outcomes after hip replacement. *Medical Care*, *31*(2), 141–154.

Greenfield, S., Aronow, H. U., Elashoff, R. M., & Watanabe, D. (1988). Flaws in mortality data: The hazards of ignoring comorbid disease. *Journal of the American Medical Association, 260*, 2253–2256.

Hornbrook, M. C. (1985). Techniques for assessing hospital case mix. *Annual Review of Public Health, 6*, 295–324.

Hosmer, D. W., & Lemeshow, S. (1980). Goodness-of-fit test for the multiple logistic regression model. *Communications in Statistics in Theoretical Methods, 10*, 1043–1069.

Iezzoni, L. I. (1996). 100 apples divided by 15 red herrings: A cautionary tale from the mid-19th century on comparing hospital mortality rates. *Annals of Internal Medicine, 124*(12), 1079–1085.

Iezzoni, L. I. (2003). *Risk adjustment for measuring health care outcomes* 3rd edition. Ann Arbor, MI: Health Administration Press.

Jencks, S. F., Daley, J., Draper, D., Thomas, N., Lenhart, G., & Walker, J. (1988). Interpreting hospital mortality data: The role of clinical risk adjustment. *Journal of the American Medical Association, 260*, 3611–3616.

Kaplan, M. H., & Feinstein, A. R. (1974). The importance of classifying initial co-morbidity in evaluatin the outcome of diabetes mellitus. *Journal of Chronic Diseases, 27*(7–8), 387–404.

Kelly-Hayes, M., Robertson, J. T., Broderick, J. P., Duncan, P. W., Hershey, L. A., Roth, E. J., . . .Trombly, C. A. (1998). The American Heart Association Stroke Outcome Classification: executive summary. *Circulation, 97*(24), 2474–2478.

Knaus, W. A., Draper, E. A., & Wagner, D. P. (1985). APACHE II: A severity of disease classification system. *Critical Care Medicine, 13*, 818–829.

Li, B., Evans, D., Faris, P., Dean, S., & Quan, H. (2008). Risk adjustment performance of Charlson and Elixhauser comorbidities in ICD-9 and ICD-10 administrative databases. *BMC Health Services Research, 8*(12), 1–7.

Linn, B. S., Linn, M. W., & Gurel, L. (1968). Cumulative illness rating scale. *Journal of the American Geriatrics Society, 16*(5), 622–626.

Pacala, J. T., Boult, C., & Boult, L. (1995). Predictive validity of a questionnaire that identifies older persons at risk for hospital admission. *Journal of the American Geriatrics Society, 43*, 374–377.

Romano, P. S., Roos, L. L., Luft, H. S., Jollis, J. G., & Doliszny, K. (1994). A comparison of administrative versus clinical data: coronary artery bypass surgery as an example. Ischemic Heart Disease Patient Outcomes Research Team. *Journal of Clinical Epidemiology, 47*(3), 249–260.

CHAPTER 12

Methods for Collecting Health Outcomes and Related Data

The data for health outcomes research can derive from various sources. Overall, data for conducting outcomes research fall into one of the three categories:

1. Self-report

2. Clinical data

3. Administrative data

Like all forms of measurement, each of the sources of outcomes data has strengths and limitations, as well as potential sources of error. Self-reported data can come from surveys, personal interview, and Web surveys. The subjects' perception of their health can only truly be obtained through self-report. The health surveys discussed in earlier chapters are examples of these measures.

Clinical data, on the other hand, represent information gathered in the course of managing the individual's health care. They are not collected systematically. In the past, clinical data were stored in paper charts. Provider notes regarding the patient's condition and their clinical progress were recorded loosely along with laboratory values, diagnostic test results, and regulatory documentation, such as HIPPA (Health Insurance Portability and Accountability Act) authorizations and consents for procedures. In recent years, these clinical data are more likely recorded and stored in electronic formats. The electronic medical record (EMR) has served to make the documentation of clinical data, its storage, and retrieval more convenient; however, the EMR has some of the same problems as paper records (e.g., it does not always provide the information needed and is not recorded in a standardized format). In addition, there are substantial costs and complexity associated with EMR roll out, as well as continued difficulty with the retrieval of data. For many, the EMR may represent much of the same data but in a more legible and more easily shared system.

Administrative data are collected for billing of medical services, hospitalizations, and pharmaceuticals. Although these data are widely used by epidemiologists and health services researchers for outcomes research, they are limited in the level of detail provided about research subjects' health risks and outcomes, such as functioning. Much of these latter data can be captured only through self-report or chart review.

SELF-REPORT

Survey instruments intended to collect data from individual subjects must avoid the following errors: (1) coverage error, (2) sampling error, (3) nonresponse error, and (4) measurement error (Dillman, Smyth, & Christian, 2009). Precision and accuracy of surveys depend on minimizing these four sources of error.

Before discussing the four reasons for error, several terms should be defined. First, the *population* represents the individuals the outcomes researcher wants to study. The population is not limited to individual persons; it might include households, clinics, and hospitals. The population serves as the *frame* (i.e., the list of subjects or objects available for selection) for drawing a *sample* (i.e., those selected from the frame for study). The sample could be based on a known probability of selecting units from the frame, in which case it is considered probabilistic. Otherwise, lacking knowledge about the likelihood for selection, the sample is nonprobabilistic, or a convenience sample. The sample frame might not include everyone in the population. The outcomes researcher lacks a complete listing of individuals eligible for study or logistically it could be onerous to create a list of eligible individuals. This leads to the first type of error.

Coverage error is the result of all members in a study not having a known likelihood of being included. In other words, our approach to collecting data needs to be systematic. If data collection is not systematic, it might exclude some individuals from the sample or increase or decrease the likelihood of including them in the study. For example, a health plan wants to survey families to measure the prevalence of smoke detectors in the home. Data used to create the sample units consists of individual beneficiaries. Since more than one beneficiary can live within a given household, households with more members will be over represented.

Sampling error concerns selecting only some units from the population studied. This is a consequence of studying only a portion of the population of research interest. For example, a physician group wants to assess its patients' satisfaction with visits over the past 6 months. There were approximately 1000 visits to the practice. To control costs, they use a single mailing to 50 patients without any additional follow-up. Only 20 surveys are returned. This is too small a sample to reliably estimate satisfaction of patients with the care provided; moreover, a poor response to the survey might not represent the population of patients.

The effect of sample size on sampling error is illustrated graphically in Figure 12-1 (Constantine & Rockwood, 2009b). The figure shows that as sample size increases the sampling error, or the level of precision of the estimate, decreases asymptotically. For sample sizes above 400, the expected sampling error is approximately 3–4%, whereas a sample of 20 provides estimates of little practical value. A simplified formula for calculating the sampling error is shown.

$$Sampling\ Error = \pm 1.96 \sqrt{\frac{P(1-P)}{n}}$$

Figure 12-1   Sampling error (± %) according to sample size

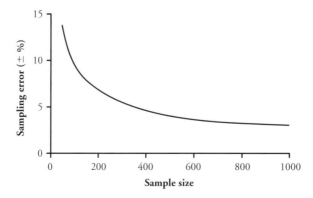

For a prevalence estimate of 50% and a sample size of 400, the estimated sampling error is ± 4.9%. This value can be interpreted as follows. For samples of 400, 95% of the time the sample estimate ± the sampling error will include the true mean for the population. Evaluating sampling error is an important step in estimating the statistical power of an outcomes study.

When persons responding to surveys differ from those not responding, the results are susceptible to *nonresponse error*. An aphorism concerning outcomes research data collection is "outcomes data will be missing." One source of missing data is the subject's nonresponse to self-reported data collection. Nonresponse occurs whenever the unit sampled does not respond to a self-reported survey or fails to answer some survey questions (Groves, 2006). This type of error is common in all outcomes studies involving mailed surveys, but is especially prevalent in studies of elderly study subjects (Hebert, Bravo, Korner-Bitensky, & Voyer, 1996).

In most outcomes studies, the effects of nonresponse are summarized in terms of a response rate. Unfortunately, the response rate is frequently miscalculated and misrepresented. The American Association for Public Opinion Research (AAPOR) has prepared standard definitions for calculating response rates and classifying survey responses (AAPOR, 2009). The guidelines provided by AAPOR are useful for evaluating self-reported information derived from different modes of data collection. Several respondent characteristics associated with nonresponse include being male, being younger, being African American, having less formal education (or social economic status), and having poorer health status.

Based on the AAPOR standard definitions, the following are several of the statistics for computing the response and participation rates for surveys. The response rate is the number of complete surveys divided by the number of eligible participants in the sample. The minimum response rate, using the AAPOR standard definition, is given as follows:

$$Response\ Rate = \frac{Completed}{(Completed + Partial) + (Refusals + Nonresponse) + Other}$$

The cooperation rate is another measure of nonresponse. To calculate this statistic, the completed and partial surveys are divided by the number of eligible participants in the sample. The cooperation rate is calculated as follows:

$$Cooperation\ Rate = \frac{Completed + Partial}{(Completed + Partial) + (Refusals + Nonresponse) + Other}$$

Refusal rates are used to summarize the proportion of individuals refusing to complete the survey. The refusal rate is calculated as follows:

$$\textit{Refusal Rate} = \frac{\textit{Refusals}}{(\textit{Completed} + \textit{Partial}) + (\textit{Refusals} + \textit{Nonresponse}) + \textit{Other}}$$

Nonresponse error represents a problem to the health outcomes research only when the outcomes based on the sample fail to accurately depict the population (Groves, Dillman, Eltinge, & Little, 2002). Two hypothetical examples illustrate that the problem of nonresponse can be present in studies with low response rate, as well as with a high response rate (Constantine & Rockwood, personal communication, December 15, 2009). In the first example (see Figure 12-2), the response rate to a study was 25% (or more accurately when discussing nonresponse error, a nonresponse rate of 75%). The solid line curve (labeled population) represents the *true* distribution for the population. The curve labeled scenario 1 shows a response distribution that is different (lower on the x axis) than the population, and thus, the nonresponse error results in an incorrect inference about the distribution of the characteristic. Alternatively, the curve labeled scenario 2 is a mirror of the population curve and thus accurately reflects the population. Just as it is possible for a study with a response rate of 25% to fail to accurately reflect the population accurately, Figure 12-3 demonstrates that it is also possible when the response rate to the study is 75% (nonresponse of 25%).

Figure 12-2 Nonresponse error for a 25% response rate

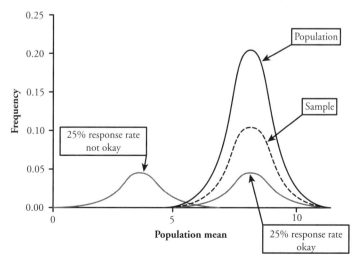

Figure 12-3   **Nonresponse error for 70% response rate**

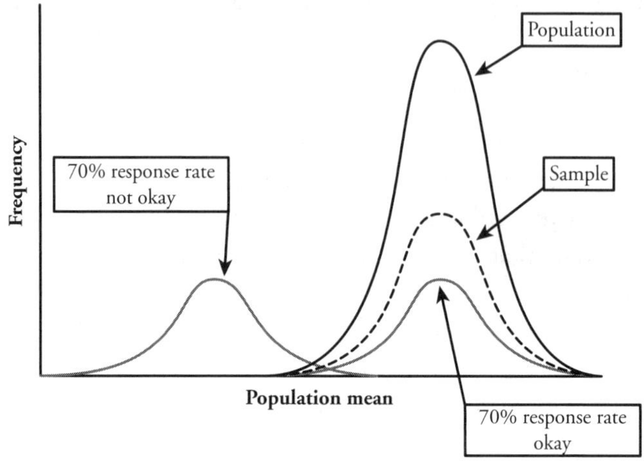

As with the first example, in scenario 1, the distribution is shifted to the left and does not accurately reflect the population, and, in scenario 2, the distribution does accurately reflect the population. Research on nonresponse has shown us what common sense tells us: that when the response rate to a study is 25%, we should be more concerned about nonresponse error than when the response rate to a study is 75% (Groves, 2006). But, this same research has shown us that just because a response rate is low, does not mean that nonresponse error is a problem (Groves & Peytcheva, 2008) and, in fact, in some instances, there is no difference between high and low response rates (Keeter, Kennedy, Dimock, Best, & Craighill, 2006).

Measurement error could derive from multiple sources; for example, individuals providing the information, the persons collecting the data, the questions used to collect the data, design of the questionnaire, and the mode of administering the questionnaires. Measurement error can result from poor wording of survey questions leading to inaccurate and uninterpretable responses. For example, a survey uses the following question: On a scale of 1 to 10, how much pain and swelling do you have in the fingers of your hands? This is a poor question for several reasons. First, the question asks for a rating along two dimensions: pain and swelling. Second, the question is unclear whether more of the symptom is rated high or low. Measurement error compromises the reliability of the measurement scale. Measurement errors result in uninterpretable results.

TAILORED DESIGN

Most strategies attempt to reduce nonresponse and measurement error. There has been too much emphasis placed on trivial factors for improving surveys (e.g., font selection, check boxes, and the color of paper used for surveys). The foundation for enhancing responses to surveys is respondent trust that the rewards of responding outweigh any anticipated costs. The basis of this principle is social exchange, which motivates the individual to return mailed self-administered surveys and complete the questions asked. Much of exchange concepts must be communicated visually through the organization of information. The *Tailored Design* is a method developed by Don Dillman and his colleagues to reduce the sources of error in self-administered surveys and encourage the responses to surveys by building positive regard (Dillman et al., 2009).

> Tailored design involves using multiple motivational features in compatible and mutually supportive ways to encourage high quantity and quality of response to the surveyor's request. It is developed from a social exchange perspective on human behavior, which suggests that respondent behavior is motivated by the return that behavior is expected to bring, and it fact, usually does bring, from others. It assumes that the likelihood of responding to a self-administered questionnaire, and doing so accurately, is greater when the respondent trusts that the expected rewards will outweigh the anticipated costs of responding. (Dillman et al., 2009, p. 16)

Some of the basic principles of *Tailored Design* are worth highlighting here. The techniques for influencing the evaluation of rewards, costs, and trust are built into *Tailored Design*. To provide <u>rewards</u>, the health outcomes research should do the following:

- Show positive regard to the survey respondent by saying thank you and providing a callback number;
- Ask the individual for help or for advice in the cover letter;
- Support group values of the community with whom they are affiliated;
- Give tangible rewards (e.g., monetary incentive, coffee cards, pens, etc.);
- Make the survey interesting; in other words, create a well-designed survey; and
- Give social validation communicating that others in their community are participating and this is a rare opportunity to respond.

To reduce the costs of participation, Dillman recommends the following:

- In designing the questionnaire, avoid embarrassing and demeaning language.
- Increase the convenience of responding by including a self-addressed stamped envelope and a callback telephone number.
- The design of the survey should be short and easy to complete.
- Minimize requests for personal information on the survey.

Finally, trust is built by the following:

- Providing a token of appreciation in advance for participating; this could include a monetary incentive.
- Establishing the sponsorship of the survey (e.g., government, university, or hospital).
- Ensuring the confidentiality and privacy of information provided.

DESIGNING A SURVEY IMPLEMENTATION SYSTEM

Mailed surveys should include a copy of the survey, a personalized cover letter, and a stamped, self-addressed envelope for return. Adhere to good principles of design; use special contacts as telephone contacts or registered mail as needed. Finally, monetary incentives can be used to increase the reward and trust in participating.

PRETESTING

Pretesting is a critical stage of survey design. In general, pretests involve: (1) review by an expert panel, (2) cognitive interviews, (3) a small pilot study using a small number of cases, and (4) a final review and proofreading.

The first stage, review by an expert panel, is conducted as part of the face validation and content validation. The second stage, cognitive interviews, seeks information about the understanding of words on the survey, the interpretation of items across respondent subjects, whether response choices fit what the respondent subject is thinking, moving about the questionnaire (e.g., skip patterns), and the overall design of the questionnaire. There are two approaches to cognitive interviewing. The first is the concurrent approach, in which individuals are asked to think aloud as they are completing the survey. This approach often takes the form of a one-on-one personal interview or small focus group. The following is the script used for typical concurrent interview.

> I am going to read you some questions (from the survey). And I would like you to tell me everything you are thinking and feeling from the moment I begin. That includes your telling me anything you like or don't like about the questions. Remember to tell me what you find enjoyable and what you find frustrating. It is important that you tell me what you are thinking and feeling while you are coming up with your best answer.

After the introduction, the individual is given a practice question followed by an item-by-item reading of the survey. The investigator uses general affirming and reflecting probes and reinforcements, such as, "What are you thinking," "Tell me more," and "Okay, good." Follow-up questions include:

> What did you like? ...dislike?
>
> What was confusing about the survey?
>
> Were you embarrassed by certain questions on the survey? ...not knowing the answer to questions on the survey?

Compared with the concurrent approach, the retrospective approach asks for the respondents' reaction by asking them complete self-reported questions about the survey, such as, "How long did it take to complete the questionnaire?"

The results from the cognitive interviews are incorporated into a revision of the survey and pilot tested. Typically, pilot testing includes at least 10 or more subjects who have characteristics similar to those anticipated to participate in the actual survey. If the pilot study has a sufficient sample, it should provide information regarding expected response rates, reliability of scales, and implementation methodology. A constraining factor for pilot testing is insufficient budget as a part of the survey development process. Before preparing the final version of the survey, it is good practice to read the survey to someone else. This permits identification of any last minute corrections, grammatical errors, dropped words, and misused terms.

CLINICAL DATA

The last decade has witnessed a dramatic move from clinical data being recorded and stored on paper medical records to electronic records for documentation, storage, and retrieval of these data. Many healthcare organizations have gone "paperless" but not without significant costs and resources. The electronic clinical records have proven a superior source of information about the patient by enabling easy retrieval of patient data and access to clinical information by all providers. Although superior to administrative data (which will be described later), the electronic clinical record has failed to advance outcomes research. Much like the paper record, not all needed data are recorded or, if they are recorded, they are recorded in a nonstandard format. These records remain "second hand" (Iezzoni, 2003a). From the vantage point of the outcomes researcher, clinical data in medical records and EMRs is often in a free text format, it is nonparameterized. So, for outcomes research, these data require evaluation and transcription by a medical records abstractor before use in outcomes research.

There are five major challenges to using medical records:

1. Medical records vary in terms of their accuracy and completeness. Charts often lack the information needed for the research.

2. Charts are often missing or the information sought is missing (e.g., a surgical record could be missing).

3. It is common to find wide variations in the medical records across facilities and types of facilities. For example, nonteaching hospitals tend to focus on acute presenting symptoms, whereas teaching hospitals focus on all problems. Hospital records tend to be superior to primary care records, which tend to be superior to nursing home records.

4. Information from paper and EMRs requires transcription from a professional staff person. The information is in a form that does not lend itself to research. The information requires some level of parameterization for purpose of analysis.

5. In medical records there is no standard way for coding and recording information. Information is inconsistently organized.

As medical records become integrated into a digital format, privacy concerns have been raised. Whole medical records may be critical for many research studies (Melton, 1997); there are risks associated with this research in the absence of strict safeguards for privacy and confidentiality (Norsigian & Whelan, 1997).

Administrative Data

Administrative data result "from running the healthcare system—enrolling people in health plans, paying claims, determining reimbursement amounts, certifying coverage, approving expenditures, tracking service utilization, and monitoring costs and performance." (Iezzoni, 2003b, p. 83). There are a number of advantages to administrative data. Among those advantages, administrative data provide:

- Large numbers of study subjects. In the case of health systems research, administrative data include the entire population of individuals.
- More representative data.
- Linkable records that facilitate tracking individuals over time.
- Standardized data content and formats.
- Using preexisting data means no additional data collection is necessary.

Although administrative data have been widely used in health outcomes research, they have a number of limitations.

1. In order to produce a medical encounter that can be accessed, the individual must have public or private health insurance. Individuals who are uninsured fail to produce a detectable and traceable administrative record.

2. There are variations in coding for diagnoses, procedures, and certain key risk factors that make it difficult for comparisons across groups of patients, hospitals, and physician practices.

3. Some administrative databases lack unique identifiers for combining and merging patient data sets.

4. Public and private insurers might not cover a service that is of interest to study. For example, patient education for chronic condition might not be reimbursable; consequently, it would not appear on patient records.

Administrative data are derived from four sources: (1) the federal government, (2) state governments, (3) private insurers, and (4) regulatory organizations. The major sources for federal data are Medicare and the US Department of Veterans Affairs (VA). For these sources, coverage is relatively complete for hospitalization, outpatient encounters, and, most recently, pharmaceutical use. In the case of Medicare, there is a standard format for submitting hospital claims (the UB-92) and outpatient encounters (the HCFA-1500). The VA has a better integrated system that links four of their national databases into a computerized National Patient Care Database.

Medicaid is a state and federal program that insures coverage for low-income individuals; it provides a broad range of coverage, which is shaped by the person's other insurance. For example, for those eligible for Medicare, Medicaid pays only what Medicare does not cover. People can be eligible for coverage based on income or they can spend down to medical poverty. These alternative routes can influence what data is available. Moreover, because this is essentially state data, it is influenced by the variation in coverage and definitions across states, leading to significant variability in the completeness (Steinwachs et al., 1998) and consistency (Ku, Ellwood, & Klemm, 1990) of these data.

Administrative databases are also built and maintained by all private insurers to evaluate utilization and cost. Distinct from federal and state data, private insurer data is more representative of the younger, working population, most of whom are healthy. These data are less accessible to outcomes researchers than federal and state data. However, certain private insurers, such as Kaiser Permanente California and Group Health Cooperative of Puget Sound have exhaustively mined their administrative database for epidemiological and health services research. Coupled with these organizations' EMRs, these integrated databases are a rich source of information on working adults and their children.

For this reason, administrative data have been particularly useful in evaluating procedures that are infrequent (Finlayson & Birkmeyer, 2009). It is for this reason that administrative data have been widely adopted for use in surgical research and other population based outcomes research. Large administrative databases are available nationally covering hospitalizations for Medicare enrollees through the Centers for Medicare and Medicaid Services (CMS, 2010) and cancer incidence and cancer-directed surgery through the Surveillance, Epidemiology and End Results (SEER; National Cancer Institute, 2010). Along with other administrative databases, these can be linked with provider information, death certificate information through the National Death Index, and cost information.

Working with these databases is not without major challenges. The data sets are large and often do not include the information required for the study. Since most administrative databases are first and foremost used for billing, some clinical information rarely appears in these records. For example, clinical information about the patient's functional status or pain is unlikely to be present in billing records. One challenge in using administrative data for measuring outcomes is that information about these nonfatal outcomes is limited (Finlayson & Birkmeyer, 2009).

Further, billing practices vary across providers and practice settings. Since bills submitted for reimbursement generate revenue for the practice, one could argue that there is an inherent tendency to maximize reimbursement. These variations in practice patterns and billing point out another major challenge in working with these types of data for assessing treatment effectiveness. Observational studies used in outcomes research are threatened by selection bias. Certain analytical techniques can minimize the impact of selection, such as propensity methods (Shadish, Cook, & Campbell, 2002) and instrumental variables (IV; Heckman, 1997). Both analytical techniques attempt to account for the likelihood of selection in the intervention condition, creating a sort of randomization of patients. Although both techniques have been used in outcomes research, there is some evidence that instrumental variables methods better account for selection bias when comparing treatment effectiveness (Stukel et al., 2007). That is particularly the case when the outcomes research is focused on making policy decisions.

To maximize the utility of administrative databases, individual patient records have to be linked using a common identifier. Except for the individual's social security number, there are no other unique identifiers available for linking records across administrative databases. In the absence of unique identifiers, records have to be linked using names, dates of birth, and so on.

To further challenge the outcomes investigator, research data has to de-identified and stripped of protected health information (PHI) in order to safeguard the individual's right to privacy under HIPAA guidelines. Unfortunately, PHI, as defined under HIPAA, includes information such as date of birth, residence, and health beneficiary numbers, all of which are needed for answering the study question or linking the administrative data. Often, the investigator is faced with working with de-identified data sets, which are once or twice removed from the original data set.

These data represent unique challenges for cleaning or scrubbing the data before proceeding to the research analysis. At a minimum, testing the data at this stage includes: (1) assessment for missing data, (2) evaluation of the data records for out of range values, and (3) data that is internally inconsistent with other characteristics found in the data record. Since it is impossible to go back and check the source data, the outcome researcher is faced with identifying anomalous findings and incorporating those into the analysis.

SUMMARY

Although the perfect may be the enemy of the good, there are no perfect sources for outcomes data. The methods for collecting outcomes data are driven by a number of factors: (1) budget and resources available, (2) the outcomes, intervention, and additional variables of interest, and (3) access to the necessary data. Each of the methods is accompanied by particular challenges. There are particular outcomes, such as pain and functioning, that the investigator will need to go directly to the patient to collect. Other individual patient data, such as laboratory tests, may be accessed through medical record abstraction, the EMR, or laboratory data systems. Despite its own unique set of challenges, administrative data may provide a more inclusive look at the population of the study interest.

REFERENCES

American Association for Public Opinion Research. (2009). *Standard definitions: Final dispositions of case codes and outcome rates for surveys* (6th ed.). Deerfield, IL: The American Association for Public Opinion Research.

Centers for Medicare and Medicaid Services. (2010). Research, statistics, data and systems. Available at: http://www.cms.hhs.gov/home/rsds.asp. Accessed May 3, 2010.

Constantine, M., & Rockwood, T. (2009a). Nonresponse error. Minneapolis, MN.

Constantine, M., & Rockwood, T. (2009b). Sampling error according to sample size. Minneapolis, MN.

Dillman, D. A., Smyth, H. D., & Christian, L. M. (2009). *Internet, mail, and mixed-mode surveys: The Tailored Design Method.* Hoboken, NJ: John Wiley and Sons, Inc.

Finlayson, E., & Birkmeyer, J. D. (2009). Research based on administrative data. *Surgery, 145*, 610–616.

Groves, R. M. (2006). Nonresponse rates and nonresponse bias in household surveys. *Public Opinion Quarterly, 70*(5), 646–675.

Groves, R. M., Dillman, D. A., Eltinge, J. L., & Little, R. J. A. (2002). *Survey nonresponse.* New York: Wiley.

Groves, R. M., & Peytcheva, E. (2008). The impact of nonresponse rates on nonresponse bias: A meta-analysis. *Public Opinion Quarterly, 72*(2), 167–189.

Hebert, R., Bravo, G., Korner-Bitensky, N., & Voyer, L. (1996). Refusal and information bias associated with postal questionnaires and face-to-face interviews in very elderly subjects. *Journal of Clinical Epidemiology, 49*(3), 373–381.

Heckman, J. (1997). Instrumental variables: A study of implicit behavioral assumptions used in making program evaluations. *Journal of Human Resources, 32*(3), 441–462.

Iezzoni, L. I. (2003a). Clinical data from medical records or providers. In L. I. Iezzoni (Ed.), *Risk adjustment for measuring healthcare outcomes* (3rd ed., pp. 139–162). Chicago: Health Administration Press.

Iezzoni, L. I. (2003b). Coded data from administrative sources. In L. I. Iezzoni (Ed.), *Risk adjustment for measuring healthcare outcomes* (3rd ed., pp. 83–138). Chicago: Health Administration Press.

Keeter, S., Kennedy, C., Dimock, M., Best, J., Craighill, P. (2006). Gauging the impact of growing nonresponse on estimates from a national RDD telephone survey. *Public Opinion Quarterly, 70*(5), 737–758.

Ku, L., Ellwood, M. R., & Klemm, J. (1990). Deciphering Medicaid data: Issues and needs. *Health Care Financing Review, Supplement*, 35–45.

Melton, L. J. (1997). The threat to medical-records research. *New England Journal of Medicine, 337*(20), 1466–1470.

National Cancer Institute. (2010). Surveillance, epidemiology and end results (SEER). Available at: http://www.seer.cancer.gov/. Accessed May 4, 2010.

Norsigian, J., & Whelan, S. (1997). Privacy and medical-records research. *New England Journal of Medicine*, *338*(15), 1076–1078.

Shadish, W. R., Cook, T. D., & Campbell, D. T. (2002). *Experimental and quasi-experimental designs for generalized causal inference*. Boston: Houghton Mifflin Company.

Steinwachs, D. M., Stuart, M. E., Scholle, S., Starfield, B., Fox, M. H., & Weiner, J. P. (1998). A comparison of ambulatory Medicaid claims to medical records: A reliability assessment. *American Journal of Medical Quality*, *13*(2), 63–69.

Stukel, T. A., Fisher, E. S., Wennberg, D. E., Alter, D. A., Gottlieb, D. J., & Vermeulen, M. J. (2007). Analysis of observational studies in the presence of treatment selections bias: Effects of invasive cardiac manaagement on AMI survival using propensity score and instrumental variable methods. *Journal of the American Medical Association*, *297*, 278–285.

CHAPTER 13

Analysis and Visual Display of Health Outcomes Research Data

Health outcomes research addresses the relationship between the treatment and the outcome. This question concerns whether the treatment and the outcome covary and the strength of association between them.

CONSIDERATIONS FOR ANALYZING HEALTH OUTCOMES DATA

A humorous anecdote is often used in introductory epidemiology to illustrate the difference between epidemiologists and statisticians.

> Two guys are in a hot air balloon, completely lost in a desert. Finally, the guys in the balloon spot a man walking on the sand below. The men shout to him, "Where are we?!"
>
> And the man in desert answers, "In a hot air balloon!"
>
> The guys in the balloon must be *epidemiologists*, because they formulate a correct question, but one that does not address the problem.
>
> The guy in the desert must be a *statistician*, because his answer—although correct—is totally useless.

Conducting health outcomes research requires both epidemiological and statistical skills. Formulating a correct question and conceptualizing the problem is a critical precursor to analyzing the data.

There are a number of considerations for analyzing health outcomes data.

- Select the appropriate analytical method
- Deal with threats to validity
  - Low statistical power
  - Fishing and error rates
- Employ acceptable methods for handling missing data
- Create a database and a data dictionary
- Operationalize study variables and structure the data for analysis

Select the Analytic Method

As discussed earlier (see Chapter 3), one threat to internal validity is statistical conclusion validity. This involves selecting an inappropriate statistical test to answer the study question and violating the assumptions for the statistical tests being used. Although a discussion of the full range of statistical tests applicable to health outcomes research is beyond the scope of this chapter, there are some general principles to keep in mind. First, the nature of the outcome variables affects what statistical tests are used. Different statistical tests are appropriate for categorical or a continuous variables and for nominal, ordinal, interval, or ratio scales. These tests distinguish statistical methods that handle normally distributed and nonnormally distributed data.

A variety of techniques could be used for analyzing outcomes. For categorical outcomes, such as death, morbidity, and hospitalization, the rigorous assumptions of normally distributed errors can be relaxed. In the biomedical literature, logistic regression[1] is widely used to analyze categorical outcomes (Allison, 2001; Hosmer & Lemeshow, 2002; Kleinbaum & Klein, 2002; Le, 1998). This technique permits the simultaneous adjustment for covariates and the analysis of ordered categorical end points. The latter approach is referred to as ordered logit. In biomedical studies, multivariate logistic regression is one of the more frequently used methods for analyzing categorical outcomes data. Results yield an odds ratio as the measure of association between the treatment of interest and the outcome (Szklo & Nieto, 2000).

---

[1] Logistic models usually employ a dichotomous outcome, but multinomial logistic models can compare outcomes with more than two states.

Analysis of categorical outcomes can be further strengthened if the investigator knows about the timing of occurrence of the outcome. Time-to-event analysis, also called survival analysis, improves statistical power for analyzing categorical outcomes by using the time to occurrence of an event as the outcome of interest (Allison, 1995; Hosmer & Lemeshow, 1999; Kleinbaum, 1996; Le, 1997). However, many categorical outcomes have onsets that are difficult to determine precisely or are impossible to obtain. An outcomes investigator might procure death records to determine the date of death for a subject or administrative data to ascertain the date of hospitalization, but the onset of an acute myocardial infarction (MI) can be clouded by an uncertain history of previous MIs, misdiagnosis, and a failure to seek medical care needed to record the event. Finally, one rarely knows the specific date of onset of some conditions, such as disability, or chronic diseases, such as diabetes mellitus.

Much of biomedical research is driven by examining the occurrence of events over time. For example, physicians look at the occurrence of infections among hospitalized patients and death rates associated with surgical or medical treatments. Operationally, these involve the investigation of event occurrences. The microprototype for this type of evaluation was the mortality and morbidity (M and M) conference, in which physician peers challenge one another attempting to ascertain what accounted for the poor outcome in a patient. In the context of health outcomes studies, this is referred to as time-to-event analysis, also called survival analysis. The outcomes could be expressed as either a rate or a proportion. The interval of time to occurrence of the outcome is the outcome of interest.

Two survival analytical methods are used in health outcomes research. The simplest is the Kaplan-Meier life table method. This method uses product moment calculations to construct a life table representing the survival, or time, from first observation until the outcome of interest. Survival analysis has several advantages over other statistical methods. First, it takes advantage of censored data, where subject data are lost or discontinued before the event occurs. Study subjects could withdraw from the study, or the outcome event of interest never occurs during the course of observation. Using the Kaplan-Meier method, the effects of separate treatments could be compared using tests for underlying differences in the survival curves.

The second method uses the Cox proportional hazards model. Also known as the Cox model, the approach incorporates explanatory covariates into the final risk for the outcome. It provides a multivariate adjusted result similar to the logistic regression method mentioned earlier. Compared with the logistic regression, the Cox model provides a relative risk as the measure of association. For a complete discussion of these approaches, the reader is referred to excellent resources by Allison (1995); Hosmer and Lemeshow (1999); Kleinbaum (1996); Le (1997); and Singer and Willett (2003).

Continuous outcome variables require a different analytical approach from these mentioned earlier. General linear regression is the simplest approach for analysis of continuous outcomes, such as health status scale scores, blood pressures, and laboratory values. These are also called fixed effects models. However, for the analysis of health outcomes data, traditional least squares are limited in several ways. First, it tends to inflate Type I errors by ignoring other sources of variability. One of the more troublesome sources of variability is repeated outcomes measures. In a basic outcomes research study, there is a baseline and follow-up health measure. The correlated nature of these repeated measures undermines using traditional fixed-effects models. Using general linear regression fails to account for the correlated nature of the outcomes measure, thereby artificially increasing the Type I error rate for the statistical test (Murray, 1998).

Mixed-model methods have become widely used to handle correlated data (Liang & Zeger, 1993; Littell, Milliken, Stroup, & Wolfinger, 1996; Murray, 1998; Singer & Willett, 2003). This analytic method has two applications in outcomes studies. Mixed model methods are used in the analysis of data from studies with repeated outcomes measures. This is equivalent to repeated measures analysis and is the basic design for the pretest/posttest outcomes study. Outcome study participants are repeatedly measured (e.g., serial blood pressure readings), completing a health status survey at regular intervals.

Mixed-model methods are appropriate when the units of assignment or sampling include factors other than the individual, a frequently encountered problem in health services, and public health research. Public health services are frequently delivered at the level of the community. Individuals within communities are more similar than individuals outside the community. The community as a source of variability, called a random effect, is nicely handled using mixed-model methods. By extension, random effects can be hospitals, schools, clinics, health plans, or any other type of grouping. These mixed-model methods can be applied to categorical or continuous outcomes.

Some sources of random error beyond the individual participant occur within study designs that draw participants from other units of interest, such as hospitals, clinics, health plans, and communities. These are often referred to as hierarchical or nested outcomes designs in which the treatment or intervention may be influenced by the level of the group, such as hospital, clinics, and so on. In effect, the care a patient receives (or a clinician delivers) may be influenced by the setting in which it is given. These designs lend themselves to mixed-model methods because of the correlated nature of their data within the level of the group (Murray, 1998). These are called mixed models because there two or more random effects, random effects at the level of the participant, and random effects at the level of the group. Table 13-1 summarizes the appropriate types of analytic approaches for different combinations of distributions, random effects, and data types. Table 13-2 gives recommended guidelines for analyzing outcomes study data.

Selection of an analytic method involves choosing a method that answers the study question and a method that is appropriate for the audience. All health outcomes analysis involves the examination of changes in outcomes with time. Conveniently, the analysis of outcomes data involves an examination of: (1) changes in the occurrence of events, such as death or disease, or (2) changes in the outcome status, for example, functional

Table 13-1   Classification Scheme for Statistical Approaches Useful in Analyzing Health Outcomes Data

Design Characteristics	Distribution	
	Normal Distribution	Distribution
One random effect	General linear model—ordinary least squares linear regression	Generalized linear model— logistic regression
Two or more random effects/replicate outcomes measures	General linear mixed model	Generalized linear mixed model—nonlinear mixed models
Time-to-event	Survival analysis—Kaplan-Meier life table methods and Cox proportional hazards regression	

Table 13-2   Recommended Guidelines for Analyzing Health Outcomes Study Data

1. What is the nature of the study outcome? a. Categorical outcomes can be either nominal, dichotomous, or ordered categorical. b. Continuous variables are in a raw form or require a transformation (e.g., cost data is highly skewed and should log transformed). c. Time-to-event analysis
2. Is the data highly correlated? Aside from random errors within the subject, are there different sources of random error? a. Correlated outcomes data and data with multiple sources of error are best handled using some form of mixed-model method. Linear mixed and nonlinear mixed-model methods are useful along with generalized estimating equation approaches. b. Noncorrelated data might use a general linear model or logistic regression.
3. Adopt generally acceptable standards for statistical power. a. Type I error less than 5% b. Type II error less than 20% c. Lowest common denominator for comparison d. Plan for available data: response rates, eligibility, missing data

status or pain levels. Survival analysis or logistic regression would be a reasonable choice for former scenario, whereas one of the mixed-model methods would be appropriate for analysis of the latter.

Threats to Validity

There are a number of threats to validity frequently encountered during the planning and analysis of outcomes research studies. A few that hold particular relevance include low statistical power, fishing and error rate problems, violated assumptions of statistical tests, and handling of missing data.

Low Statistical Power

All too often the first question asked by researchers is: How many subjects do I need for my study? Although this is important, the question is premature before developing a study question, designing the study, and preparing an analysis strategy. Planning for statistical power begins by addressing the following questions:

- What is the research question?
- Who is the target population?
- How am I going to recruit study subjects?
- How large an effect is expected?
- How much variation in the outcome is anticipated?
- What analysis strategy is needed to answer the question?
- Is the question feasible to study?

All health outcomes studies need to be designed to detect differences between persons receiving the treatment and those not receiving the treatment. In planning the study, the goal is to detect a true effect. Formally stated, the primary concern of statistical power analysis is detecting the truth about the treatment outcome relationship. It is important to appreciate that, with a sufficient sample, any difference can be statistically significant. The salient question is whether the effect size is large enough to be clinically important. Hence, retroactive power calculations based on numbers needed to treat to create a difference may be as valuable (Fletcher & Fletcher, 2005; Haynes, Sackett, Guyatt, & Tugwell, 2006).

The determinants of sample size can be best understood in the context of hypothesis testing. For example, in a study to investigate the difference between the risk of occurrence of adverse outcomes between a "new" medical treatment e and usual care signified by c, one sets up a hypothetical test scenario as follows.

Hypothesis	$P_e > P_c$
Null Hypothesis:	$P_e = P_c$
Alternative Hypothesis:	$P_e \neq P_c$

Where P_e represents the probability of the event among experimental subjects and P_c the probability of the event among controls.

Statistics test the likelihood that an observed difference occurred by chance. In a study designed to test for differences in the adverse event rates between the "new" treatment and usual care, the determinant of the sample size is the statistical significance level, also called the Type I error rate (α); it reflects the likelihood that one sees a difference that could

Figure 13-1   **How Threats to Validity Impact on Statistical Power**

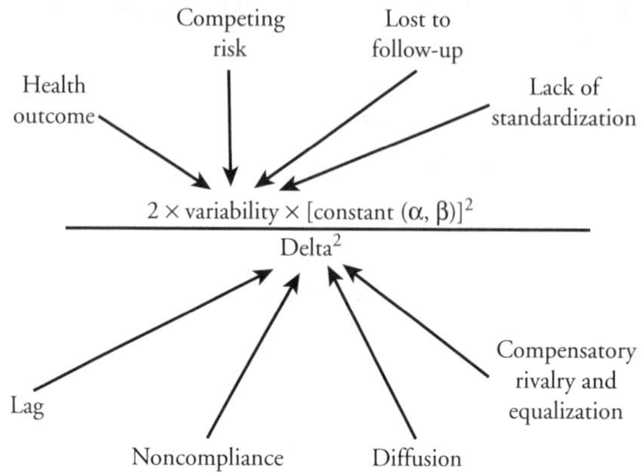

simply have occurred by chance. This is equivalent to the risk of drawing a false conclusion that there is a difference between P_e and P_c. By contrast, a Type II error claims no difference when in fact one exists.[2] Statistical power, or 1 minus the Type II error (β), is the probability of discovering a true difference between P_e and P_c. Next, the size of difference considered important is considered. The latter is defined in terms of the effect size, a standardized difference, which reflects how large a difference one wants to be able to demonstrate statistically. Finally, one considers the number of subjects or the number of groups necessary. Examining the interrelationship of the Type I error rate, the Type II error rate, and the magnitude of the effect being sought is referred to as statistical power analysis.

Many factors under the direct control of the outcomes researcher directly affect the statistical power of outcomes studies. Figure 13-1 shows the impact of various threats to validity on statistical power. In the center of the figure, there is general function for estimating sample size (Friedman, Furberg, & DeMets, 1996). Delays in implementing a treatment intervention (lag), individuals not taking prescribed study medications (nonadherence), and treatments spilling over to individuals assigned to the control group (diffusion, compensatory rivalry, and equalization), all increase the number of individuals needed to detect differences between

---

[2]Look carefully at the first table in almost any article. You will see that the authors have likely tested for the wrong type of error. They test for a Type I error, and finding none, incorrectly declare success.

treatment and control groups. In the numerator, poor standardization of the study, individuals being lost to follow up (attrition), persons dying from causes other than target condition (competing risk), and selecting a health outcome measure with poor responsiveness characteristics all inflate the needed sample size. Low statistical power is a recurring threat to the validity of health outcomes research study designs.

Planning and implementing a health outcome study is a collaborative endeavor. The best advice is to seek the counsel of an expert, preferably someone who will conduct the analysis. This expert advice should be sought at the **outset** of the study, while there is still an opportunity to improve the design. Bringing data from a poorly designed study to a statistician in hopes of finding a solution is a little like trying to reanimate a corpse.

Because statistical power is critical to the design and planning of an outcomes study, it should always be specified in advance through an a priori power analysis. Sometimes you can use the work of others; sometimes you will need to do some pilot work to get a feel for the distribution and covariation of the key variables. Using the results from published studies and the knowledge regarding the outcomes measure, it is possible to make an "educated guess" regarding the likely size of the effect of the intervention. This is quantified in terms of an effect size or detectable difference. It may be asked another way: How big a difference is needed to convince the target audience that the treatment effect is meaningful? Although this enhances the efficiency of study designs and eliminates frivolous outcomes studies, most statistical power analysis is done at the end of the study. This post hoc power analysis is helpful in assessing the results and informing readers about how big a sample would have been needed to detect a difference, but it is not statistical transubstantiation; it cannot redeem a poorly designed study. Post hoc power analysis should always be done where no statistically significant differences were found in the analysis to be sure a real difference has not been overlooked. The sample size needed to support a claim of no difference is usually much larger than that needed to show a difference.

The following are some guidelines for statistical power analysis:

- Consult with an expert during the planning phase; remember that statistical power analysis and estimating sample size is a collaborative endeavor.
- Sample size should be specified in advance.

- Set standards for considering statistical power.
  - Type I error less than 5%
  - Type II error less than 20%
  - Establish a lowest common denominator for comparison.
  - Plan for available data considering response rates, subject eligibility, missing treatment and available outcomes data.
- Be guided by research objectives; consider monetary and indirect costs.
- Be conservative in estimates of statistical power.

Design a study for the smallest subgroup analysis planned and available data. Guided by the study objectives, always consider the monetary and nonmonetary costs of a study and be conservative in estimates. It is generally a good idea to continuously evaluate the study assumptions as the research unfolds.

Most analysts perform statistical power analysis using any one or a combination of three resources. (1) Formulas for the direct calculation of statistical power can be found in a number of different sources (Friedman et al., 1996; Murray, 1998; Schlesselman, 1982). In general, most formulas incorporate measures of the type I error, type II error, and the effect size. The arithmetic expression in the center of Figure 13-1 provides a conceptual depiction of the interrelationship of these elements. (2) Tables for frequently used statistical tests can be found in resources such as Cohen (1988). (3) Shareware over the Internet and commercial software, such as nQuery Advisor (Elashoff et al., 2000) are available.

Statistical power analysis calculations are more involved when it comes to multivariate analysis. Because these frequently involve complex computations and multiple design parameters, these are best left to skilled biostatisticians, epidemiologists, and health services researchers. Failing to detect a hypothesized effect, the outcomes investigator needs to consider the lack of statistical power as the underlying problem. At the very least, any lack of statistically significant results should result in a post hoc power analysis.

Fishing and Error Rate Problems

There are different styles of outcomes research. One can cast a wide net and essentially trawl through the data to see what is hauled in; or one can aim precisely at a target, like harpooning. Harpooning is far more elegant and persuasive. Post hoc testing of a diverse data haul is generally less rewarding and provides a weaker basis for claiming causation.

Most people can intuitively recognize that if a researcher conducted 100 tests of statistical significance, 5 would be statistically significant (at the 5% level) by chance. Yet frequently, outcomes studies are designed to make multiple comparisons and ignore chance in interpreting the statistical tests.[3] These are collectively referred to as "fishing and error rate" problems. The inflation of Type I errors is particularly troublesome in outcomes studies, especially in studies using multiple outcomes and multidimensional scales.

This threat to validity arises when investigators fail to specify their end points in advance of conducting their study or the primary outcomes are ill defined. In the absence of specifying primary end points, the investigator incorporate multiple outcomes measures in their study. When analyzing their results, each of the outcomes is treated as having primary importance to answering the study question, thereby converting the study to one that is more exploratory than hypothesis driven.

A second threat involves the use of multidimensional measures; for example, a new treatment is hypothesized to improve the quality of life of participants. The investigator chooses a multidimensional scale to measure quality of life, such as the Medical Outcomes Study 36-Item Short Form Health Survey (SF-36) (Ware, 1991; Ware & Sherbourne, 1992; Ware, Snow, Kosinski, & Gandek, 1993) or the Sickness Impact Profile (Bergner, 1989; Bergner, Bobbitt, Carter, & Gilson, 1981). Without specifying a specific subscale from these measures, the investigator increases the likelihood of Type I errors by treating all the subscales as equally important to confirming the hypothesis.

Various methods have been devised to adjust for an inflated Type I error rate: (1) the least significant difference (LSD) approach, (2) Bonferroni correction, (3) Tukey's method, and (4) Scheffé's method (Rosner, 2005; Shadish, Cook, & Campbell, 2002). A thorough discussion of these techniques can be found in most biostatistics texts (Rosner, 2005) and epidemiology texts (Last, 2001). In general, the approaches adjust the Type I error rate downward, making it more difficult to reject the null hypothesis (no difference) and thereby reducing spurious associations. A related problem occurs when an investigator addresses one of the simpler techniques, such as the Bonferroni technique, which adjusts the alpha level downward by dividing the critical value (i.e., the significance level)

---

[3]It is not always possible to distinguish fishing or exploratory studies when they are ultimately presented. A lot depends on how the narrative is told.

by the number of tests. In the case of the eight outcomes derived from the multidimensional SF-36, the critical value of 5% is adjusted to 0.63% for reporting a statistically significant finding.

Strategies for minimizing error rate problems in health outcomes research studies include:

- Recognizing the problem of making multiple comparisons.
- Establishing the primary outcomes for the study.
- Incorporating greater specificity in outcomes measures.
- Making adjustments for multiple comparisons selecting one of the accepted statistical techniques, such as Bonferroni, Tukey, or Scheffé.

Employ Acceptable Methods for Handling Missing Data

In outcomes studies, data will always be missing. The best way to minimize threats posed by missing data is good quality control. This includes careful study management, well-defined project protocols, and clear and well-thought-out operations. Continuous monitoring of quality minimizes missing data. Murphy's Law for outcomes research could read: "If there are any ways in which data can be missing, they will be" (Cohen, Cohen, West, & Aiken, 2002). Observations needed for conducting outcomes research could be missing for a number of reasons. Attrition, which was discussed previously, is one reason for missing data, but there are lots of others. Individuals answering questionnaires may skip questions either accidentally or deliberately. In other cases, information requested might be difficult or impossible for the participant to provide (e.g., questions are too personal or difficult), data systems crash and cannot be recovered, or measuring instruments, such as automatic blood pressure machines, fail.

Missing data threatens the integrity of outcomes research and greatly complicates statistical analysis. It threatens the validity of statistical conclusions drawn, particularly if the method for handling missing data is unacceptable and introduces systematic bias. Missing data effectively reduces data for analysis by attenuating statistical power, thereby reducing the likelihood of detecting differences. Nonetheless, it is always best to use available data rather than discarding study variables or cases. Missing data is positive information. In order to effectively reduce problems posed by missing data, it is critical to distinguish between the types of missing data (Cohen et al., 2002). Is the data missing for the outcome or the treatment? If the outcome is missing, the investigator is faced with dropping the subject from the study. This can lead to a comparison of unbalanced groups, less representative samples, and a loss of statistical power.

Is data randomly or selectively missing? Health survey researchers expect a certain amount of random nonresponses in every study. If the pattern of nonresponse is equally distributed across all subjects, it should not introduce a systematic bias. Selectively missing data poses a more serious problem. Selectively missing data is frequently encountered in studies of special populations, such as the elderly or persons with mental health problems. In studies of the elderly, those with cognitive deficits are less likely to provide risk factor data than those with full cognitive function (Radosevich, 1993), but individuals who are unable to provide requested information about their baseline status may be at higher risk for poor health outcomes.

Are many versus few items missing? As a general rule, no more than 1–2% of values should be missing for outcomes study variables. If the pattern of missing values shows that certain data is missing more frequently, then questionnaires and data collection forms should be revised.

Dropping variables with high rates of missing values may be safer than dropping subjects. Some investigators elect to drop variables from their analysis if extensive data is missing. If the data being dropped makes no material contribution to the outcomes study, dropping it is of little consequence. In that case, the investigator might reconsider why the variable was included in the study. Resources were wasted and information is being lost.

On occasion, the investigator chooses to drop participants from the study. In many advanced statistical packages used for analyzing health outcomes data, this procedure is referred to as listwise deletion. If the data is an outcome, as noted earlier, dropping participants might be perfectly justified. However, beyond 1–2% of participants, this could introduce significant attrition bias into studies. The outcomes study overall loses statistical power and becomes less representative of the target population. This selective loss of subjects is an unacceptable strategy for handling missing data.

Pairwise deletion of participants is generally found in studies using correlation methods or bivariate techniques. Associations are examined only for the paired observations in which the study factor of interest and outcome are both present. If data is randomly missing, this approach might work, but the investigator is unclear as to the study population.

A number of acceptable methods for handling missing data in outcomes studies have been suggested. First, use dummy variable codes for missing values. This means that in the place of a missing value for a variable, one employs a dummy code that flags the variable as missing. In the analysis, this strategy has the effect of creating an additional variable for the missing factor and quantifying potential bias introduced by the absence of a value for that variable.

A second group of techniques involves the interpolation of outcomes values: (1) carrying the last observed outcome forward, (2) interpolation between known outcomes, and (3) assuming the worst outcome. Different assumptions underlie each of these approaches. For example, in a study of the long-term follow up of mechanical heart valve recipients, individuals lost to follow up are assumed to have died from a heart valve related condition. This involves assuming the worst case scenario. As an alternative, one might assume the individual was still alive because that was his or her status at the time of his or her last contact.

Finally, mean substitution is an extension of linear regression techniques and frequently used where the outcome variable is derived from a multi-item scale. The basis for this approach is that the best predictor for a missing value is the other values for the same individual. For multi-item scales such as the 10-item Physical Functioning Scale (PF-10) score (McHorney, Kosinski, & Ware, 1994; Ware, 1991; Ware & Sherbourne, 1992; Ware et al., 1993), a mean scale score is computed on the basis of available items. If the individual completes seven of the ten items comprising the PF-10, the scale score is based on the available seven items. This approach underscores an additional advantage of using multi-item scales.

One approach to choosing the best method for handling missing data is to analyze the data using each of the methods. Using sensitivity analysis, the outcomes investigator analyzes the data using each of the three techniques mentioned earlier. If the conclusions are unaffected by the missing value technique, then you have a greater level of certainty that missing data technique had an impact on your results. However, if your results were negative using one of the techniques, say assuming the worst outcome, then this conclusion is a useful and possibly insightful conclusion for the study.

CREATE A DATABASE AND A DATA DICTIONARY

More time is spent in the management of data sets than in the statistical analysis of data. Analysis begins with an end in mind. The creation of databases for outcomes needs to be done with an eye to the types of analyses and the variables needed for analysis.

Database design begins with identification of the data elements needed for the research and their relationship. For data collected prospectively, it is likely that a relational database will need to be constructed in order to accommodate the entry of data manually or electronically and the extraction of data. Relational database design and their construction can be resource intensive and require the help of an expert if the research is complex. For FDA compliant clinical trials, the database must adhere to Part 11 regulations, called FDA 21 Part 11 compliance. Briefly, Part 11 compliance must have study procedures, administrative controls and electronic systems that meet the FDA regulations. On the electronic systems side, a few of the features of the database include: (1) password protection, (2) electronic signatures, (3) logging options, and (4) audit trails. For a complete discussion of the regulations, the reader is referred to the FDA Web site (http://www.fda.gov/downloads/Drugs/GuidanceComplianceRegulatoryInformation/Guidances/UCM072322.pdf).

For most outcomes studies, a relational database is suitable for the storage, management, and retrieval of study data. It is considered essential that a data dictionary be constructed as part of the management and retrieval of study data. The data dictionary includes information about the contents of the data repository. It might include any of the following: (1) variable names, (2) descriptions, (3) data format, (4) data source, (5) response values, (6) labels, (7) response distributions/marginal frequencies, and (8) position or locations in the data repository. Table 13-3 gives an example of "bare bones" dictionary from the first National Health and Nutrition Examination Epidemiologic Follow-up Study (NHEFS I).

Table 13-3   Data Dictionary for the NHANES Epidemiologic
Follow-up Study

NHEFS Data Dictionary			
Name	**Description**	**Frequency Mean ± SD**	**Position**
SEQNUMB			1
SEX	Gender		2
	Value Label		
	1 Male	1210	
	2 Female	1580	
AGE1	Age at NHEFS1 Interview		3
	Value Label		
	0 65–69 years	601	
	1 70–74 years	576	
	2 75–79 years	995	
	3 80–84 years	584	
	4 85 years and older	34	
RACE	Racial Background		4
	Value Label		
	0 White	2431	
	1 Black	359	
PYNHEFS1	Years to NHEFS I	10.07 ± 1.20	5
PYNHEFS2	Years to NHEFS II	2.82 ± 0.35	6
NEWCESD	Center for Epidemiologic Studies Depression Scale (CES-D)	9.08 ± 7.95	7

NHEFS, NHANES Epidemiologic Follow-up Survey; SD, standard deviation; NHANES, National Health and Nutrition Examination Survey

OPERATIONALIZE STUDY VARIABLES AND STRUCTURE DATA FOR ANALYSIS

Defining study variables, coding variables, and scoring measurement scales can be a labor-intensive process requiring the expertise of epidemiologists, health services researchers, and statisticians. Dummy codes are frequently used in outcomes research. Reference coding is the most common type of dummy code used in biomedical research. To implement dummy coding, the attribute of research interest is coded as a 1 with all other cases coded 0. For example, the study variable "current smoker" is coded 1 for current smokers and 0 for former smokers and nonsmokers. In the analytical model, the effect of current smoking is expressed as a magnitude of difference compared with all current nonsmokers. Although other coding systems are used, most see limited application in the outcomes research.

Scoring measurement scales is conceptually simple but technically complex to carry out. Scoring most scale scores involves making provisions for recoding response choices, attributing weights to items and responses, implementing rules for missing data, and creating scale scores through some arithmetic process. Along with creating the data necessary for determining reliability and validating the use of the measure, computer macros are required for scoring even the simplest health status scale score. Unless you are an experienced programmer, the health outcomes researcher should seek the counsel of an expert.

There are multiple steps involved in structuring data for eventual analysis. First, data has to be structured for the type of analysis. Outcomes data analysis, discussed earlier, fits neatly into three types of data structures: (1) univariate file structures, (2) multivariate file structures, and (3) time-to-event file structures. The differences between the data structures are best illustrated using simple outcomes studies. In the first example, the investigator wants to evaluate two different surgical hip replacement techniques (cemented versus uncemented). Outcomes were measured using the Physical Functioning Scale score from the SF-36. The following example in Table 13-4 of a *univariate file structure* was required to answer the question.

This file structure would be needed for one of the mixed model methods discussed. In setting up the analysis, time, technique, and time × technique interaction predict Physical Functioning score. One strength of this mixed methods approach is that analysis is nested within each individual subject, so it accounts for the correlated nature of the data. It is of importance to note that results from the time × technique interaction answer

Table 13-4   Univariate File Structure

ID Code	Time	Technique	Physical Functioning Score
01	1	Cemented	50
01	2	Cemented	75
01	3	Cemented	90
02	1	Uncemented	65
02	3	Uncemented	86
03	1	Cemented	25
03	2	Cemented	50
03	3	Cemented	100
.	.	.	.
.	.	.	.
.	.	.	.

Physical Functioning Scores over 3 time points ← (pointing to scores 50, 75, 90)

the question: Are physical functioning outcomes superior in cemented or uncemented hip replacements?

The *multivariate file structure* depicts the study subjects as a single record rather than multiple records as shown earlier. The same data set, restructured as a multivariate file, follows in Table 13-5.

Table 13-5   Multivariate File Structure

ID Code	Technique	Physical Functioning Score at Time 1	Physical Functioning Score at Time 2	Physical Functioning Score at Time 3
01	Cemented	50	75	90
02	Uncemented	65	.	86
03	Cemented	25	50	100
.	.	.	.	.
.	.	.	.	.
.	.	.	.	.

Table 13-6   Time-to-Event File Structures

ID Code	Technique	Surgery Date	Hip Failure Date
01	Cemented	07/16/2003	.
02	Uncemented	02/28/2002	10/17/2008
03	Cemented	12/01/2005	.
.	.	.	.
.	.	.	.
.	.	.	.

In restructuring the data, it becomes readily apparent that subject 01 is missing a physical functioning score at time point 2. This file structure permits analytical comparisons between measures of physical functioning at different time points (e.g., Time 1 versus Time 2). A paired *t* test could be used to compare outcomes at different points in time.

Finally, *time-to-event file structures* are used for survival analysis, such as Kaplan-Meier and Cox models. For these analyses, the basic record has a single record for each subject a start time (e.g., a surgery date) and an event date (e.g., a hip failure date). Using the example for hip replacement surgical techniques, Table 13-6 has a time-to-event file structure.

For each subject record, follow-up status is determined. Hip failures are coded as a 1 and study subjects with a functioning hip are coded as 0. The number of days between the surgery date and the hip is calculated for each study subject. Since those with a functioning hip do not have a failure date, they are censored using an end of observation date. In this example, 5 years after the hip replacement surgery (or the end of 2009) might seem reasonable for analysis.

Outcomes researchers should develop some facility for manipulating the structure of data files. One size does not fit all when it comes to analysis. Within the scope of many outcomes studies, all three file structures could be necessary.

VISUAL DISPLAY OF HEALTH OUTCOMES INFORMATION

"Data display is critical to data analysis" (Cleveland, 1994, p. 9). Formal preparation for analytical work emphasizes the arithmetic processes for computing test statistics and the mathematics that serve as the foundation for statistical theory. Much less attention is given to exploratory data analysis (Tukey, 1977) and the graphical display of information (Cleveland, 1994). The visual display of health outcomes information should be guided by a few easy to grasp principles. The following set of guidelines is compiled from a number of authoritative sources on the visual display of information (Cleveland, 1994; Tufte, 1990, 1997, 2001; Tukey, 1977).

Figures should tend toward the horizontal. Since the time of the ancient Greeks, it has been recognized that rectangles with particular dimensions were more aesthetically pleasing. A rectangle with the dimensions of 1 unit height for every 1.61 units of width was preferred and called the golden rectangle. Always plot the cause along the horizontal axis and the outcome along the vertical axis. Table 13-7 gives some guidelines for graphing based on the works of Edward Tufte (1990, 1997, 2001).

REGULATORY DEMANDS ACCOMPANYING HEALTH OUTCOMES RESEARCH

An institutional review board (IRB) is a committee that formally approves, monitors, and reviews biomedical and behavioral research. Universities, hospitals, and health systems involved in research are required to establish and maintain an IRB. Unless an outcomes research study is conducted under guise of quality improvement or quality monitoring, it is likely that the research must be approved by the IRB at the organization in which the research is conducted.

IRBs are federally mandated under Title 45 CRF (Code of Federal Regulations) Part 46 (NIH, 2005) and regulated by the Office of Human Research Protection (OHRP), an office within Health and Human Services (HHS). IRBs were created in response to ethical abuses in the early 20th century. The Tuskegee Syphilis Study provided the greatest impetus for change in the conduct of clinical trials. In the Public Health Service study, African American men were untreated for syphilis decades after validating the effectiveness of penicillin as a cure.

For health studies, studies of new drugs, and medical devices, IRB approval must be obtained. The purpose of the IRB is to:

- Review, in advance, study protocols;
- Periodically monitor the study; and
- Protect the rights and welfare of individuals participating in the research.

Table 13-7   Additional Guidelines or Dos and Don'ts for Graphing Health Outcomes Information

1. Make the data on the graph stand out. Avoid data and information that is unnecessary and gratuitous to the graph. Edward Tufte refers to this as "chartjunk." Do not clutter the interior of the graph.
2. Use visually prominent graphical elements to show the data. If lines are used to connect the data points, then these graphical elements should appear prominently.
3. Visually point tick marks outward. Inward point tick marks tend to create clutter.
4. Do not overdo tick marks. Three to 10 tick marks is a useful rule of thumb.
5. It is better to use upper and lowercase letters. DO NOT USE ALL CAPITALS.
6. It is better to use **serif** not **sans serif** fonts. This is especially true for individuals with visual deficits.
7. Avoid using red and green next to each other. Even for individuals not color blind, these colors are difficult to distinguish.
8. Do not print words vertically.
9. Use a reference line when there is an important value that must be seen across the entire graph, but do not let the line interfere with the data.
10. Do not allow the data labels to interfere with the quantitative data. Superfluous labels can create chart clutter. Avoid putting an abundance of notes or keys inside the graph.
11. Give the source of the information and identity of who produced the graph.
12. Provide a key or legend if more than one group or time period is depicted.
13. Be sure that overlapping plotting symbols are visually distinguishable.
14. Clearly explain error bars. They might represent a standard deviation of the data, a standard error, a confidence interval for a statistical quantity, or an interquartile range.
15. Mute or completely remove grids.
16. Appropriate use of scales: (1) the range of tick marks should include all or nearly all the range of data; (2) do not graph on the scale lines (i.e., x-axis and y-axis); (3) include a zero value unless it is a waste of space; (4) when making comparisons among different groups or time periods for the same measure, keep the scaling the same among different panels; and (5) when the line segments are being used to judge the rate of change, bank the line segments to 45 degrees—this is based on psychological research done in the 1980s.

(continues)

Table 13-7 *(continued)*

17. When comparing two or more groups and the number of observations differ between the groups, report percentages rather than counts.
18. If an object is used to represent numbers, its size should be directly proportional to the numerical quantities represented (Tufte, 2001). If it is either larger or smaller proportionally, it is has a lie factor.
19. Avoid "pop charts" and three-dimensional representations of the data.

Chiefly, IRBs are responsible for reviewing the ethics of the research and research methods, ensuring that the subject is informed and voluntarily consents to participate in the research, and the guaranteeing safety of subjects once enrolled in the study. For the latter, a Data Safety Monitory Board (DSMB) is set up to independently monitor the safety of the study for participants, progress of the study, and the reporting and evaluation of adverse events. All FDA, cancer studies, and projects that pose an increased risk to the subjects require a DSMB.

Although requirements for IRB approval will differ between organizations, for prospective studies, approval by the governing human subjects' protection office will be involved and time consuming. Subjects might be required to complete an informed consent, which adds to the resources necessary to complete the project and time required to recruit study subjects. For outcomes studies that use existing data, such as medical records, administrative data, and registries, it is possible to get IRB approval that is more expedited.

SUMMARY

Successful analysis involves selecting the correct method to answer the study question for the intended audience. Analysis needs to address any number of common threats to validity. Fishing and error rate problems, low statistical power, violated statistical assumptions, and handling missing data were several threats discussed here. It is important to recall that the greatest threat to the validity of quasi-experimental designs is selection bias. To handle this threat, risk adjustment is critically important, along with multivariate statistical methods, propensity analysis, or the use of instrumental variables. Finally, the regulatory demands of the project need to be considered. In most outcomes studies, these are part and parcel of the planning process.

REFERENCES

Allison, P. D. (1995). *Survival analysis using the SAS® System: A practical guide.* Cary, NC: SAS Institute Inc.

Allison, P. D. (2001). *Logistic regression using the SAS® System: Theory and application.* Cary, NC: SAS Institute Inc.

Bergner, M. (1989). Quality of life, health status, and clinical research. *Medical Care, 27*(Suppl), S148–S156.

Bergner, M. B., Bobbitt, R. A., Carter, W. B., & Gilson, B. S. (1981). The Sickness Impact Profile: Development and final revision of a health status measure. *Medical Care, 19*, 787–805.

Cleveland, W. S. (1994). *The elements of graphing data.* Summit, NJ: Hobart Press.

Cohen, J. (1988). *Statistical power analysis for the behavioral sciences.* Hillsdale, NJ: Lawrence Erlbaum Associates, Publishers.

Cohen, P., Cohen, J., G., W. S., & Aiken, L. S. (2002). *Applied multiple regession/correlation analysis for the behavioral sciences* (3rd ed.). Mahwah, NJ: Lawrence Earlbaum Associates, Inc.

Elashoff, J. D., Oliver, M. R., Yeghiazarian, K., Zheng, M., Jamshidian, M., & Koyfman, I. (2000). Query Advisor (Version 4.0). Los Angeles, CA.

Fletcher, R. H., & Fletcher, S. W. (2005). *Clinical epidemiology: The essentials* (4th ed.). Philadelphia, PA: Lippincott Williams and Wilkins.

Friedman, L. M., Furberg, C. D., & DeMets, D. L. (1996). *Fundamentals of clinical trials.* St. Louis, MO: Mosby.

Haynes, R. B., Sackett, D. L., Guyatt, G. H., & Tugwell, P. (2006). *Clinical epidemiology: How to do clinical practice research* (3rd ed.). Philadelphia, PA: Lippincott, Williams & Wilkens.

Hosmer, D. W., & Lemeshow, S. (1999). *Applied survival analysis: regression modeling of time to event data.* New York: Wiley-Interscience.

Hosmer, D. W., & Lemeshow, S. (2002). *Applied logistic regression* (2nd ed.). New York: John Wiley and Sons, Inc.

Kleinbaum, D. G. (1996). *Survival analysis: A self-learning text.* New York: Springer-Verlag.

Kleinbaum, D. G., & Klein, M. (2002). *Logistic regression: A self-learning text.* New York: Springer-Verlag.

Last, J. M. (Ed.). (2001). *A dictionary of epidemiology* (4th ed.). New York: Oxford University Press.

Le, C. T. (1997). *Applied survival analysis.* New York: Wiley-Interscience.

Le, C. T. (1998). *Applied categorical data analysis.* New York: John Wiley and Sons, Inc.

Liang, K.-Y., & Zeger, S. L. (1993). Regression analysis for correlated data. *Annual Review of Public Health, 14*, 43–68.

Littell, R. C., Milliken, G. A., Stroup, W. W., & Wolfinger, R. D. (1996). *System for mixed models.* Cary, NC: SAS Institute, Inc.

McHorney, C. A., Kosinski, M., & Ware, J. E. (1994). Comparisons of the costs and quality of norms for the SF-36 survey collected by mail versus telephone iInterview: Results from a national survey. *Medical Care, 32*(6), 551–567.

Murray, D. M. (1998). *Design and analysis of group-randomized trials* (Vol. 27). New York: Oxford University Press.

National Institutes of Health. (2005). Regulations and ethical guidelines: Title 45 CRF. Available at: http://ohsr.od.nih.gov/guidelines/45cfr46.html. Accessed May 4, 2010.

Radosevich, D. M. (1993). *Factors associated with disability in the elderly.* Minneapolis: University of Minnesota.

Rosner, B. (2005). *Fundamentals of biostatistics* (5th ed.). Belmont, CA: Duxbury Press.

Schlesselman, J. J. (1982). *Case-control studies: Design, conduct, analysis*. New York: Oxford University Press.

Shadish, W. R., Cook, T. D., & Campbell, D. T. (2002). *Experimental and quasi-experimental designs for generalized causal inference*. Boston: Houghton Mifflin Company.

Singer, J. D., & Willett, J. B. (2003). *Applied longitudinal data analysis: Modeling change and event occurrence*. New York: Oxford University Press.

Szklo, M., & Nieto, E. J. (2000). *Epidemiology: Beyond the basics*. Gaithersburg, MD: Aspen Publishers.

Tufte, E. R. (1990). *Envisioning information*. Cheshire, CT: Graphics Press.

Tufte, E. R. (1997). *Visual explanations: Images and quantities, evidence and narrative*. Cheshire, CT: Graphics Press.

Tufte, E. R. (2001). *The visual display of quantitative information*. Cheshire, CT: Graphics Press.

Tukey, J. W. (1977). *Exploratory data analysis*. Reading, MA: Addison-Wesley Publishing Company.

Ware, J. E. (1991). Conceptualizing and measuring generic health outcomes. *Cancer, 67*(3), 774–779.

Ware, J. E., & Sherbourne, C. D. (1992). The MOS 36-Item Short-Form Health Survey (SF-36). *Medical Care, 30*(6), 473–483.

Ware, J. E., Snow, K., K, Kosinski, M., & Gandek, B. (1993). *SF-36 Health Survey: Manual and interpretation guide*. Boston: The Health Institute, New England Medical Center.

Making Sense of It All: Interpreting the Results

ORGANIZING ONE'S THINKING

Given the enthusiasm for evidence-based medicine, the demand for solid outcomes research will grow even faster. Outcomes research can be considered as the intersection of careful clinical reasoning and strong research design. It is infeasible and impractical to expect that all clinical questions will be addressed by randomized controlled trials (RCTs). Even if it was possible to conduct RCTs on all the topics of interest, we could never cover all the variations in possible treatments. Much of the knowledge that powers the field will have to come from prospective observational studies; it is essential that they be done well. Observational studies require more planning and analysis than do RCTs precisely because they cannot control factors by design. They demand more thoughtful and insightful interpretation.

Earlier in this book, we urged the importance of developing a conceptual model that could inform the analysis. That model should indicate which variables are thought to influence the outcomes and how that effect is brought about. A conceptual model need not be equivalent to a theoretical model in the sense that it does not have to draw upon some grand general theory. Instead, it can be based on one's clinical experience or even beliefs about what is going on and what factors are likely to influence the outcomes of interest. Its major role is to clarify the expected relationships. Indeed, the clearer the conceptual model, the easier it will be to convince clinicians of the value of the research and the need for the results. Often, drawing a model illuminates the analytic problems. Such diagrams can distinguish the primary risk factors from the intervening events (including both treatments and complications of treatment) and can make clear the temporal relationships among the variables.

The capacity to statistically account for variance has become a passion in some quarters, but it is important to appreciate that the more temporally proximal a variable is to the outcome, the more variance for which it will usually account. (At the extreme, cessation of respiration predicts death very well.) However, explaining variance is not always helpful. For example, absence of a heartbeat will undoubtedly explain much of the variation in mortality rates, but so what?

In many instances we seek to create complex causal models that use explanatory variables actively to isolate the main effects of those of greatest interest. But this strategy can backfire. You do not want to adjust away important differences that may be the basis for differences in performance. In some cases, accounting for variation may lead to false conclusions. For example, a study of the utilization of medical care by the informal caregivers for Alzheimer's disease patients showed that they appeared to use less care than controls. The investigators had earlier identified that depression was more common among caregivers and hence controlled for this difference in their analysis to render the two groups more comparable. However, a causal model might well suggest that the development of depression was a result of caregiving and a determinant of medical care use. Controlling for such a step would dramatically dampen the effects of giving this stressful care and hence misstate the effects of care giving.

The conceptual model needs to make clear not only the relationship between various antecedents and the outcomes but also the relationship among the various outcomes themselves. In some instances, the outcomes may be seen as parallel, but in many cases, they will assume some sort of hierarchical form, where one may be expected to lead to the next. The discussion of this measurement hierarchy and its role in relating outcomes to interventions (covered in Chapter 4 on measures) is very relevant here (Spiegel et al., 1986).

In planning an outcomes study, it is important to identify in advance which outcome is the primary one, the basis on which success or failure can be ultimately judged. Many interventions can be expected to achieve a variety of results, but in the end, one outcome must be identified as the most significant. This decision will, among other things, affect the choice of what variables to use in calculating the necessary sample size to obtain statistical power.

A priori identification of the major outcome does not preclude retrospective insight, but it should cast it in a different light. It is reasonable—even desirable—that greater understanding about the relationship between treatments and outcomes occurs after one has systematically studied the problem. There is nothing wrong with postulating new relationships or embellishing the prior models, but one must appreciate that such post hoc reasoning is not causal; it represents hypothesis formulation, not hypothesis testing. It should be pursued, but it should be recognized for what it is. One cannot generate a hypothesis to apply to data after it has been analyzed, but the insights gained from such thought (and the exploratory analyses associated with it) can be usefully applied in planning (or recommending) the next series of studies. Unfortunately, there is no absolute protection against misrepresentation. Except for those instances where hypotheses are on file (e.g., grant proposals), it is impossible to know with certainty when in the course of a study a hypothesis was generated.

THE SEARCH FOR SIMPLE MEASURES

Many clinicians (and policy makers) long for a single simple outcome. Is there a number that can be said to summarize all the outcomes of concern, akin to the Dow Jones average or the percent of GNP spent on health care or even the infant mortality rate? Most outcome measures are too complex. The best ones usually offer a profile of results, where a provider (or a treatment) can excel in one area and fall short in another. Just as some prefer a GPA as the summary of a student's academic success, others look for the profile of areas of success and failure. However much some may wish it, most of life cannot be summed up in a single statistic.

Economists are fond of using quality-adjusted life years (QALYs) as a health outcome. Such a measure weights survival with function. Some view this process of imposing external fixed values on a highly personal area an act of hubris. Is the quality of a year lived really judged by one's functional level? Certainly one can be very active and still have a very bad year. Conversely, some people have had very meaningful lives despite severe functional limitations. Imagine Helen Keller's QALYs. If quality of life is very intimate and subjective, perhaps each person could rate his or her own. Leaving aside the problems of retrospectively assessing those who died, such an approach would produce a great deal of interrater variation. Similar problems arise with so-called health-related quality of life (HRQL).

Moreover, providing a complex summary measure that represents the weighted average of many outcome variables may not be illuminating either. Such indexes are not immediately understandable. They lack a frame of reference. They have no clinical relevance. What does it mean to have a score of x or to have improved by y points? When such scale scores are used, it is very useful to provide some sort of guide that can allow the reader to translate the numerical value into something more tangible and familiar. For example, "someone with a score of x cannot do the following. . .or is similar to someone who is in y condition." (The importance of anchoring such measures in the context of life events is discussed more thoroughly in Chapter 4.) Some clinicians are more comfortable with more categoric scores, rather than summed scales. They think in terms of discrete events.

ADJUSTING FOR CASE MIX

"Always plan for the worst." Outcomes research is the most interesting when it challenges previously held beliefs. It is always, then, the most controversial. Anyone presenting the results of a study that contradict firmly held dicta should expect a hard time. Every doctor treats the most difficult patients. Comparisons among practitioners will inevitably raise questions about comparability of caseloads. Thus, assessing severity and comorbidity is especially salient. If in doubt, it is better to err on the side of excess measurement of patient characteristics.

Much of the technical literature on outcomes research addresses the search for measures of outcomes. However, particularly in observational studies, the more crucial questions pertain to measuring the variables that describe the subjects of the study. Precisely because the cases cannot be randomly allocated, credibility of the results depends on the audience believing that the groups were comparable. Those whose oxen are being gored are likely to grasp for whatever straws they can. Being unable to answer the question "Did you control for serum zinc levels?" makes the research vulnerable to such attacks.

For this reason, researchers should collect even more descriptive information than they might think necessary. It is always better to be able to say that one looked at a given aspect and found it made no difference than to have to argue that it should not make a difference but went unmeasured. At the same time, there must be some finite limits to what data can be realistically collected. One strategy to provide anticipatory protection and still remain affordable is to recruit an advisory committee that includes skeptics. Encourage them to raise as many questions as possible during the design phase. It will be annoying, but it should pay off.

DATA QUALITY

The bane of many clinical studies is data quality. There is a basic conviction that real data comes from clinicians; patient reports cannot be relied on. This medicocentric bias needs to be attacked on two grounds. First, patient perceptions can provide extremely useful information. In some instances, they may be the only (or certainly the best) source. They may not be technically accurate in areas that require clinical expertise, but they may be the most valid sources for information about how they feel and how disease affects them. Filtering such information through a clinician does not always improve the noise-to-signal ratio. Information on activities of daily living, for example, sounds more professional from a clinician, but unless there has been specific formal testing, the information is based on patient reports. Some clinicians believe that they can sort out inconsistencies in patient reports or detect areas of exaggeration, but there is little hard evidence to support such a contention. In most cases, the data is psychometrically sounder when it comes through fewer filters.

Secondly, clinician reports are not universally useful or accurate. Often elaborate systems are devised to review records reliably. Record abstractors are trained and monitored closely to comparable work. However, the quality of the review can be only as good as the substrate on which it is based. Most medical records leave much to be desired. Some years ago, Lawrence Weed, the creator of the Problem-Oriented Medical Record, observed that if clinician scientists kept their lab books in the same manner that they completed clinical records, science would be in turmoil (Weed, 1968a, 1968b). Not only is medical information recorded in incomplete ways, it is impossible to infer what an omission means. Does the lack of a comment on a physical finding or a symptom imply that nothing of interest was found or that nothing was looked for? What does it mean when a record says a body system was "within normal limits?" What type of examination was actually done? What does "no history of x" mean? What questions were asked? Few clinicians systematically record all the pertinent information needed to adjust for risk factors, nor do they provide complete data on which to establish outcomes.

For many variables, especially those that require judgment or interpretation, clinicians are the best source of information, even when their interrater (and perhaps even their intertemporal) reliability has not been established. The challenge is to collect such information in a systematic and consistent manner (Feinstein, 1977, 1987). Getting useful data from clinicians usually means setting up some type of prospective data collection apparatus. Some means of querying the clinicians is needed to be sure that they make the complete set of observations sought and record the information consistently.

Clinicians do not generally respond well to such demands for structured information collection. Many have a strong aversion to forms, which they deprecate as some type of "cookbook medicine." In order to gain their cooperation, it is often necessary to involve them proactively in designing the data collection forms or at least identifying the relevant material to be included.

This proactive strategy is especially important in the context of quality improvement projects. Although purists will worry (justifiably) that such active involvement will bias clinician behavior, such a bias is precisely what quality improvement seeks. Moreover, those being judged are more likely to accept the results of the outcomes analysis if they have had some role in developing the criteria and the way the data are collected.

In some cases, the bias toward clinician-generated information may be misplaced. Clinicians serve as mere conduits; the data can be better collected directly from patients, who may provide more and better information without the clinician filter. For example, data on patient functioning is usually better collected directly from the patients (or their proxies). Even information on key symptoms can often be obtained more easily and better directly from patients. In some cases, office (or hospital) personnel can be trained (and induced) to collect questionnaires (or even conduct short interviews) with patients when they present themselves for care.

GETTING FOLLOW-UP DATA

Good observational studies should be conducted with the same rigor used in RCTs. While it may not be feasible to standardize the intervention, its description should use a standard format. The schedule of data collection should be the same for everyone. The baseline data and follow-up information should be consistently collected. Consistency means not only collecting the same information but collecting at the same time for all study participants.

Although it is at least theoretically possible to structure baseline and risk factor data collection into ordinary clinical activities, obtaining follow-up information is more complicated. Even if clinicians were cooperative, problems would arise. Patients are not usually seen for follow-up appointments on a consistent schedule. Some patients are lost to follow up. Because biased data can be extremely dangerous, some form of systematic data collection that does not rely on patients returning to the clinic or hospital is in order. Although such a step adds cost and represents an added dimension, its value in providing adequate unbiased coverage justifies the expense.

Many physicians who participate in research studies are used to having a research nurse who collects the data. They have developed systems by which the nurse collects designated data when patients present themselves for care. But systematic data collection cannot rely on patients returning to the clinic. The timing of return visits may vary. Some patients may not show up. (Often they are the most interesting ones.)

Follow-up data can be collected by various means. The most expensive is in-person interviews. Such a step is generally not required unless the patients are especially unreachable (e.g., nursing home patients) or data must be physically collected (e.g., blood samples, blood pressure, weight). Most times the data can be reduced to patient reports of symptoms and behaviors, which can be collected by either mailed questionnaires or telephone interviews. The choice of which approach to use is based on money and expected compliance. Often a mixed approach will be needed, with nonrespondents to the mailed survey contacted by phone or even visited.

Response rates are very important. The basic concern is about response bias (where those responding are systematically different from those who do not). Follow ups evoke images from the Sherlock Holmes story,

The Hound of the Baskervilles. The dog not barking may be more interesting than his barking. Those who return for follow up are likely to be different from those who do not. Failure to return may reflect a great success or a great dissatisfaction. It may also simply mean that the patient came from a distant referral and is returning to their primary physician. In some cases, the source of the bias is obvious (e.g., those returning for follow-up care). In most cases, the reasons for nonresponse are not evident, even when interviewers ask why the patient refused to participate. The best way to avoid such a bias is to plan in advance for proactive follow up and to go all out to collect data on all subjects who are eligible. It is a great temptation to stint at the end game; it is also a great mistake. Inevitably, the last group to be reached will require the majority of the overall follow-up effort, but they are likely the most interesting cases as well.

Those not familiar with research methods sometimes confuse large numbers of respondents with adequate response rates. Whereas sample size is important in determining the statistical power of an analysis, large numbers of respondents cannot compensate for poor response rates. It is usually better to use the available resources to ensure that one collects a high proportion of those targeted than just a lot of cases. A high response rate from a smaller sample is by far preferable to a larger but more incomplete sample.

In some instances, patients may not be able to respond because they are too sick or cognitively compromised. Proxy respondents can be used to obtain information, but they should be employed with caution. Often, family members will try to protect patients from such contacts, even when the patients can and want to participate. In some cases, those responsible for the patient may not want them to participate or may view the data collection activity as another nuisance. For example, nursing homes may find it inconvenient to get patients to a telephone to answer questions. Persistence and creativity will be needed to counter these ploys.

In some cases, proxies are inevitable. Care and common sense should be used in deciding when a proxy can accurately represent the patient. At least two criteria should apply: (1) the proxy should have recent and adequate exposure to the patient to be able to report on his or her status (e.g., family members listed as the responsible party in a hospital or nursing home may not have visited frequently enough to know what is really happening); and (2) the domains that proxies can address should make sense; for example, it is unrealistic to expect a proxy to report on a patient's degree of pain or the patient's state of mind. At a minimum, proxy responses should be identified in the analysis with a dummy variable. In some cases, it may be prudent to analyze them separately. A good first step is to compare the overall patterns of proxy responses and direct subject responses.

The timing of follow ups is important. Particularly when treatments may extend over long periods (e.g., outpatient therapy), the effects of dating follow ups from the beginning or the end of treatment can make a huge difference. If follow up is dated from the beginning of the treatment and some patients remain in treatment substantially longer than others, the differences in outcomes may be attributable to the time between the end of treatment and the follow up. Thus, it is usually safer to date follow up from the end of treatment. On the other hand, if treatment extends for a long time and there is a natural course to recovery, those with longer treatments will have had more time to recover. For example, an RCT of geriatric evaluation units found differences at discharge between those treated and not, but failed to recognize that these differences might simply be attributable to natural recovery, especially since they disappeared with time (Cohen et al., 2002). Thus a crucial data point may be the status at the end of treatment. However, even this precaution will not eliminate the need to pay careful attention to the duration of the treatment. As noted in Chapter 10, duration and intensity are important attributes of treatment that must be considered in the analysis of its effects.

The duration of treatment can thus have several effects—for instance, it can mask the effects of the natural course of a disease. If the disease in question has a natural history independent of treatment, a longer duration of treatment may simply allow the problem to run its course. Remaining in prolonged treatment may reflect patients' motivation and hence influence their recovery. If those who become discouraged drop out of treatment, it is hard to separate the effects of less treatment from inherent characteristics of the patients. Because those who drop out may also be harder to contact at follow up, there may be a selective attrition bias.

USING EXTANT DATA SOURCES

In some cases, outcomes information can make use of extant secondary data sources. Many large national studies are restricted to data that can be gleaned from administrative records. Such studies have policy value but they have serious limitations. The outcomes are usually limited to death, and healthcare utilization and the databases have little clinical information that permits strong case-mix adjustments. For example, Medicare records can be used to trace when a person is rehospitalized or when a given operation is revised. Using secondary data sources, especially administrative databases, can be limiting and challenging. It is no coincidence that the most common outcomes addressed are death and rehospitalization. They are the two items that most administrative databases can yield. In some circumstances, such follow-up data can provide useful adjunctive information. For example, a study of hip replacement may address short-term benefits in terms of pain and mobility, but it may also be useful to see how long the prostheses lasted.

It is important to distinguish studies that rely exclusively on secondary data and those that use it in conjunction with primary data. The former faces problems of limited information, especially when it comes to adjusting for risk factors, most of which cannot be found in administrative data sets. Thus, outcomes studies derived from administrative data, while they can relatively inexpensively compare the results of large heterogeneous groups of providers, are often harshly criticized as being unfair and biased. For example, the Medicare mortality studies, which found widely varied death rates among hospitals serving Medicare patients, were actively challenged as inadequately correcting for case-mix (Greenfield, Aronow, Elashoff, & Watanabe, 1988; Jencks et al., 1988; Kahn et al., 1988).

On the other hand, it may be possible to link clinical information from medical records and even patient interviews with administrative data. For example, a study of the outcomes of hip replacements used data from record abstracts and Medicare administrative data to link baseline severity and comorbidity with outcomes to show a difference across genders (Holtzman, Saleh, & Kane, 2002).

BASIC ANALYSIS ISSUES

Although data analysis is an integral component of a successful outcomes system, this book cannot explore this topic in great depth. Many good texts and commentaries are available (see Shadish, 2002; and Feinstein, 1977). Nonetheless, a few basic suggestions and cautions are offered. The first and most important is to recognize the complexities of this area and to get the necessary assistance. Outcomes analysis can often be a subtle process. The potential statistical pitfalls are numerous. It is crucial to consult with a statistician while developing the study ideas. Few statisticians like to be approached after everything has been decided. Statistical concerns can directly affect decisions about sample size, instruments, and overall design.

An important step in designing an analytic strategy is to link each hypothesis or research question with a specific analysis. This translation needs to be done in considerable detail. The concepts alluded to in the hypothesis need to be translated into specific variables and the type of analysis specified. It is often helpful to create dummy tables that show just how the results will be displayed. Going through the exercise of designing those tables can help investigators (especially neophytes) clarify just how they will organize their data and what form each variable will take.

Most analyses involving outcomes will eventually use some type of multivariate analysis, most of which will fall into one or another type of regression model. Many regression models provide two types of information: the amount of variance explained (R^2) and the relationship of each independent variable to the dependent variable (regression coefficient). These two factors may not be related. It is possible to explain a substantial amount of the variance without a single significant coefficient, and significant variables need not contribute much to explaining the overall variance. Each item connotes something different. It is important to decide which piece of information is most salient. The explained variance can be thought of as comparable to, in epidemiologic terms, attributable (or absolute) risk. Attributable risk reflects how much added risk for developing a condition a given factor poses. The individual variable coefficient is comparable to relative risk; how does the risk of developing the condition with the factor compare without it? In rare events, one may encounter a very high relative risk but a small attributable risk.[1] Likewise, with outcomes, the goal may be to identify factors

---

[1]To appreciate the difference between attributable risk and relative risk, imagine two interventions: one reduces the risk of the common cold from 1 in 2 to 1 in 4; the other prevents a rare leukemia, reducing the risk from 1 in 2 million to 1 in 4 million. Both have a relative risk of 0.5, but the attributable risk for the common cold is 1 in 4, whereas the attributable risk for leukemia is 1 in 4 million.

that influence outcomes even if they do not explain much of the overall risk of the outcome occurring.[2]

In one respect, treatment can be viewed as one of a series of risk factors[3] that affect the outcomes of care. In most instances, the goal of the analysis is to separate the effect of treatment from the effects of the other risk factors. It is also possible, however, to use outcomes analyses to directly examine the effect of other risk factors.

In some cases, one may want to see how a risk factor performs after the effects of other factors have been controlled. (i.e., what is the specific contribution of a given factor). In other situations, the effect of other factors may be thought to have an effect on the factor interest (i.e., there is an interaction). For example, hospital length of stay may be influenced by whether a patient is discharged to a nursing home and whether that person is covered by Medicaid. One could examine the individual contributions of each variable in a regression model. However, the effect of a nursing home discharge might be modified by the patient's Medicaid status. To test this possibility, one could look at the effect of the interaction of these two variables on the dependent variable or one could form two subgroups (those on Medicaid and those not) and compare the effects of nursing home discharge on each.

Different types of variables will require different types of analyses. The differences may be based on the assumptions about the normality of the distribution of the variables (i.e., is the curve bell-shaped). In general, researchers talk about two classes of analyses: parametric and nonparametric. The former are appropriately used when the dependent variable is assumed to be normally distributed. In some cases, it is possible to transform the dependent variable into a normal distribution to make

---

[2]To be accurate, we should note that in many studies, the explained variance and regression coefficients do not precisely correspond to predictive variables because they describe associations that have been gathered retrospectively. Hence, they should be interpreted more cautiously. When a study uses what epidemiologists call a "case-control" model (i.e., it begins by identifying those with and without the outcome and looks for factors that are associated with one or the other), the best an investigator can do is to identify factors (i.e., treatments) that are likely to be more strongly associated with the outcome than its absence. These relationships are more appropriately expressed as odds ratios, which do not imply causal assumptions.

[3]The term "risk factor" is used here in a generic sense to include all of the factors that can affect the outcomes of care. In some discussions of disease severity (see Chapter 7), risk factor is used interchangeably with "severity." In this book, we have tried to use it consistently in the larger context.

such analyses more feasible. Some variables have unusual distributions. Variables, like healthcare cost and utilization data, may show a large peak near zero use and a thin, long tail of high users (i.e., there may be a large number of cases in which there is no event during the observation period; many people use few, if any, services in a given year). For example, approximately 20% of Medicare enrollees will use no services in a given year. Using regular regression techniques will result in biased coefficients. Special analytic techniques have been developed to handle such cases. Categorical-dependent variables (including dichotomous or polytomous) variables require different analytic techniques, usually termed "nonparametric." Special regression techniques (e.g., logistic regression) that avoid the problem of biased coefficients are available for these circumstances.

A note of caution is in order. Care should be used in interpreting the results of regression analyses. A variety of problems can haunt such efforts, including using too many variables for the number of observations, colinearity among the variables, endogeneity (i.e., reciprocal relationships among the dependent and independent variables), and unusual distributions that bias the coefficients or render them uninterpretable. Statistical assistance is invaluable, both when designing a study and in interpreting the results.

ETHICS

Outcomes investigators may encounter some ethical issues. There is still debate about how much informed consent must be obtained from patients. In general, when an outcomes project is done as part of an ongoing quality of care process that is incorporated into a medical care system's regular activities, no special permission is required. It is assumed that the patient who initially agreed to be treated accepts the outcomes work as part of that treatment. However, if outside agencies are used to collect the data or if it is used for more scientific purposes (or any purpose beyond direct quality improvement for the clinicians involved), then patients must first give their permission to be interviewed or even to have their records examined.

Confidentiality is an important ethical consideration. Some institutional review boards (who must adjudicate the ethical aspects of a study) will not even permit an outside research agency to contact patients directly to request their permission to participate in a study. Simply releasing their names is seen as a breach of confidentiality and a HIPAA violation. Instead, the patients' physicians must first seek their permission to be contacted. Such a step rigorously enforced can put an end to outcomes research. Few care providers have the resources to persist in following up the substantial numbers of patients who simply fail to respond to an invitation to participate. Although it would be wrong to coerce a patient into participating, it is also dangerous to eliminate from a study those who simply fail to indicate whether or not they are willing to participate. Somehow the investigators need to be deputized to act in the physicians' stead if the study is to be conducted.

Both patients and providers need to be clear about how the material around an outcomes study will be used. When anonymity is promised, it must be complete. Under such cases, the results about a given patient cannot be shared with that patient's doctors. On the other hand, some patients may want the information shared; they should be given an opportunity to indicate such a preference. In general, outcomes information is obtained under the promise that it will be used only in aggregate form and no identifiers will be attached.

Providers also need to know in advance when they will be identified with the results. In cases where the outcomes information may be useful to consumers in making informed choices, anonymity would be disadvantageous. However, providers may be rightfully concerned that adequate case-mix adjustments have been made before data is released. On the other hand, failure to release identifying information can be viewed with suspicion, as if the providers had something to hide. Careful prior arrangements need to be established about how and when data will be released.

DISEASE MANAGEMENT

The rise of chronic disease has spawned enthusiasm for disease management. This term applies to various efforts to pay closer attention to the status of patients in such a way as to intervene before their deteriorating clinical course becomes a crisis. A number of commercial programs have been developed but the science underlying their efficacy, assessed either economically or in terms of actual changes in disease state, is still underdeveloped.

Outcomes research has only a limited amount to offer to disease management. They share common needs for measures that reflect clinical status and a need for strong information systems. Outcomes research can make an important contribution by testing the effectiveness of disease management. By comparing groups that do and do not receive such attention, one can ascertain if the clinical trajectories are affected.

QUALITY IMPROVEMENT

Quality actions can be considered at several levels. The most basic is quality assessment, which implies simply measuring the quality of care (perhaps expressed in terms of outcomes). Assessment, per se, assumes no responsibility for what is done with the information. By contrast, quality assurance implies a commitment to ensure that at least a certain level of quality is reached. It is a much heavier responsibility.

In the middle of those poles lies quality improvement (QI). In essence, QI rejects the idea of meeting some fixed standard to strive for an ever higher goal. At the same time, this philosophy can be construed as performing positively when very bad care becomes only bad care. The basic approach to QI consists of a cycle that includes assessing the situation, designing an intervention, implementing the intervention, and assessing the outcome. Outcomes research methods are thus congruent with the goals of QI; they are frameworks on which it is based. However, the standard of precision normally applied to outcomes research may be more relaxed for QI (Berwick, 2008). In many instances, it is sufficient to create the sense of a problem as a spur to action. Likewise, the perception of improvement may be a motivation for continued efforts to improve. Ultimately, however, stringent standards of evidence will be needed to justify sustained QI efforts.

OPERATIONAL STEPS

Perhaps the best way to illustrate the various issues around conducting an outcomes study is to offer an example.[4] Consider the case of a study done with a large number of Minnesota hospitals to assess the outcomes of

---

[4]For a practical guide to implementing quality improvement projects, see Radosevich Kalambokidis, and Werni (1996).

Table 14-1 **Variables Used in Cholecystectomy Study**

Outcomes	Risk Adjustment	Treatment
Concordance with classic cholecystitis pain	Severity measures (duration, x-ray findings, symptoms)	Open versus laparoscopic
Symptom score	Comorbidity (Charlston scale)	Hospital
Functional status	Demographics (age, gender)	Surgeon
Satisfaction (three factors)	Prior history	

elective cholecystectomy (Kane et al., 1995). The study was sponsored by a consortium of hospital and medical associations at the state and county levels. The group had originally been organized to develop guidelines or protocols for care management under the assumption that it was preferable to develop one's own than to have someone else's thrust upon one. In the course of the guidelines work, questions were raised about the quality of the database available on which to base determinations of appropriate care. It was decided that the study should be expanded to include the collection of outcomes. A study design was developed to identify the potential risk factors that should be considered in assessing the effect of treatment on the outcomes of cholecystectomy. Table 14-1 summarizes the major categories of variables used in this study according to the classification scheme used in this book.

In this case, the treatment variable of interest was initially the surgeon and the hospital where the operation was performed. The question posed was not whether performing a cholecystectomy was better than using some sort of medical treatment or even watchful waiting. Rather, the question was: Did the operation performed by one person lead to better outcomes than if done by another, and which characteristics of a case predicted better outcomes? Just as the study was being designed, a new approach to cholecystectomy, laparoscopic surgery, was introduced. The study was quickly emended to include a comparison of the results of the two approaches: conventional open surgery versus laparoscopic.

Clinical teams worked with outcomes researchers to establish the conceptual model. Literature reviews and meetings with clinicians were used to identify the potential risk factors that could influence the outcomes. The outcomes themselves were derived from several sources. Condition-specific measures included symptoms that were associated with indications for performing the procedure (e.g., pain, nausea). In effect, the appropriateness criteria were adapted as outcome measures under the assumption that the main purpose of the treatment was to alleviate the factors that suggested a need for care in the first place. In addition, pertinent generic measures of quality of life (e.g., the ability to perform daily activities and self-rating of health status) were added. These were reviewed to that the clinicians believed that good care would actually influence them.

A series of risk factors was established based on such aspects as severity and duration of the problem. Certain physiological and laboratory tests were used as criteria. After a preliminary review of some sample charts, it became quickly evident that much of the information deemed pertinent would not be available from the hospital record. The nursing departments from each of the participating hospitals were contacted to see if they would be willing to implement a special data collection activity at the time of admission. The data collected at baseline would include both specific symptom information and more generic measures; it would also be an opportunity to obtain informed consent to be contacted subsequently to ascertain follow-up status. Although the nursing staffs proved willing to undertake this added work (some were sold on the basis that this study would prove an opportunity to demonstrate the value of good nursing care as well), logistical problems did occur. As same-day surgery increased, it proved harder to obtain the baseline data: Patients were not available in advance.

The follow-up data was collected by a special survey research unit. The primary data collection mode was by mail, but telephone follow ups were used if responses were not received within the time frames allocated. This sort of follow-up plan required that patients' names and addresses be known; special procedures were used to keep the records confidential. All completed follow ups were coded with a specific code number linked to an index. All subsequent analyses were done with only that code number. The linking of the several components of data (the baseline interviews, the follow-up questionnaires, and the medical record abstracts) was done by a small team that was part of the sponsoring organization. Careful monitoring was required to ensure that the 6-month follow ups were collected within the time window. As soon as cases were enrolled and baseline data collected, a file was opened and the case tracked.

The medical records of each case were reviewed using a specially designed abstraction form. Interrater reliability was checked and monitored to be sure that the same information was interpreted consistently. The results of this step were combined with the baseline and follow-up data to create a single analytic file. This file had no identifiers for patients, surgeons, or hospitals. Instead, code numbers were substituted for each.

The analysis used regression models to examine the effects of the potential risk factors on the various outcomes of interest. When potential risk factors were shown to play an active role, they were retained in the models when the independent variables of major interest were introduced. The effects of laparoscopic surgery were examined by both using a dummy variable to represent the type of surgery and by examining the outcomes separately for those undergoing laparoscopic and open cholecystectomies.

SUMMARY

The demand for outcomes information is growing. For clinicians and academics, outcomes information is needed to support and grow the underlying information base that will help the field to base its actions on strong evidence. It is potentially useful to consumers as the basis for choosing providers of care. Although it might be too optimistic to believe that healthcare decisions will be any more rational than most consumer purchases, at least some subset of the population will welcome better information, especially if it can be presented in a useful way. For many decisions, however, the number of cases in a given clinician's portfolio over a finite period may be too small to allow adequate analysis.

Outcomes research has the potential to add considerably to the empiric basis of medical practice. It will never be feasible to base all (or even a large proportion) of medical care on randomized clinical trials. On the other hand, it is irrational to assume that simply intuitively assembling the lessons of clinical experience serves as an adequate basis for scientific practice. The immediate response to the recognition of substantial variation in practice has been the institution of guidelines based largely on professional judgments about what constitutes good care. The next step is to amass the empirical database that those looking for a more scientific basis to establish guidelines have not found.

Careful observations developed as part of well-designed studies will go a long way toward providing the insights needed. One may never be able to say with absolute certainty that a given treatment works in a given situation, but one will have come a lot closer to making informed statements. Simply collecting data is not the answer. Studies must be carefully designed. Conceptual models must be created that combine the best of clinical and social science insights. These models should form the basis for deciding what information is to be collected and how it will be analyzed. The technology of outcomes research has come a long way in the last decades and promises to go much further. Sophisticated analytic and measurement methods are available. Like any other powerful tools, they must be handled carefully by persons skilled in their use. The best outcomes research is likely to come from partnerships of technically proficient analysts and clinicians, each of whom is sensitive to and respectful of the contributions others can bring.

REFERENCES

Berwick, D. M. (2008). The science of improvement. *JAMA, 299*(10), 1182–1184.

Cohen, H. J., Feussner, J. R., Weinberger, M., Carnes, M., Hamdy, R. C., Hsieh, F., . . .Lavori, P. (2002). A controlled trial of inpatient and outpatient geriatric evaluation and management. *New England Journal of Medicine, 346*(12), 905–912.

Feinstein, A. R. (1977). *Clinical biostatistics.* St. Louis, MO: C. V. Mosby.

Feinstein, A. R. (1987). *Clinimetrics.* New Haven, CT: Yale University Press.

Greenfield, S., Aronow, H. U., Elashoff, R. M., & Watanabe, D. (1988). Flaws in mortality data: The hazards of ignoring comorbid disease. *Journal of American Medical Association, 260*, 2253–2256.

Holtzman, J., Saleh, K., & Kane, R. (2002). Gender differences in functional status and pain in a Medicare population undergoing elective total hip arthroplasty. *Medical Care, 40*(6), 461–470.

Jencks, S. F., Daley, J., Draper, D., Thomas, N., Lenhart, G., & Walker, J. (1988). Interpreting hospital mortality data: The role of clinical risk adjustment. *Journal of the American Medical Association, 260*, 3611–3616.

Kahn, K. L., Brook, R. H., Draper, D., Keeler, E. B., Rubenstein, L. V., Rogers, W. H., & Kosecoff, J. (1988). Interpreting hospital mortality data. How can we proceed? *Journal of the American Medical Association, 260*, 3625–3628.

Kane, R. L., Lurie, N., Borbas, C., Morris, N., Flood, S., McLaughlin, B., . . .Schultz, A. (1995). The outcomes of elective laparoscopic and open cholecystectomies. *Journal of the American College of Surgeons, 180*(2), 136–145.

Radosevich, D. M., Kalambokidis, T. L., & Werni, A. (1996). *Practical guide for implementing, analyzing, and reporting outcomes measures.* Bloomington, MN: Health Outcomes Institute.

Shadish, W. R., Cook, T. D., Campbell, D. T. (2002). *Experimental and quasi-experimental designs for generalized causal inference.* Boston: Houghton Mifflin Company.

Spiegel, J. S., Leake, B., Spiegel, T. M., Paulus, H. E., Kane, R. L., Ward, N. B., & Ware, J. E. Jr. (1986). What are we measuring? An examination of self-reported functional status measures. *Arthritis and Rheumatism, 31*(6), 721–728.

Weed, L. L. (1968a). Medical records that guide and teach. *New England Journal of Medicine, 278*(11), 593–600.

Weed, L. L. (1968b). Medical records that guide and teach. *New England Journal of Medicine, 278*(12), 652–657 (concl).

INDEX

Note: Page numbers followed by *f, t,* or *n* indicate figures, tables, and footnotes, respectively.

A

AAPOR. *See* American Association for Public Opinion Research
absolute risk (AR), 27–29, 29*t*
A-CAHPS. *See* Ambulatory CAHPS
activities of daily living (ADLs), 91, 92*t*, 93, 107
ADLs. *See* activities of daily living
administrative data, collectio n methods
  advantages, 291
  challenges, 292–294
  databases, 292–293
  EMR, 292
  government, federal, 291–292
  government, state, 291–292
  insurers, private, 291
  limitations, 291
  Medicaid, 292
  Medicare, 291–292
  organizations, regulatory, 291
  PHI, 293
  VA, 291–292
Agency for Healthcare Research and Quality (AHRQ), 2
AHA. *See* American Heart Association
AHCA. *See* American Health Care Association
AHRQ. *See* Agency for Healthcare Research and Quality
Ambulatory CAHPS (A-CAHPS), 182
American Association for Public Opinion Research (AAPOR), 284
American Health Care Association (AHCA), 184*t*, 186–187
American Heart Association (AHA), 263
American Heart Association (AHA) Stroke Outcome Classification, 263

analysis, health outcomes data, 297
  analytic method selection, 298–302
  Bonferroni correction, 307–308
  considerations, 297–301, 301*t*, 302, 302*t*, 303–304, 304*f*, 305–311
  Cox proportional hazards model, 299–300, 301*t*
  expert advice, 305
  fixed effect model, 300
  general linear regression, 300
  hierarchical or nested outcomes designs, 301
  Kaplan-Meier life table method, 299, 301*t*
  logistic regression, 298, 302
  LSD approach, 307
  M and M conference, 299
  missing data, handling method, 308–311
  mixed-model method, 300
  problems, fishing/error rate, 306–308
  random effect, 300, 301*t*
  random error, 300–301
  retroactive power calculations, 303
  sample size, determinant, 303
  Scheffé's method, 307
  statistical power, 302–304, 304*t*, 305–306
  statistical significance level, 303–304, 307
  survival, 299–300, 302
  time-to-event analysis, 299, 301*t*
  true effect, 303
  Tukey's method, 307
  Type I error rate, 303–304, 307
  Type II error rate, 304
  validity threat, 302, 304*f,* 307
analysis, recommended guidelines, 302*t*
analysis, statistical approach scheme, 301*t*

analysis issues, basic, 332
  attributable *vs.* relative risk, 333*n*
  multivariate analysis, 333
  nonparametric, 334
  parametric, 334
  regression analysis, 334
  regression model, 333
  risk factors, 333–334
  variables, 334–335
analysis of variance (ANOVA) technique,
    67, 67*t*, 69
analysis/visual display, outcomes
    research data
  analysis considerations, 297–301, 301*t*,
    302, 302*t*, 303–304, 304*f*, 305–311
  database/data dictionary creation,
    311, 312*t*
  regulatory demands, 316, 317*t*–318*t*, 318
  study variables, structure data,
    313–314, 314*t*, 315, 315*t*
  visual display, outcomes information,
    315–316
analyst clinician partnership, 341
analytic method selection
  Cox proportional hazards model,
    299–300, 301*t*
  fixed effect model, 300
  general linear regression, 300
  hierarchical, nested outcomes
    designs, 301
  Kaplan-Meier life table method,
    299, 301*t*
  logistic regression, 298, 302
  M and M conference, 299
  mixed-model method, 300
  random effect, 300, 301*t*
  random error, 300–301
  statistical conclusion validity, 298
  survival, 299–300, 302
  time-to-event analysis, 299, 301*t*
  validity threat, 302, 304*f*
Andersen–Aday model, 33, 34*f*
ANOVA. *See* analysis of variance technique
anxiety, psychologic factors, 216
  Anxiety Adjective Checklist, 217
  EMAS, 217
  PGC Morale Scale, 217
  STAI, 217

Anxiety Adjective Checklist, 217
AR. *See* absolute risk
Area Resource File, 202
association *vs.* causation, 27–29, 29*t*
attrition bias, 46, 47

B
bandwidth, 80
Behavioral Risk Factor Surveillance
    Survey, 202
bias, 12*n*
  attrition, 46, 47
  compliance, 46
  conceptual models, 32*f*, 39
  contamination, 46
  intention to treat rule, 47
  mortality, 47
  mortality attrition, 47
  selection bias control, 270, 271*f*
  therapeutic personality, 46
Bonferroni correction, 307–308
Bowling, A., 152
Bradford-Hill criteria, 27*t*
Brief Pain Inventory, 211
British Medical Research Council, 26
burden, measures selection, 62, 77

C
CAHPS. *See* Consumer Assessment of
    Healthcare Providers
CAHPS Nursing Home Survey
    (NH-CAHPS), 184*t*, 186
calibration levels, 79
CAM. *See* complementary and alternative
    medicine
Canadian Neurological Scale (CNS),
    264, 265*t*
case mix adjustment, 327
  morbidity, 326
  severity, 326
causation, 25–26
  association *vs.*, 27–29, 29*t*
  Bradford-Hill criteria, 27*t*
ceiling effects, 79
Center for Epidemiologic Studies
    Depression Scale (CES-D), 213, 216
CES-D. *See* Center for Epidemiologic
    Studies Depression Scale

Charlson Comorbidity Index, 266, 266*t*–269*t*
cholecystectomy study, 338*t*
classical test theory (CTT), 56–57
clinical data, collection methods
  advantages, administrative data, 291
  challenges, 290
  databases, 292–293
  electronic, 290
  EMR, 290
  limitations, administrative data, 291
  Medicaid, 292
  Medicare, 291–292
  sources, administrative data, 291–292
  VA, 291–292
CNS. *See* Canadian Neurological Scale
Cochrane Collaborating Centers, 1
cognitive function, psychologic factors
  Mental Status Questionnaire, 218
  MMSE, 218
  Short Portable Mental Status
    Questionnaire, 218
collection methods
  AAPOR, 284
  administrative data, 281–282, 291–294
  clinical data, 281–282, 289–294
  cooperation rate, 284
  cooperation rate formula, 284
  coverage error, 282–283
  design, tailored, 287–288
  EMR, 282
  frame, 282
  HIPAA, 281, 293
  measurement error, 282, 286
  nonresponse error, 282, 284–285,
    285*f*, 286, 286*f*
  population, 282
  pretesting, 288–289
  refusal rate, 285
  refusal rate formula, 284
  response rate, 284
  response rate formula, 284
  sample, 282
  sampling error, 282–283
  sampling error formula, 283
  self-report, 281–286
  system, survey implementation,
    design, 288

comorbidity, risk adjustment, 262–263
  analysis, subgroup, 271–272, 272*f*
  bias, selection control, 270, 271*f*
  Charlson Comorbidity Index, 266,
    266*t*–269*t*
  data sources, 272–273
  generic measures, 264, 266,
    267*t*–269*t*, 270
  outcome prediction, improvement,
    271, 271*f*
comparative scaling methods, 58–60
complementary and alternative medicine
  (CAM), 238, 241*n*
compliance bias, 46
conceptual models, modeling, 29–30
  basic, 31*f*
  interactive, 31*f*
  literature review, 17–18
  model development, 17
  model variables, 19*t*
  research plan, 18–20
  researchable question, 17
  selection bias, congestive heart
    failure, 32*f*
  treatment/outcomes, congestive heart
    failure, 32*f*
  variable operationalization, 18
condition-specific measures, 85
  alternatives, 140–142, 142*t*
  cataract surgery study, 137, 148
  choice, 143–148, 151–153
  clinical, 133
  clinimetrics, 137
  conceptual model, 143–146, 148
  disease *vs.* case definition, 140
  experiential, 133
  generic measures *vs.*, 133–135,
    140–142, 148–151
  hierarchy of measurement, 146–148
  importance, 136–137
  physiological measures, 137–138,
    138*t*, 139–140
  SF-36, 134–136
condition-specific measures, types
  function test, 143, 144*t*, 146
  signs, 143, 144*t*, 145
  symptoms, 143–144, 144*t*
  test, 143, 144*t*, 145–146

Consolidated Standards of Reporting
Trials (CONSORT), 13
CONSORT. *See* Consolidated Standards
of Reporting Trials
Consumer Assessment of Healthcare
Providers (CAHPS), 177, 177*t*, 178
Consumer Satisfaction Survey (CSS), 178
contamination bias, 46
content validity, 62–63
COOP. *See* Cooperative Information
Project Charts
Cooperative Information Project (COOP)
Charts, 86–87, 112–114, 124*t*
Cox proportional hazards model,
299–300, 301*t*
CPX. *See* symptoms/problems
Cronbach's alpha coefficient, 68–69
CSS. *See* Consumer Satisfaction Survey
CTT. *See* classical test theory

D
DALYs. *See* disability adjusted life
expectancy
Dartmouth Primary Care Cooperative
Information Project (COOP), 112
data follow-up
adequate response rate, 330
consistency, 329
proxies, 330–331
response rates, 329–330
timing, 331
treatment duration, 331
data quality, 327–328
Data Safety Monitory Board (DSMB), 318
database/data dictionary creation
FDA compliant clinical trials, 311
NHEFS I, 311, 312*t*
relational database, 311
Deficit Reduction Act of 2005, 1
demographic, psychologic, social factors
control variables, 199–200, 200*f*, 201
dependent variables, 199–200, 200*f*, 201
independent variables, 199–200,
200*f*, 201
demographic factors, 199, 201
age, 202
Area Resource File, 202
Behavioral Risk Factor Surveillance
Survey, 202

dwelling characteristics, 203
genetics, 202–203
marital status, 204–205
race, 203–204, 204*t*
residence, 202–203
SES, 203, 205, 205*t*, 206
depression, psychologic factors
CES-D, 216
*Diagnostic and Statistical Manual of
Mental Disorders*, 216
Geriatric Depression Scale, 216
Self-Rating Depression Scale, 216
design, measures selection, 62, 78
design, tailored
costs, 287–288
Dillman, 287
rewards, 287
trust, 287–288
diagnosis *vs.* treatment, 241
Diagnosis-Related Grouping (DRG), 263
Diagnostic and Statistical Manual of
Mental Disorders, 216
Dillman, Don, 287
disability adjusted life expectancy
(DALYs), 126
disease management, 336–337
Donabedian model, 164
dosage, 242
DRG. *See* Diagnosis-Related Grouping
DSMB. *See* Data Safety Monitory Board

E
EBM. *See* evidence-based medicine
econometric methods, 60–61
effect size (ES), 27–28
electronic medical record (EMR), 282,
290, 292, 294
EMAS. *See* Endler Multidimensional
Anxiety Scales
EMR. *See* electronic medical record
Endler Multidimensional Anxiety Scales
(EMAS), 217
epidemiological approach, 40
errors
nonresponse, 25% rate, 285*f*
nonresponse, 70% rate, 285*f*
relationship, measurement, 64*f*, 65*f*
sampling, 283*f*
ES. *See* effect size

ethics
anonymity, 336
confidentiality, 335–336
data release conditions, 336
HIPAA, 336
informed consent, 335
EuroQol, 87, 120, 120*t*, 121
evidence-based medicine (EBM), 3, 6
evidence-based practice, 1
expectancy–disconfirmation model,
160–161
explanatory models, 35
Andersen–Aday model, 33, 34*f*
Health Belief Model, 33, 35*f*
health resource utilization, 33, 34*f*
external validity, 41

F
face validity, 62–63
FACIT. *See* Functional Assessment of
Chronic Illness Therapy
FACT. *See* Functional Assessment of
Cancer Therapy
FACT-G. *See* Functional Assessment of
Cancer Therapy-General
FDA. *See* US Food and Drug
Administration
fidelity, 80
fixed effect model, 300
floor effects, 79
Functional Assessment of Cancer Therapy
(FACT), 109, 110*t*–111*t*
Functional Assessment of Cancer Therapy-
General (FACT-G), 109, 110*t*
Functional Assessment of Chronic
Illness Therapy (FACIT), 108–109,
111*t*–112*t*

G
General Well-Being Schedule, 210
generic measures
advantages/disadvantages, 88, 88*t*
choice, 98–99
condition-specific measures *vs.*,
133–135, 148–151
considerations, 96–98
COOP, 86–87, 97–98
domain, 89–95
EQ-5D, 87

EuroQol, 87
Health Utilities Index Mark 3, 87
HRQL, 87, 89–90
importance, 86–88
mortality/morbidity, 90, 98–99
profiling, 87–88
proxy response, 87
Quality of Well-Being Scale, 87
risk adjustment, 87
selection criteria, 88, 89*t*
seven generic domains of health, 90,
91–95, 91*t*
SF-36, 85–86, 93
SIP, 85
6 Ds, 90
unidimensional scales, 90, 92*t*
utilization, 98–99
World Health Organization, 86
Geriatric Depression Scale, 216
graph guidelines, outcomes information,
317*t*–318*t*

H
HAQ. *See* Stanford Health Assessment
Questionnaire
H-CAHPS. *See* Hospital CAHPS
HCSM. *See* Home Care Satisfaction
Measure
HCTC. *See* Home Care and Terminal
Care
Health Belief Model, 33, 35*f*
health domains, seven generic, 90
cognitive functioning, 91*t*, 92*t*, 94–95
overall well-being, 91*t*, 95
pain, 91*t*, 94
physical functioning, 91*t*, 92*t*, 93
psychological well-being, 91*t*, 92*t*, 93
social functioning, 91*t*, 92*t*, 93–94
vitality, 91*t*, 95
Health Insurance Portability and
Accountability Act (HIPAA), 281
health resource utilization, 33, 34*f*
Health Utilities Index (HUI), 3, 87,
121–123, 124*t*
health-related quality of life (HRQL), 210
ADLs, 107, 121, 126, 126*t*
applications, 108–128
components, 106*t*
conceptual model, 107*f*

health-related quality of life *(continued)*
  condition-specific, 108–109
  COOP, 112–114, 124*t*
  DALYs, 126
  distal–proximal continuum,
    implications, 107–108
  EuroQol, 120, 120*t*, 121
  FACIT, 108–109, 111*t*–112*t*
  FACT, 109, 110*t*–111*t*
  FACT-G, 109, 110*t*
  HUI, 121–123, 124*t*
  IADLs, 126, 126*t*
  Karnofsky Scale, 109, 112, 113*t*, 124*t*
  QALYs, 118–119, 123, 125–126
  QOL, 106, 118, 121
  QOL coverage, 123, 124*t*
  QWB, 118–120, 124*t*
  short-form measures, 114–115, 115*t*
  SIP, 115–116, 117*t*, 118, 124*t*
  US population, healthy life years,
    127*t*–128*t*
  utility assessment, 123, 125–126, 126*t*,
    127*t*, 128*t*
  WHO, 105–106, 121
  WHOQOL-BREF, 121, 122*t*–123*t*
Heckman, James, 40
Henle, Jakob, 26
Henle-Koch's postulates, 26
HIPAA. *See* Health Insurance Portability
  and Accountability Act
Home Care and Terminal Care (HCTC),
  185*t*, 187
Home Care Satisfaction Measure
  (HCSM), 184*t*, 187
Hosmer and Lemeshow Goodness-of-Fit
  Test, 277
Hospital CAHPS (H-CAHPS), 178,
  179*t*, 180
HRQL. *See* health-related quality of life
HUI. *See* Health Utilities Index
Hume, David, 25

I
IADLs. *See* instrumental activities of daily
  living
ICC. *See* intraclass correlation coefficient
Illness Behavior Questionnaire, 212
Index of Well-Being, 210

informed choice, 1
institutional review board (IRB), 316, 318
instrumental activities of daily living
  (IADLs), 91, 93, 126, 126*t*
instrumental variables (IVs), 40
intention to treat rule, 47
interactive conceptual model, 31*f*
internal validity threats, 41, 42*t*
interval measurement, 55, 55*t*
intervention effect, isolation
  epidemiological approach, 40
  instrumental variables, 40
  propensity score, 41
  selection bias, 39
intraclass correlation coefficient (ICC),
  67–68
IRB. *See* institutional review board
item response theory (IRT)
  Rasch model, 61
  unidimensional models, 61
IV. *See* instrumental variables

K
Kaplan-Meier life table method,
  299, 301*t*
Karnofsky Scale, 109, 112, 113*t*, 124*t*
Keller, Helen, 325
Koch, Robert, 26

L
latent constructs, 51–52
least significant difference (LSD), 307
Life Stressors and Social Resources
  Inventory, 212
Likert-type scale, 57–58
locus of control, psychologic factors
  MHLC, 211
  MHLCS, 211
Low Back Classification, 264
Low Back Pain Disability
  Questionnaire, 212
LSD. *See* least significant difference

M
M and M. *See* mortality and morbidity
managed care, 2
McDowell, I., 151–152
McGill Pain Questionnaire, 211–212

measurement
  calibration levels, 79
  conceptualization, 49
  errors relationship, 64*f,* 65*f*
  latent constructs, 51–52
  multiple- *vs.* single-item measure,
    78–79
  operationalization, 49
  overview, definition, 49–52
  phenomena, observable/unobservable, 51
  scaling, 52–56
  scaling methods, 56–61
  strategic questions, health outcomes
    measures, 61–78
  useful terms, 79–80
measurement levels, conceptual/
  operational/variable, 53*t*
measurement methods, satisfaction,
  167–168
  issues, 169–170
  psychometric testing, 170–172
  rating *vs.* reporting, 173
  reference group, 173
  surveys, 172–173
  utilization patterns, 172
*Measuring Disease: A Review of
  Disease-Specific Quality of Life
  Measurement Scales* (Bowling), 152
*Measuring Health: A Guide to Rating Scales
  and Questionnaires* (McDowell),
  151–152
Medicaid, 292
Medicare, 291–292
medications, 242
Mental Health Locus of Control
  (MHLC), 211
Mental Status Questionnaire, 218
MHLC. *See* Mental Health Locus of
  Control
MHLCS. *See* Multidimensional Health
  Locus of Control scale
Mini-mental State Exam (MMSE), 218
missing data, handling methods
  attrition, 308
  dummy variable codes, 310
  mean substitution, 310
  Murphy's Law, 308
  outcome value interpolation, 310

  selective, 309
  sensitivity analysis, 310–311
  types, 308–309
MMSE. *See* Mini-mental State Exam
MOB. *See* Mobility scale
Mobility scale (MOB), 119
model variables, 19*t*
models, causal thinking
  Bradford-Hill criteria, 27*t*
  causation, 25–29
mortality and morbidity (M and M), 47,
  90, 98–99, 299
MOS Pain Measure, 212
Multidimensional Health Locus of
  Control scale (MHLCS), 211
multiple- *vs.* single-item measure, 78–79
multivariate file structure, 313–314,
  314*t*
Murphy's Law, 308

N
National Drug Code (NDC), 272–273
National Health Examination
  Epidemiologic Follow-up Study
  (NHEFS I), 311, 312*t*
National Health and Nutrition
  Examination Survey
  (NHANES), 312*t*
NDC. *See* National Drug Code
NHANES. *See* National Health and
  Nutrition Examination Survey
NH-CAHPS. *See* CAHPS Nursing
  Home Survey
NHEFS I. *See* National Health
  Epidemiologic Follow-up Study
NHRSS. *See* Nursing Home Resident
  Satisfaction Scale
Nightingale, Florence, 261
nominal measurement, 52, 55*t*
NRS. *See* numerical rating scale
numerical rating scale (NRS), 57, 58*t*
Nursing Home Resident Satisfaction
  Scale (NHRSS), 184*t*, 186

O
odds ratio (OR), 27–29, 29*t*
Office of Human Research Protection
  (OHRP), 316

OHRP. *See* Office of Human Research
   Protection
One-Group Pretest–Posttest Design,
   45, 45*t*
operational steps
   abstraction form, 340
   cholecystectomy study variables,
      337–338, 338*t*, 339–340
   conceptual model, 338–339
   condition-specific measures, 339
   follow-up data, 339
   generic measures, 339
   regression model, 340
   risk factors, 339–340
   study design, 338
OR. *See* odds ratio
ordinal measurement, 54, 55*t*
outcome *vs.* prediction, dichotomous, 276*f*
outcomes research, 2, 7
   accountability, 3–5
   conceptual modeling, 16–20
   cross-tabulated data, 29*t*
   data collection, 5
   data issues, 5–6
   EBM and, 3, 6
   explanatory models, 33, 34*f*, 35
   market decisions, 3
   marketing and, 4
   measurement, 15–16
   model variables, 19*t*
   pseudo-equation, 8
   purpose, 3–8
   QI and, 3
   RCT and, 3, 11–14
   remedial action and, 5
   risk adjustment, 9–10
   study designs, 11–14
   treatment, 10–11

P
pain, psychologic factors
   Brief Pain Inventory, 211
   Low Back Pain Disability
      Questionnaire, 212
   McGill Pain Questionnaire, 211–212
   MOS Pain Measure, 212
   VAS, 211
PAS. *See* Physical Activity Scale

patient clinical characteristics, 9
Patient Judgments on Hospital Quality
   (PJHQ), 180
patient satisfaction, theoretic models
   attribution, 162–163
   care process, 166
   cognitive–affect model, 160
   determinants, psychosocial, 163
   dimensions, 163–164, 164*t*, 165*f*, 166
   Donabedian model, 164
   element importance, 173–174, 174*t*
   evidence-based medicine, 160
   existing measures, 174, 175*t*–176*t*,
      177, 177*t*, 178, 179*t*, 180, 181*t*,
      182–183, 184*t*–185*t*, 186–188
   expectancy–disconfirmation model,
      160–161
   expectations, 161–163
   literature reviews, 188
   measurement axes, 168*f*
   measurement methodology, 167–173
   outcomes, 166–167, 189
   ratings interpretation, 161–167
Patient Satisfaction Questionnaire III
   (PSQ-III), 182–183
Patient Satisfaction Questionnaire (PSQ),
   182–183
Perceived Stress Questionnaire, 212
PGC Morale Scale, 217
PHI. *See* protected health information
Physical Activity Scale (PAS), 119
physiological measures, condition-specific
   clinimetrics, 137
   disease state, 138–140
   intermediate/surrogate, 138–139
   outcome types, 137, 138*t*
   in vitro, 138–139
PJHQ. *See* Patient Judgments on
   Hospital Quality
Pragmatic–Explanatory Continuum
   Indicator Summary (PRECIS), 40
PRECIS. *See* Pragmatic–Explanatory
   Continuum Indicator Summary
pretesting, collection methods
   interviews, cognitive, 288–289
   pilot study, 288–289
   review, expert panel, 288–289
   review, proofreading, 288–289

Pretest–Posttest Control Group Design, 44, 44*t*
propensity score, 41
protected health information (PHI), 293
PSQ. *See* Patient Satisfaction Questionnaire
PSQ-III. *See* Patient Satisfaction Questionnaire III
psychologic factors, 199, 200*f*, 201
  affect, 213
  anxiety, 216–218
  behavioral medicine, 206
  Brief Pain Inventory, 211
  change stages, 212
  cognitive function, 218
  depression, 216
  Illness Behavior Questionnaire, 212
  locus of control, 207*t*–208*t*, 210–211
  Low Back Pain Disability Questionnaire, 212
  McGill Pain Questionnaire, 211–212
  MHLC, 211
  MHLCS, 211
  mind–body connection, 206, 207*t*–210*t*
  MOS Pain Measure, 212
  other, 210*t*, 212
  pain, 208*t*, 211–212
  Perceived Stress Questionnaire, 212
  placebo effect, 206
  Social Adjustment Schedule, 223
  social function, 218–219
  social function, adjustment, 219, 220*t*–222*t*, 223
  Social Maladjustment Schedule, 223
  Social Readjustment Rating Scale, 212
  social support, 219, 220*t*
  stress, 209*t*–210*t*, 212
  well-being, 207*t*, 210

Q
QALYs. *See* Quality Adjusted Life Years
QI. *See* quality improvement
QOL. *See* quality of life
Quality Adjusted Life Years (QALYs), 4, 118–119, 123, 125–126
quality improvement (QI), 3, 337
quality of life (QOL), 106, 118, 121

Quality of Well-Being (QWB) Index, 124*t*
  CPX, 118–120
  MOB, 119
  PAS, 119
  SAC, 119
QWB. *See* Quality of Well-Being Index

R
randomized-controlled trials (RCT), 3, 11–14, 26, 39–40
Rasch model, 61
rating scales, 57–58
ratio measurement, 55*t*, 56
RCT. *See* randomized-controlled trials
receiver operating characteristic (ROC)
  analysis, 76, 76*f*, 77
  curve, 277
Reed, Lawrence, 327
regulatory demands
  DSMB, 318
  IRB, 316, 318
  OHRP, 316
  Tuskegee Syphilis Study, 316
relative risk (RR), 27–29, 29*t*
reliability, measures selection, 62
  ANOVA, 67, 67*t*, 69
  bias, random/nonrandom, 63
  ICC, 67–68
  internal consistency, 65, 68–69
  interrater/interobserver, 65–66, 70
  intrarater, 65
  split-half, 65
  test–retest, 65, 68
  validity *vs.*, 63–65
research designs, basic, 43
  One-Group Pretest–Posttest Design, 45, 45*t*
  Pretest–Posttest Control Group Design, 44, 44*t*
  Solomon Four-Group Design, 44, 44*t*
  time-series experiments, 45, 45*t*
  untreated control group design, 46*t*
responsiveness, measures selection, 62, 74–77
  ROC analysis, 76, 76*f*, 77
result interpretation
  analysis issues, basic, 332–335
  case mix adjustment, 326–327

result interpretation *(continued)*
    causal model, 324–325
    conceptual model, 323–324
    data quality, 327–328
    data source, extant, use, 331–332
    disease management, 336–337
    ethics, 335–336
    follow-up data, acquisition, 329–331
    HRQL, 326
    interrater variation, 325–326
    Keller, 325
    operational steps, 337–338, 338*t*,
        339–340
    organization, mental, 323–325
    QALYs, 325
    QI, 337
    RCT, 323, 329
    simple measures, search, 325–326
    statistical power, 324
    variance, 324
rheumatoid arthritis, hierarchy of
        measure, 147–148
risk adjustment, 261
    AHA Stroke Outcome Classification,
        263
    analysis, subgroup, 271–272, 272*f*
    APACHE II, 263
    bias, selection control, 270, 271*f*
    Charlson Comorbidity Index, 266,
        266*t*–269*t*
    CNS, 264, 265*t*
    comorbidity, 262–263
    considerations, data-related, 273–274
    c-statistic, 277
    data sources, 272–273
    diagnosis, relative importance, 273
    DRG, 263
    generic measures, comorbidity, 264,
        266, 266*t*–269*t*, 270
    Hosmer and Lemeshow Goodness-
        of-Fit Test, 277
    logit function, 276
    Low Back Classification, 264
    NDC, 272–273
    outcome prediction, improvement,
        271, 271*f*
    outcome *vs.* prediction, dichotomous,
        276*f*

    performance, statistical, 275–276,
        276*f*, 277
    purpose, 273
    regression, logistic, 276
    ROC curve, 277
    selection, consideration, 273–275
    severity, 262
    severity, diagnosis-specific, 263
ROC. *See* receiver operating characteristic
RR. *See* relative risk

S
SAC. *See* Social Activity Scale
sampling error
    formula, 283
    sample size effect, 283, 283*f*
    self-report collection methods,
        282–283, 283*f*, 284
SAQs. *See* Satisfaction Assessment
        Questionnaires
Satisfaction Assessment Questionnaires
        (SAQs), 184*t*, 186–187
satisfaction measures, 174
    A-CAHPS, 182
    AHCA SAQs, 184*t*, 186–187
    ambulatory care, 180, 181*t*, 182–183
    CAHPS, 177, 177*t*, 178
    CSS, 178
    H-CAHPS, 178, 179*t*, 180
    HCSM, 184*t*, 187
    HCTC satisfaction scale, 185*t*, 187
    health plan, 174, 175*t*–176*t*, 177–178
    hospital, 178, 179*t*, 180
    long-term care, 183, 184*t*–185*t*, 186–188
    NH-CAHPS, 184*t*, 186
    NHRSS, 184*t*, 186
    PJHQ, 180
    PSQ, 182–183
    PSQ-III, 182–183
    VSQ, 182
    Women's Primary Care Satisfaction
        Survey, 180
scaling
    definition, 52
    interval measurement, 53*t*–54*t*, 55, 55*t*
    nominal measurement, 52, 53*t*–54*t*, 55*t*
    ordinal measurement, 53*t*–54*t*, 54, 55*t*
    ratio measurement, 53*t*–54*t*, 55*t*, 56

scaling methods
  comparative, 58–60
  CTT, 56–57
  econometric, 60–61
  IRT, 61
  Likert-type scale, 57–58
  NRS, 57, 58*t*
  rating, 57–58
  VAS, 57, 57*t*
Scheffé's method, 307
selection bias
  conceptual models, 32*f*, 39
  congestive heart failure, 32*f*
  control, 270, 271*f*
Self-Rating Depression Scale, 216
self-report, collection methods, 282
  AAPOR, 284
  cooperation rate formula, 284
  coverage error, 282–283
  formula, sampling error, 283
  frame, 282
  measurement error, 284, 286
  nonresponse error, 284–285, 285*f*,
    286, 286*f*
  population, 282
  refusal rate formula, 284
  response rate formula, 284
  sample, 282
  sampling error, 282–283, 283*f*, 284
sensibility, measures selection
  content validity, 62–63
  face validity, 62–63
SES. *See* social economic status
severity, risk adjustment, 262
  AHA Stroke Outcome Classification,
    263
  APACHE II, 263
  CNS, 264, 265*t*
  comorbidity, generic, 264, 266,
    266*t*–269*t*, 270
  diagnosis-specific, 263
  DRG, 263
  Low Back Classification, 264
SF-36. *See* Short-Form Health Survey
Short Portable Mental Status
  Questionnaire, 218
Short-Form Health Survey (SF-36),
  85–86, 93, 134–136

Sickness Impact Profile (SIP), 85,
  115–116, 117*t*, 118, 124*t*
single- *vs.* multiple-item measure, 78–79
SIP. *See* Sickness Impact Profile
6 Ds, 90
Social Activity Scale (SAC), 119
Social Adjustment Schedule, 223
social economic status (SES), 203, 205,
  205*t*, 206
social factors, 199–200, 200*f*, 201
Social Maladjustment Schedule, 223
Social Readjustment Rating Scale, 212
Solomon Four-Group Design, 44, 44*t*
STAI. *See* State-Trait Anxiety Inventory
Stanford Health Assessment
  Questionnaire (HAQ), 90
State-Trait Anxiety Inventory (STAI), 217
statistical power, validity threat impact, 304*t*
strategic questions, health outcomes
    measures, 61
  burden, 62, 77
  design, 62, 78
  reliability, 62–70
  responsiveness, 62, 74–77
  sensibility, 62–63
  validity, 62–65, 70–74
stress, psychologic factors
  Life Stressors and Social Resources
    Inventory, 212
  Perceived Stress Questionnaire, 212
  Social Readjustment Rating Scale, 212
study variables/structure data, analysis
  dummy codes, 313
  follow-up status, 315
  multivariate file structure, 313–314, 314*t*
  scoring measurement scales, 313
  time-to-event file structures, 313,
    315, 315*t*
  univariate file structure, 313–314, 314*t*
survival analysis
  Cox proportional hazards model,
    299–300, 301*t*
  Kaplan-Meier life table method, 299, 301*t*
symptoms/problems (CPX), 118–120

T

therapeutic personality bias, 46
time-series experiments, 45, 45*t*

time-to-event file structures, 313, 315, 315*t*
treatment, intervention, 235–236
    CAM, 238, 241*n*
    comparisons, 239–240, 240*t*
    components, 237–242
treatment, intervention *(continued)*
    counseling/education, 243
    diagnosis *vs.*, 241
    elements, 239*t*
    medications, 242
    medicine, allopathic, 241
    procedures, 242–243
    quality improvement, 254
    taxonomy, 238, 239*t*
    variation, 248, 249*t*–250*t*, 250,
        251*t*–252*t*, 252–254
treatment and outcomes, conceptual
    models, 32*f*
Tukey's method, 307
Tuskegee Syphilis Study, 316
Type II error rate, 304

U
univariate file structure, 313–314, 314*t*
untreated control group design, 46*t*
US Department of Veterans Affairs (VA),
    291–292
US Food and Drug Administration
    (FDA), 311
US population, years of healthy life,
    127*t*–128*t*

V
VA. *See* US Department of Veterans Affairs
validity, measures selection, 62

confirmatory factor analysis, 74
    construct, 70–72, 74
    content, 70–71
    convergent, 73
    criterion-related, 70–72, 72*f*, 73*t*
    discriminant, 73
    multitrait–multimethod matrix, 73
    reliability *vs.*, 63–65
validity threats, 41, 42*t*, 43, 318
VAS. *See* visual analog scale
Visit-Specific Satisfaction Instrument
    (VSQ), 182
visual analog scale (VAS), 57, 57*f*, 211
visual display, outcomes information, 315
    guidelines, 316, 317*t*–318*t*
VSQ. *See* Visit-Specific Satisfaction
    Instrument

W
well-being, psychologic factors
    General Well-Being Schedule, 210
    Index of Well-Being, 210
WHO. *See* World Health Organization
WHOQOL-BREF. *See* World Health
    Organization Quality of Life-BREF
Women's Primary Care Satisfaction
    Survey, 180
World Health Organization Quality of
    Life-BREF (WHOQOL-BREF),
    121, 122*t*–123*t*
World Health Organization (WHO),
    105
    health definition, 86
    QOL, 106
    WHOQOL-BREF, 121